Elsevier's Integrated
Physiology

Elsevier's Integrated
Physiology

Robert G. Carroll PhD

Professor of Physiology
Brody School of Medicine
East Carolina University
Greenville, North Carolina

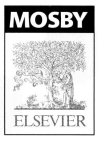

1600 John F. Kennedy Blvd
Suite 1800
Philadelphia, PA 19103-2899

ELSEVIER'S INTEGRATED PHYSIOLOGY

ISBN-13: 978-0-323-04318-2
ISBN-10: 0-323-04318-6

Notice

Knowledge and best practice in this field are constantly changing. As new research and experience broaden our knowledge, changes in practice, treatment and drug therapy may become necessary or appropriate. Readers are advised to check the most current information provided (i) on procedures featured or (ii) by the manufacturer of each product to be administered, to verify the recommended dose or formula, the method and duration of administration, and contraindications. It is the responsibility of the practitioner, relying on their own experience and knowledge of the patient, to make diagnoses, to determine dosages and the best treatment for each individual patient, and to take all appropriate safety precautions. To the fullest extent of the law, neither the Publisher nor the Author assumes any liability for any injury and/or damage to persons or property arising out or related to any use of the material contained in this book.

The Publisher

Library of Congress Cataloging-in-Publication Data

Elsevier's integrated physiology.
    p. cm.
  ISBN 0-323-04318-6
    1. Human physiology.

QP34.5.E47 2007
612—dc22

2006043013

Acquisitions Editor: Alex Stibbe
Developmental Editor: Andrew Hall

Printed in China

Last digit is the print number: 9 8 7 6 5 4 3 2 1

Preface

At a conference, I was asked to summarize physiology in twenty-five words or less. Here is my response: "The body consists of barriers and compartments. Life exists because the body creates and maintains gradients. Physiology is the study of movement across the barriers." Twenty-five words exactly.

This book is organized along those lines. Most chapters begin with an anatomic/histologic presentation of the system. Function does indeed follow form, and the structure provides limitations on physiology of a system. Physiology, however, is the study of anatomy in action. If anatomy is the study of the body in three dimensions, physiologic function and regulation extend the study of the body into the fourth dimension, time.

Robert G. Carroll, PhD

Editorial Review Board

Contents

Series Preface

How to Use This Book
The idea for Elsevier's Integrated Series came about at a seminar on the USMLE Step 1 exam at an American Medical Student Association (AMSA) meeting. We noticed that the discussion between faculty and students focused on how the exams were becoming increasingly integrated—with case scenarios and questions often combining two or three science disciplines. The students were clearly concerned about how they could best integrate their basic science knowledge.

One faculty member gave some interesting advice: "read through your textbook in, say, biochemistry, and every time you come across a section that mentions a concept or piece of information relating to another basic science—for example, immunology—highlight that section in the book. Then go to your immunology textbook and look up this information, and make sure you have a good understanding of it. When you have, go back to your biochemistry textbook and carry on reading."

This was a great suggestion—if only students had the time, and all of the books necessary at hand, to do it! At Elsevier we thought long and hard about a way of simplifying this process, and eventually the idea for Elsevier's Integrated Series was born.

The series centers on the concept of the *integration box*. These boxes occur throughout the text whenever a link to another basic science is relevant. They're easy to spot in the text—with their color-coded headings and logos. Each box contains a title for the integration topic and then a brief summary of the topic. The information is complete in itself—you probably won't have to go to any other sources—and you have the basic knowledge to use as a foundation if you want to expand your knowledge of the topic.

You can use this book in two ways. First, as a review book . . .
When you are using the book for review, the integration boxes will jog your memory on topics you have already covered. You'll be able to reassure yourself that you can identify the link, and you can quickly compare your knowledge of the topic with the summary in the box. The integration boxes might highlight gaps in your knowledge, and then you can use them to determine what topics you need to cover in more detail.

Second, the book can be used as a short text to have at hand while you are taking your course . . .
You may come across an integration box that deals with a topic you haven't covered yet, and this will ensure that you're one step ahead in identifying the links to other subjects (especially useful if you're working on a PBL exercise). On a simpler level, the links in the boxes to other sciences and to clinical medicine will help you see clearly the relevance of the basic science topic you are studying. You may already be

confident in the subject matter of many of the integration boxes, so they will serve as helpful reminders.

At the back of the book we have included case study questions relating to each chapter so that you can test yourself as you work your way through the book.

Online Version
An online version of the book is available on our Student Consult site. Use of this site is free to anyone who has bought the printed book. Please see the inside front cover for full details on the Student Consult and how to access the electronic version of this book.

In addition to containing USMLE test questions, fully searchable text, and an image bank, the Student Consult site offers additional integration links, both to the other books in Elsevier's Integrated Series and to other key Elsevier textbooks.

Books in Elsevier's Integrated Series
The nine books in the series cover all of the basic sciences. The more books you buy in the series, the more links are made accessible across the series, both in print and online.

 Anatomy and Embryology

 Histology

 Neuroscience

 Biochemistry

 Physiology

 Pathology

 Immunology and Microbiology

 Pharmacology

 Genetics

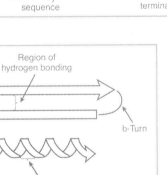

Figure 3-1. The peptide bond linking α-carbons and their side chains together into a polypeptide. The *trans* conformation is favored, producing a rigid structure that restricts freedom of movement except for rotation around bonds that join to the α-carbons.

Artwork:

The books are packed with 4-color illustrations and photographs. When a concept can be better explained with a picture, we've drawn one. Where possible, the pictures tell a dynamic story that will help you remember the information far more effectively than a paragraph of text.

Integration boxes:

Whenever the subject matter can be related to another science discipline, we've put in an Integration Box. Clearly labeled and color-coded, these boxes include nuggets of information on topics that require an integrated knowledge of the sciences to be fully understood. The material in these boxes is complete in itself, and you can use them as a way of reminding yourself of information you already know and reinforcing key links between the sciences. Or the boxes may contain information you have not come across before, in which case you can use them a springboard for further research or simply to appreciate the relevance of the subject matter of the book to the study of medicine.

Figure 3-3. Secondary structure includes α-helix and β-pleated sheet (β-sheet).

MICROBIOLOGY

Prion Diseases

Prions (PrP^{Sc}) are formed from otherwise normal neurologic proteins (PrP) and are responsible for encephalopathies in humans (Creutzfeldt-Jakob disease, kuru), scrapie in sheep, and bovine spongiform encephalopathy. Contact between the normal PrP and PrP^{Sc} results in conversion of the secondary structure of PrP from predominantly α-helical to predominantly β-pleated sheet. The altered structure of the protein forms long, filamentous aggregates that gradually damage neuronal tissue. The harmful PrP^{Sc} form is highly resistant to heat, UV irradiation, and protease enzymes.

Since proline has no free hydrogen to contribute to helix stability, it is referred to as a "helix breaker." The α-helix is found in most globular proteins and in some fibrous proteins (e.g., α-keratin).

Text:

Succinct, clearly written text, focusing on the core information you need to know and no more. It's the same level as a carefully prepared course syllabus or lecture notes.

rmation

-structure) consists of

tabilized by hydrogen

f adjacent sequences.

can be the same (parallel) or opposite (antiparallel) direction. β-Structures are found in 80% of all globular proteins and in silk fibroin.

Supersecondary Structure and Domains

Supersecondary structures, or *motifs*, are characteristic combinations of secondary structure 10–40 residues in length that recur in different proteins. They bridge the gap between the less specific regularity of secondary structure and the highly specific folding of tertiary structure. The same motif can perform similar functions in different proteins.

* The four-helix bundle motif provides a cavity for enzymes to bind prosthetic groups or cofactors.
* The β-barrel motif can bind hydrophobic molecules such as retinol in the interior of the barrel.
* Motifs may also be mixtures of both α and β conformations.

Physiology: The Regulation of Normal Body Function

1

Life is not always about homeostasis and balance. The body must also adapt to changing requirements, such as during exercise. Now the normal resting values are physiologically inappropriate, since an increase in muscle blood flow, cardiac output, and respiratory rate are necessary to support the increased metabolic demands associated with physical activity. Physiology is the study of adaptive adjustments to new challenges.

Life is a state of constant change. The physiology of the body alters as we age. An infant is not a small adult, and the physiology of an octogenarian is different from that of an adolescent. Chapter 16 provides a concise summary of physiologic changes in each sex across the life span.

Finally, physiology makes sense. As a student, you need to look for the organizing principles in your study of the body. There are more details and variations than can be memorized. However, if you focus on the organizing principles, the details fall into a logical sequence. Look for the big picture first—it is always correct. The details and complex interactions all support the big picture.

●●● PHYSIOLOGY

Body function requires a stable internal environment, described by Claude Bernard as the "milieu intérieur," in spite of a changing outside world. Homeostasis, a state of balance, is made possible by negative feedback control systems. Complex neural and hormonal regulatory systems provide control and integration of body functions. Physicians describe "normal" values for vital signs—blood pressure of 120/80 mm Hg, pulse of 72 beats/min, respiration rate of 14 breaths/min. These "normal" vital sign values reflect a body in homeostatic balance.

A stable milieu interior also requires a balance between intake and output. Intake and production will increase the amount of a compound in the body. Excretion and consumption will decrease the amount of a compound in the body. Body fluid and electrolyte composition is regulated about a set point, which involves both control of ingestion and control of excretion. Any changes in ingestion must be compensated by changes in excretion, or the body is out of balance.

●●● LEVELS OF ORGANIZATION

Medical physiology applies basic principles from chemistry, physics, and biology to the study of human life. Atoms are safely in the realm of chemistry. Physiologic study begins with molecules and continues through the interaction of the organism with its environment (Fig. 1-1).

Physiology is the study of normal body function. Physiology extends to the molecular level, the study of the regulation of the synthesis of biomolecules, and to the subcellular level, details of the provision of nutrients to support mitochondrial metabolism. Physiology includes cellular function, the study of the role of membrane transport, and describes organ function, including the mechanics of pressure generation by the heart. Integrative physiology is the study of the function of the organism, including the coordinated response to digestion and absorption of the nutrients in a meal.

The components of physiology are best approached as organ systems. This approach allows all aspects of one system, e.g., the circulatory system, to be discussed, emphasizing their commonalities and coordinated function.

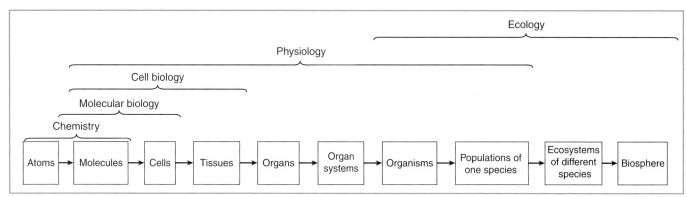

Figure 1-1. Physiology bridges the gap between chemistry and ecology. Physiology incorporates the investigational techniques from cell biology and molecular biology as well as ecology in order to better understand the function of the human body.

TABLE 1-1. Specific Examples of the Movement Theme			
Process	**Movement**	**Driving Force**	**Modulated by**
Flow	Flow	Pressure gradient	Resistance (–)
Diffusion	Net flux	Concentration gradient	Permeability (+) Surface area (+) Distance (–)
Osmosis	Water	Particle gradient	Barrier particle permeability (–) Barrier water permeability (+)
Electrochemical	Current	Ionic gradient	Membrane permeability (+)
Capillary filtration	Flow	Combined pressure and oncotic gradient	Capillary surface area (+)
Transport	Secondary active	Ion gradient	Concentration gradient (–)

+, Modulators enhance the movement; –, modulators impede the movement.

●●●● COMMON THEMES

Common Theme 1: Movement Across Barriers

Life is characterized as a nonequilibrium steady state. The body achieves homeostatic balance—but only by expending energy derived from metabolism. Although the processes listed below appear different, they share common features. Movement results from a driving force and is opposed by some aspect of resistance (Table 1-1).

Movement against a gradient requires energy. ATP is ultimately the source of energy used to move compounds against a gradient. This is important, because after the gradients are created, the concentration gradients can serve as a source of energy for other movement (e.g., secondary active transport and osmosis).

Common Theme 2: Indicator Dilution

$$\text{Amount/volume} = \text{concentration}$$

or, rearranged,

$$\text{Volume} = \text{concentration/amount}$$

If any two of the above are known, the third can be calculated. This approach is used to determine a physiologic volume that cannot be directly measured. For example, plasma volume can be estimated by adding a known amount of the dye Evans blue, which binds tightly to albumin and remains mostly in the plasma space. After the dye distributes equally throughout the plasma volume, a plasma sample can be taken. The observed concentration of the sample, together with the amount of dye added, allows calculation of the plasma volume (Fig. 1-2).

There are some assumptions in this process that are rarely met, but the estimations are close enough to be clinically useful. The indicator should be distributed only in the volume of interest. There must be sufficient time for the indicator to equilibrate so that all areas of the volume have an identical concentration. For estimation of plasma volume with Evans blue, those assumptions are not met. Some albumin is lost for the plasma volume over time, so an early sampling is desirable. But some plasma spaces have slow exchange rates, and Evans blue dye requires additional time to reach those spaces. In practice, a plasma sample is drawn at 10 or 20 minutes after indicator injection, and the plasma volume is calculated with the knowledge that it is an estimate and with awareness of the limitations of the technique.

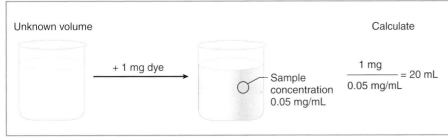

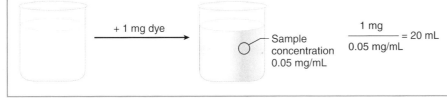

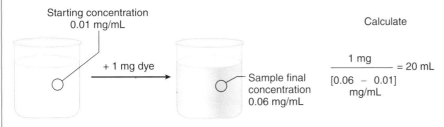

Figure 1-2. Indicator dilution allows calculation of unknown volumes and flows. **A,** The indicator dilution technique uses addition of a known quantity of a marker, and the final concentration of that marker, to calculate the volume in which it was distributed. **B,** The procedure is the same even if some of the marker is already present in the volume. The only alteration is that the final concentration is subtracted from the starting concentration to determine the change in concentration caused by adding the marker. **C,** An equivalent procedure can be used to calculate flows. If you know the amount of O_2 absorbed across the lungs per minute, and the change in blood O_2 concentration that resulted from that absorption, you can calculate the blood flow through the lungs, or the cardiac output.

TABLE 1-2. Application of Indicator Dilution		
Volume or Flow	**Indicator (The Tracer)**	**The Change**
Total body water	Iothalamate	Iothalamate concentration
Extracellular fluid volume	Inulin	Inulin concentration
RBC volume	^{51}Cr-labeled RBC	^{51}Cr-labeled RBC concentration
Residual lung volume	N_2	N_2 washout
Cardiac output	Temperature (a volume of cold saline)	Change in blood temperature over time
Cardiac output	Rate of O_2 uptake in the lungs	Change in O_2 content in blood flowing through the lungs
Glomerular filtration rate	Inulin	Inulin excretion rate
Renal blood flow	Para-aminohippuric acid	Para-aminohippuric acid excretion rate

In the best case, the only indicator in the system is the new indicator that was added. Alternatively, if the compound is already in the system, the term "change in amount" can be substituted for "amount" and "change in concentration" can be substituted for "concentration."

Change in amount/volume = change in concentration

A flow is actually a volume over time, so the indicator dilution technique can also be used to estimate flows. Instead of amount, the indicator is expressed as amount per time (Table 1-2).

Flow = amount per time/change in concentration

Common Theme 3: Feedback Control

Stability is maintained by negative feedback control. The system requires a set point for a regulated variable, the ability to monitor that variable, the ability to detect any error between the actual value and the set point, and an effector system to bring about a compensatory response (Fig. 1-3).

The acute regulation of arterial blood pressure by the arterial baroreceptors (the baroreceptor reflex) is a prototype for physiologic negative feedback control systems. Normal blood pressure is taken as the set point of the system. The

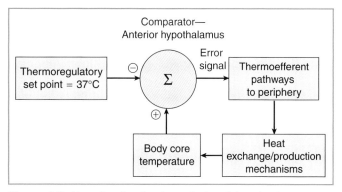

Figure 1-3. Negative feedback control matches body temperature to the thermoregulatory set point. The anterior hypothalamus compares the body core temperature against the set point. If the two do not match, an error signal is generated, which results in a compensatory change in the heat gain/heat loss balance of the body. This change should bring body core temperature back to the set point.

sensing mechanism is a group of stretch-sensitive nerve endings in the walls of the arch of the aorta and in the walls of the carotid arteries near the carotid bifurcation. These nerve endings are always being stretched, so there is always some background firing activity. The rate of firing of these receptors is proportionate to the stretch on the blood vessels. Stretch (and therefore firing) increase as blood pressure increases, and a decrease in stretch (and therefore a decrease in firing rate) accompanies a fall in blood pressure. The afferent nerves from these receptors synapse in the cardiovascular center of the medulla, where the inputs are integrated. The efferent side of the reflex is the parasympathetic and sympathetic nervous systems (PNS and SNS), which control heart rate, myocardial contractility, and vascular smooth muscle contraction.

A sudden drop in blood pressure leads to a decrease in stretch on the baroreceptor nerve endings, and the decrease in nerve traffic leads to a medullary mediated increase in sympathetic activity and decrease in parasympathetic nerve activity. Increased sympathetic activity causes vascular smooth muscle contraction, which helps increase peripheral resistance and restore blood pressure. Increased sympathetic nerve activity also increases myocardial contractility and, together with the decrease in parasympathetic activity, increases heart rate. The resultant increase in cardiac output also helps restore blood pressure. As blood pressure recovers, the stretch on baroreceptor nerve fibers returns toward normal and the sympathetic activation diminishes. Table 1-3 illustrates the wide variety of physiologic functions controlled by negative feedback.

TABLE 1-3. Some Important Negative Feedback Control Systems

Regulated Variable	Sensed by	Response Mediated by	Effector
Arterial blood pressure	Baroreceptors	SNS and PNS	Heart, vasculature
Microcirculation blood flow	Tissue metabolites		Vascular smooth muscle, precapillary sphincter
Arterial blood CO_2	Central and peripheral chemoreceptors	CNS	Respiratory muscles
Arterial blood O_2	Peripheral chemoreceptors	CNS	Respiratory muscles
Plasma osmolarity	CNS osmoreceptors	ADH	Kidneys
Glomerular filtration rate	Macula densa	Angiotensin II	Efferent arteriole
Plasma K^+	Adrenal cortex	Aldosterone	Cells, renal tubule
Plasma glucose	Pancreas	Multiple hormones	Liver, adipose, skeletal muscle, mitochondria
Muscle stretch	Muscle spindle	Motor neuron	Muscle fibers
Gastric emptying	Small intestinal chemoreceptors	Enteric nerves, GI hormones	Pyloric tone
Body fluid volume	Cardiopulmonary volume receptors	SNS, ADH	Kidney

ADH, antidiuretic hormone; CNS, central nervous system; PNS, peripheral nervous system; SNS, sympathetic nervous system.

Positive feedback provides an unstable escalating stimulus-response cycle. Positive feedbacks are rare in human physiology. Three situations in which they do occur are oxytocin stimulation of uterine contractions during labor, the LH surge before ovulation, and Na^+ entry during the generation of an action potential. In a positive feedback system, movement away from a starting point elicits a response resulting in even more movement away from the starting point. As an example, oxytocin stimulates uterine contraction during labor and delivery. Central nervous system (CNS) oxytocin release is directly proportionate to the amount of pressure generated by the head of the baby on the opening of the uterus. So once uterine contractions begin, the opening of the uterus is stretched. Stretch elicits oxytocin release, stimulating stronger uterine contractions. Pressure on the opening of the uterus is further increased, stimulating additional oxytocin release. This positive feedback cycle continues until the pressure in the uterus is sufficient to expel the baby. Delivery stops the pressure on the uterus and removes the stimulus for further oxytocin release.

Feed-forward regulation allows an anticipatory response before a disturbance is sensed by negative feedback control systems. An excellent example is the regulation of ventilation during exercise. Respiration during sustained exercise increases five-fold even though arterial blood gases (and therefore chemoreceptor stimulation) do not appreciably change. During aerobic exercise, the increased alveolar ventilation is stimulated by outflow from the CNS motor cortex and not by the normal CO_2 chemoreceptor control system. This appears to be a finely tuned response, since the ventilatory stimulus increases as the number of motor units involved in the exercise increases. The coupling of ventilation to muscle activity allows an increased ventilation to support the increased metabolic demand without first waiting for hypoxia (or hypercapnia) to develop as a respiratory drive.

Feed-forward controls are involved in gastric acid and insulin secretion following meal ingestion and behavioral responses to a variety of stresses, such as fasting and thermoregulation. The combination of feed-forward and negative feedback controls provides the body with the flexibility to maintain homeostasis but to also adapt to a changing environment.

Common Theme 4: Redundant Control

The sophistication and complexity of physiologic control systems are quite varied. For example, Na^+ is the major extracellular cation and is controlled by multiple endocrine agents, physical forces, and appetite. In contrast, Cl^- is the major extracellular anion, but in humans, Cl^- is not under significant endocrine control.

The degree of redundant regulation can be viewed as a reflection of the importance of the variable to life. For example, a drop in plasma glucose can induce shock, but hyperglycemia is not as immediately life threatening. Consequently, there are four hormones (cortisol, glucagon, epinephrine, and growth hormone) that increase plasma glucose if glucose

levels fall too low, but only one hormone (insulin) that lowers glucose should glucose levels be too high. Na^+ is an essential dietary component, and Na^+ conservation is regulated by numerous endocrine and renal mechanisms. The effectiveness of the two hormones promoting Na^+ excretion (atrial natriuretic peptide and urotensin) is limited. Arterial blood pressure control is perhaps the most redundant and includes numerous physical, endocrine, and neural mechanisms.

Disease states often provide insight into the relative importance of competing control systems. The hypertension accompanying renal artery stenosis illustrates the prominent role of the kidney in the long-term regulation of blood pressure. Plasma K^+ changes are apparent in disorders of aldosterone secretion, and plasma Na^+ changes reflect the dilutional effects of ADH regulation of renal water excretion. In each chapter of this book, emphasis is given to the more prominent or disease-related control systems.

Common Theme 5: Integration

The normal assignment of separate chapters to each organ system downplays the significant interaction among the organ systems in normal function. Provision of O_2 and nutrients by the respiratory and gastrointestinal systems is essential to the function of all cells within the body, as is the removal of metabolic waste by these systems and the kidneys. Blood flow is similarly essential to all organ function.

Coordination of body functions is accomplished by two major regulatory systems: the nervous system and the endocrine system. This level of regulation is superimposed on any intrinsic regulation occurring within the organ. The endocrine and nervous systems are often redundant. For example, the autonomic nervous system (ANS), angiotensin II, and adrenal catecholamines all regulate arterial pressure. In spite of the overlap, the systems usually work in concert, achieving the appropriate physiologic adjustments on organ function to counteract any environmental stress.

Common Theme 6: Graphs, Figures, and Equations

Graphs, figures, and equations condense and simplify explanations. Different graph formats communicate specific relationships. Understanding the strengths of each approach allows a reader to more quickly assimilate the important information.

Graphs

X-Y Graph. The most common graph format is the *x-y* plot. If a graph illustrates a cause-effect relationship, the *x*-axis represents the independent variable (cause), and the *y*-axis represents the dependent variable (effect). The same graph format is used to show observations that may not be cause-effect coupled, and in this case the graph illustrates only a correlation. In physiology, time is often plotted on the *x*-axis, allowing the graph to illustrate a change in the *y*-axis variable over time (Fig. 1-4).

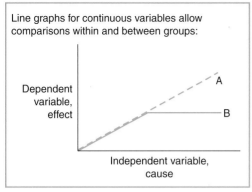

A

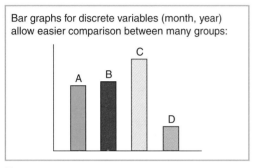

B

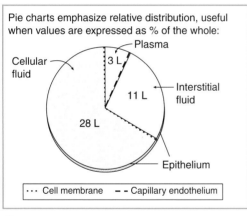

C

Figure 1-4. Different graph formats convey different types of information. **A**, The *x-y* graph allows comparison of two variables. If there is a dependent variable, it is always plotted along the *y*-axis. **B**, Bar graphs are used for comparisons between many groups. **C**, Pie charts are used to emphasize distribution relative to the total amount available.

Bar Graph. A line *x-y* graph is used when both *x* and *y* numbers are continuous, such as the plot of time versus voltage on an electrocardiogram. In some measurements, the *x*-axis is a discrete variable (month, age, sex, treatment group), and the *y*-axis measures frequency. This plotting approach allows easy visual comparison among many groups.

Pie Chart. A pie chart effectively illustrates the relative distribution. It is useful to communicate proportions. Values are expressed as percentages of the whole rather than absolute values.

Equations

Variables that have a direct or inverse relationship are summarized more quickly in equations than in graphs. This approach is used for relationships that are not constant. If there are curves in the line (other than mathematical curves resulting from power, inverse, or log functions), then a line graph will have to be used.

Equations are a quick summary of direct and inverse relationships. For Fick's law of diffusion,

$$J = -DA \frac{\Delta c}{\Delta x}$$

The text version saying the same thing as the equation is:

The net movement of a compound, or flux (J), is determined by the diffusion coefficient (D), the surface area available for exchange (A), the concentration gradient (Δc), and the distance over which the compound has to diffuse (Δx).

Compounds moving by diffusion always travel down the concentration gradient. By convention, the side with the higher concentration is considered first, and the side with the lower concentration is considered second. The convention uses a negative sign (–) to indicate that the flux is away from the area with the original higher concentration.

The ability of a compound to move is determined by the diffusion coefficient (D). This coefficient is characteristic of the individual compound and the barrier, and includes the molecular weight and size of the compound, its solubility, and the temperature and pressure conditions.

Flux is directly proportionate to the surface area (A) available for exchange. As the surface area participating in exchange increases, the flux of the compound also increases. As the surface area participating in the exchange decreases, the flux will decrease. If there is no surface area participating in the exchange, the flux will be zero.

Flux is directly proportionate to the concentration gradient (Δc). An increase in the concentration gradient will increase the flux of a compound, and conversely, a decrease in the concentration gradient will decrease the flux of a compound. If there is no concentration gradient, the flux will be zero.

Flux is inversely proportionate to the distance over which a compound must travel (Δx). As the distance to be traveled by the compound increases, the flux will decrease. As the distance to be traveled by the compound decreases, the flux will increase.

The explanation took 279 words to convey the information contained in the equation. Equations are a useful shorthand method and are particularly useful if the reader is aware of all the implications.

Common Theme 7: Autonomic Nervous System

The ANS is a major mechanism for neural control of physiologic functions. Discussions of ANS usually take one of three perspectives: (1) an anatomic perspective based on structure, (2) a physiologic perspective based on function, (3) a pharmacologic perspective based on the receptor subtypes involved. All three perspectives are valid and useful.

The anatomic perspective separates the ANS into a sympathetic and a parasympathetic branch, based in part on the origin and length of the nerves. The sympathetic nerves arise from the thoracolumbar spinal cord and have short preganglionic neurons. The preganglionic nerves synapse in the sympathetic chain, and long postganglionic nerves innervate the final target. Acetylcholine is the preganglionic nerve neurotransmitter, and norepinephrine is the postganglionic neurotransmitter, except for the sweat glands, which have a sympathetic cholinergic innervation. There is an endocrine component of the SNS. Circulating plasma norepinephrine levels come from both overflow from the sympathetic nerve terminals and from the adrenal medulla. Plasma epinephrine originates primarily from the adrenal medulla.

The parasympathetic nerves arise from the cranial and sacral portions of the spinal cord and have a long preganglionic nerve. They synapse in ganglia close to the target tissue and have short postganglionic nerves. The parasympathetic nerves use acetylcholine as the neurotransmitter for both the preganglionic and postganglionic nerves. There is not an endocrine arm to the PNS.

The physiologic perspective of the ANS is based on both homeostatic control and adaptive responses. The ANS, along with the endocrine system, regulates most body functions through a standard negative feedback process. The adaptive component of the ANS characterizes the SNS as mediating "fight or flight" and the PNS as mediating "rest and digest." This classification provides a logical structure for the diverse actions of the sympathetic and parasympathetic nerves on various target tissues.

The SNS is activated by multiple stimuli, including perceived threat, pain, hypotension, or hypoglycemia. The parasympathetic nerves are active during quiescent periods, such as after ingestion of a meal and during sleep. The specific ANS control of each organ is discussed in the appropriate chapter.

The pharmacologic division of the ANS is based on the receptor subtype activated. The SNS stimulates α- and/or β-adrenergic receptors on target tissues. The PNS stimulates nicotinic or muscarinic cholinergic receptors on the target tissues. Cells express different receptor subtypes, and the receptor subtype mediates the action of SNS or PNS on that cell.

Common Theme 8: Physiologic Research

As indicated by the volume of material contained in textbooks, much is already known about human physiology. The current understanding of body function is based on more than 3000 years of research. The presentation in this text represents the best understanding of body function. Much of the material represents models that are being tested and refined in research laboratories.

Each generation of students believes they have mastered all the physiology that it is possible to learn. They are wrong. Recent physiologic research has uncovered the mechanism of action of nitric oxide, the existence of the hormone atrial natriuretic peptide, and the nongenomic actions of steroid hormones. The sequencing of the human genome potentially has opened an entirely new clinical approach—genetic medicine. The interaction of physiology and medicine will continue. In 20 years these days may be looked upon as the "good old days" when the study of the human body was easy.

●●● APPLICATION OF COMMON THEMES: PHYSIOLOGY OF THERMOREGULATION

The anterior hypothalamic "thermostat" adjusts heat balance to maintain body core temperature. Heat exchange is determined by convection, conduction, evaporation, and radiation. Radiation, conduction, and convection are determined by the difference between the skin temperature and the environmental temperature (*common theme 1*). Behavioral mechanisms can assist thermoregulation. The rate of heat loss depends primarily on the surface temperature of the skin, which is in turn a function of the skin's blood flow. The blood flow of the skin varies in response to changes in the body's

ANATOMY

Autonomic Nervous System

The sympathetic nerves originate in the intermediolateral horn of the spinal cord and exit at the T1 through L2 spinal cord segments. The preganglionic nerve fibers synapse in either the paravertebral sympathetic chain ganglia or the prevertebral ganglia before the postganglionic nerve fibers run to the target tissue. The parasympathetic nerves exit the CNS through cranial nerves III, VII, IX, and X and through the S2 through S4 sacral spinal cord segments. The parasympathetic preganglionic nerve fibers usually travel almost all the way to the target before making the synapse with the postganglionic fibers.

PHARMACOLOGY

Adrenergic Receptor Subtypes

There are at least two types of α-adrenergic receptors. α_1-Receptors work through IP_3 and DAG to constrict vascular and genitourinary smooth muscle and to relax GI smooth muscle. α_2-Adrenergic receptors decrease cAMP, promote platelet aggregation, decrease insulin release, and decrease norepinephrine synaptic release. There are at least three subtypes of β-adrenergic receptors, all of which increase cAMP. β_1-Receptors in the heart increase heart rate and contractility, and in the kidney release renin. β_2-Receptors relax smooth muscle and promote glycogenolysis. β_3-Adrenergic receptors in adipose promote lipolysis.

core temperature and to changes in temperature of the external environment (Box 1-1).

There are two different physiologic responses to a change in body temperature. A forced change in body temperature results when an environmental stress is sufficient to overcome the body thermoregulatory systems. Prolonged immersion in cool water would result in forced hypothermia, a drop in body core temperature. Prolonged confinement in a hot room could result in forced hyperthermia, an elevation in body core temperature. A regulated change in body temperature occurs when the hypothalamic set point is shifted (*common theme 3*). A regulated hyperthermia accompanies the release of pyrogens during an influenza infection. A regulated hypothermia follows exposure to organophosphate poisons.

A forced drop in body core temperature initiates adrenergic heat conservation (*common theme 3*). Piloerection of cutaneous hair decreases conductive heat loss. Sweating is decreased to reduce evaporative heat loss (*common theme 7*). Cutaneous adrenergic vasoconstriction decreases blood flow

and therefore diminishes radiant loss of heat (*common theme 7*). These physiologic responses are augmented by behavioral responses that diminish exposure to cold, such as moving to a warmer environment or putting on additional clothes. A drop in body core temperature also stimulates heat production. Shivering and movement increase metabolic heat production. In neonates, adrenergic activity increases metabolism of neonatal brown fat. Long-term cold exposure increases thyroid hormone release and increases basal metabolic rate (*common theme 4*).

A forced increase in body core temperature initiates heat loss (*common theme 3*). A decrease in vascular sympathetic nerve activity causes an increase in cutaneous blood flow, which augments the radiant loss of heat (*common theme 7*). Sympathetic cholinergic activity increases sweating (*common theme 7*). Excessive sweating can deplete body Na^+. Aldosterone release decreases Na^+ lost in sweat in long-term heat adaptation (*common theme 5*). Increases in body core temperature also result in decreased heat production. There can be a behavioral decrease in activity, movement to a cooler environment, or removal of clothes. In the long term, basal metabolic rate can be diminished by lower thyroid hormone release (*common theme 4*).

The time course of the body thermoregulation alterations caused by influenza is shown in Figure 1-5. During the early stages of the flu, pyrogens are produced that elevate the hypothalamic thermoregulatory set point, usually to around 39°C. The body core temperature is 37°C, below the set point, generating a "too cold" error signal (*common theme 3*). The thermoregulatory balance is altered to favor heat gain mechanisms, such as shivering and reduced cutaneous blood flow, complemented by behavioral changes such as curling up in a fetal position and getting under blankets. These mechanisms persist even though body core temperature is higher than "normal." As body core temperature and set point come into balance at 39°C, there is some reduction in the heat gain mechanisms.

As the influenza infection subsides, pyrogen production ceases and the set point returns to 37°C. The hypothalamic set point is now lower than body core temperature, generating a "too hot" error signal (*common theme 3*). Heat loss mechanisms are activated, including sweating and increased cutaneous blood flow, and complemented by behavioral

Box 1-1. HEAT LOSS AND HEAT GAIN MECHANISMS

Enhance heat loss/diminish heat gain when ambient temperature is lower than body temperature

Increase cutaneous blood flow
Increase sweating (even when ambient temperature is higher than body temperature)
Remove clothing
Move to cooler environment
Decrease metabolic rate
Take sprawled posture

Diminish heat loss/enhance heat gain when ambient temperature is lower than body temperature

Decrease cutaneous blood flow
Piloerect
Huddle or take ball posture
Move to warmer environment
Increase activity and movement
Shivering
Metabolize brown adipose (infants)
Increase metabolic rate

NEUROSCIENCE

Hypothalamic Temperature Control

The preoptic area of the anterior hypothalamus is largely responsible for thermoregulatory control. The hypothalamus receives sensory information regarding temperature from central and peripheral temperature-sensitive neurons. This information is integrated in the hypothalamus, and efferent signals from the hypothalamus activate temperature regulatory mechanisms.

MICROBIOLOGY

Influenza

There are three major classes of influenza viruses: A, B, and C. Influenza A viruses are found in many different species and are subclassified based on the presence on the surface of the virus of either the hemagglutinin or the neuraminidase protein. Influenza B viruses are found almost exclusively in humans. Influenza C viruses cause only a minor respiratory infection. Small changes in the surface proteins occur each year, making it difficult to develop effective flu vaccines.

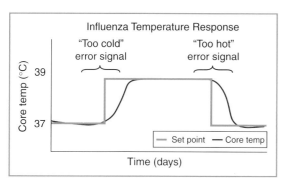

Figure 1-5. Influenza results in a transient increase in body core temperature. The increase in body core temperature is initiated following an elevation in the hypothalamic set point. Return of body temperature toward normal occurs only after the set point has returned to 37°C.

mechanisms, such as lying on top of the covers and spreading out to increase exposed surface area (*common theme 5*). The excessive heat loss continues until body core temperature returns to 37°C, "normal."

The febrile response to influenza can be blocked by aspirin, ibuprofen, and acetaminophen, all of which block prostaglandin production. The febrile response to influenza, however, is a protective physiologic response and assists the immune system in combating the infection. Individuals allowed to exhibit a febrile response have a shorter duration of infection and faster recovery (*common theme 8*). Current research is examining the protective role of regulated hypothermia in enhancing survival following hemorrhage.

●●● TOP 5 TAKE-HOME POINTS

1. The majority of compounds move in the body by diffusion down a concentration gradient, with only a small portion being transported against the concentration gradient.
2. The stability of the internal environment of the body is due to a variety of negative feedback control systems. Positive feedback control is inherently unstable and is often characteristic of disease states.
3. The endocrine and autonomic nervous systems provide coordinated, often complementary control of body function.
4. The autonomic nervous system has two mechanisms of action: shifting between sympathetic and parasympathetic activation, and altering the basal activity of the sympathetic or parasympathetic nerves.
5. Thermoregulation entails both a normal negative feedback control and a hypothalamic set point.

The Integument

2

CONTENTS

Epithelia are specialized to serve a variety of functions. Epithelia provide a physical barrier, often supplemented by epithelial cell secretions. Lipids and keratin in the skin provide a waterproof barrier. Mucous secretions protect the GI, female reproductive, and lung epithelia from abrasive damage. Cilia of the respiratory and fallopian tube epithelia move mucus and fluid lining the epithelia toward the mouth or vagina, respectively, for expulsion. Some epithelial cells are specialized for transepithelial transport of ions, nutrients, and metabolic wastes.

Epithelial membranes contain specialized transport proteins. These proteins promote absorption of nutrients into the body from luminal or duct contents, and secretion into luminal or duct fluids for excretion from the body.

●●● EPITHELIA

Epithelial cells provide a continuous barrier between the internal and external environments. Epithelial cells line the skin, sweat glands, gastrointestinal (GI) tract, pulmonary airways, renal tubules, and pancreatic and hepatic ducts. Consequently, materials in the GI lumen, respiratory airways, renal tubules, reproductive system lumens, and secretory ducts are functionally "outside" the body. Compounds that are secreted across epithelia are exocrine secretions, in contrast to endocrine secretions, which remain within the body. For example, pancreatic digestive enzymes that are secreted into the lumen of the small intestine are exocrine pancreatic secretions, in contrast to insulin and glucagon, which are secreted into the blood as endocrine pancreatic secretions.

Epithelial cells have polarity, since the tight junctions between cells separate the epithelial cell membrane into an apical and a basolateral surface (Fig. 2-1). Epithelial tight junctions allow osmotic and electrochemical gradients to exist across the epithelia. The apical surface faces the outside of the body or, for the GI tract and secretory ducts, a lumen. The basal and lateral surfaces face the inside of the body, or serosa, and are surrounded by extracellular fluid. Epithelia express different populations of protein transporters on the apical surface and the basolateral surface. The structural integrity of epithelial cells is provided by tight junctions and by desmosomes, a site of attachment for the extracellular matrix protein keratin.

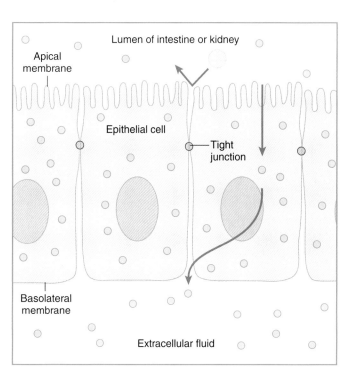

Figure 2-1. Tight junctions separate the apical membrane from the basolateral membrane of the epithelial cell. The proteins expressed on the apical membrane differ from the proteins on the basolateral surface, providing polarity or orientation for epithelia. The epithelial cell barrier allows the concentration of compounds on one side of the epithelium to be different from the concentration of that compound on the other side of the epithelium.

The common functional role of epithelia is reflected in the common transport proteins located in apparently different organs. Identical sodium-dependent amino acid and glucose transporters are found in the epithelia of the small intestine and renal proximal tubule. Identical Cl⁻ reabsorbing channels are found in epithelia of salivary glands, sweat glands, pancreatic ducts, and bile ducts. Genetic defects in these transport proteins affect all organs that express the protein. For example, defects in the Cl⁻ channel cystic fibrosis transmembrane regulator (CFTR) affect the lungs, exocrine pancreas, sweat glands, and GI tract.

Transit across the epithelial barrier occurs by two pathways—transcellular and paracellular (Fig. 2-2). Transcellular transport passes through the cell and consequently has to cross both the apical and basolateral membranes. Carrier proteins are necessary to move lipid-insoluble substances across these cell membranes. Vesicular movement, such as pinocytosis, may be necessary for larger proteins. Paracellular movement occurs through the tight junctions and water-filled spaces between cells. This is the primary pathway for water-soluble substances in some epithelia.

Transepithelial water movement occurs in response to an osmotic gradient. Movement of the solvent water causes a change in the concentration of the solutes on either side of the epithelia—solute concentration increases on the side where the water exits, and solute concentration decreases on the side where the water enters. If the tight junctions are also permeable to the solute, water movement can cause solute movement, a process called solvent drag.

Paracellular movement is restricted by the "tightness" of epithelial tight junctions. "Tight" tight junctions restrict the paracellular movement of water and electrolytes. "Loose" tight junctions allow the paracellular movement of water and electrolytes. Tight junction permeability varies between tissues and within different regions of the same tissue. Water-impermeable areas include the esophagus, stomach, and portions of the renal tubules distal to the loop of Henle. Water-permeable areas include the small intestine and renal proximal tubules.

Transport of ions across epithelium generates a transepithelial potential. This electrical force may oppose further movement of ions, analogous to the membrane potential. Transepithelial potential is important for aldosterone action in the renal distal tubule and connecting segment (see Chapter 11) (Fig. 2-3).

●●● INTEGUMENT LAYERS

The integument, or skin, is the largest organ containing epithelial cells. Skin diminishes or prevents damage from

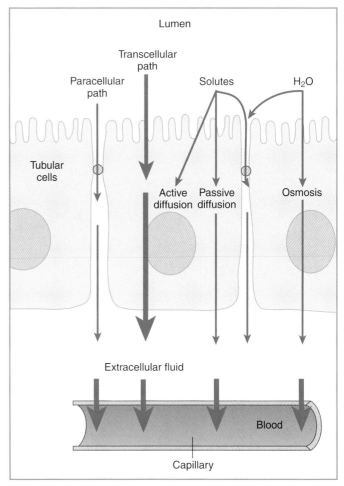

Figure 2-2. Transepithelial absorption can go across the epithelial cells in the transcellular pathway or between the epithelial cells in a paracellular pathway. Compounds absorbed by the transcellular pathway have to cross both the apical and the basolateral membranes and travel through the cytoplasm of the cell. Movement through the paracellular pathway is determined by the permeability of the tight junctions that join the epithelial cells.

PATHOLOGY

Cystic Fibrosis

Cystic fibrosis is a recessive genetic defect in the epithelial CFTR Cl⁻ channel. Cystic fibrosis occurs in approximately one of every 3500 live births, and an estimated 10 million Americans are carriers of the defective gene. The impaired Cl⁻ movement interferes with transepithelial water movement, resulting in excessively thick secretions that block the lungs, GI tract, and pancreatic and bile ducts.

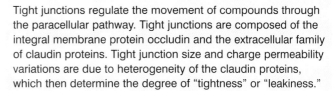

HISTOLOGY

Tight Junctions

Tight junctions regulate the movement of compounds through the paracellular pathway. Tight junctions are composed of the integral membrane protein occludin and the extracellular family of claudin proteins. Tight junction size and charge permeability variations are due to heterogeneity of the claudin proteins, which then determine the degree of "tightness" or "leakiness."

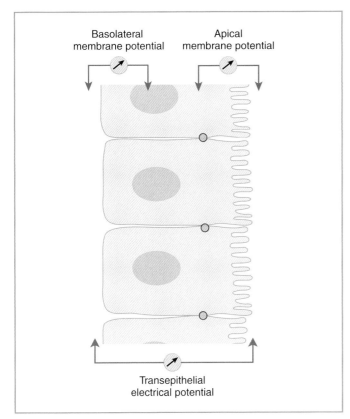

Basolateral membrane potential   Apical membrane potential

Transepithelial
electrical potential

Figure 2-3. Impermeable epithelial tight junctions are necessary to develop a significant transepithelial electrical potential. The reabsorption or secretion of ions across epithelia can establish electrical charge differences across the epithelial barrier. Leakage of ions through the paracellular pathway can dissipate the electrical charge. If the tight junctions are impermeable to ion movement, electrical potential will be maintained.

trauma. The epidermal layer provides a mechanical barrier, supplemented by cushioning by the adipose in the hypodermis. Bacteria, foreign matter, other organisms, and chemicals penetrate it with difficulty. Melanin in the epidermal layer diminishes damage from sunlight. The oily and slightly acidic secretions of skin sebaceous glands protect the body further by limiting the growth of many organisms.

Skin is impermeable to water and electrolytes, and it limits the transcutaneous loss of these compounds. Insensible loss of water and electrolytes occurs only through pores. Burns and other injuries that damage the skin eliminate this protection and cause severe dehydration.

Skin makes up 15% to 20% of body weight. Skin has three primary layers: the epidermis, the dermis, and the hypodermis. Numerous specialized structures are located in the epidermis, including eccrine glands, apocrine glands, sebaceous glands, hair follicles, and nails (Fig. 2-4).

Epidermis

The epidermis is the thin, stratified outer skin layer extending downward to the subepidermal basement membrane. The thickness of the epidermis ranges from 0.04 mm on the eyelids to 1.6 mm on the palms and soles. Keratinocytes are the principal cells of the epidermis, and produce keratin. The cells replicate in the basal cell layer and migrate upward toward the skin surface. On the surface, they are sloughed off or lost by abrasion. Thus, the epidermis constantly regenerates itself, providing a tough keratinized barrier.

Skin coloration is due to both epidermal pigment accumulation and blood flow. The primary cutaneous pigment is melanin, synthesized in granules in epidermal melanocytes and a corresponding layer of the hair follicles. Skin color differences result from the size and quantity of granules as well as from the rate of melanin production. Natives of equatorial Africa have an increase in the size and number of granules as well as increased melanin production. In natives of northern Europe, the granules are small and aggregated, producing less melanin. With chronic sun exposure, there is an increase in concentration of melanocytes as well as in size and functional activity. The presence of melanin limits the penetration of sun rays into the skin and protects against sunburn and development of ultraviolet light–induced skin carcinomas. Melanin that is produced in the epidermis can be deposited in the dermal skin layer through various processes (such as inflammation).

Melanocyte-stimulating hormone (MSH) is the primary controller of regulated melanin production. ACTH shares some sequence homology with MSH, so high ACTH can cause melanin production and increase skin pigmentation, such as in Cushing's disease (see Chapter 13).

Blood flow to skin also imparts a tint reflecting the concentration and oxygenation of hemoglobin in the blood. Normally, oxygenated hemoglobin imparts a pinkish/reddish color. Severe restriction of cutaneous blood flow causes a whitish color, such as shock states. The presence of deoxygenated hemoglobin causes a bluish color. These colors may not be apparent in skin regions with high melanin content but can be seen in areas of relatively low melanin content such as the bed of the fingernail.

The epithelial barrier function is supplemented by hair and nails and secretions from sebaceous glands, eccrine glands, and apocrine sweat glands. These structures are invaginations of epidermis into the dermis.

Nails and Hair

Nails and hair consist of keratinized and, therefore, "dead" cells. Nails are horny scales of epidermis that grow from the nail matrix at the proximal nail bed. Fingernails grow about 0.1 mm/day, and complete reproduction takes 100 to 150 days. Toenails grow more slowly than do fingernails. A damaged nail matrix, which may result from trauma or aggressive manicuring, produces a distorted nail. Nails are also sensitive to physiologic changes; for instance, they grow more slowly in cold weather and during periods of illness (Fig. 2-5).

Hair is found on all skin surfaces except the palms and soles. Each hair follicle functions as an independent unit and goes through intermittent stages of development and activity. Hair develops from the mitotic activity of the hair bulb. Hair

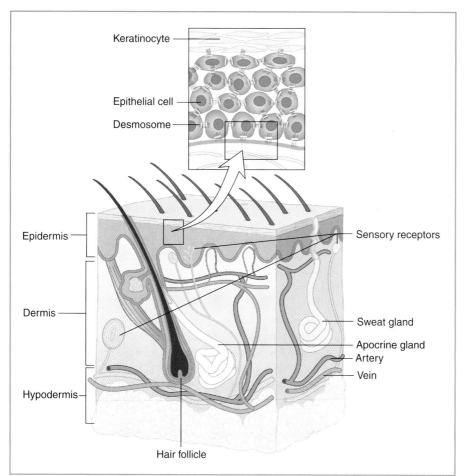

Keratinocyte

Epithelial cell

Desmosome

Epidermis

Dermis

Hypodermis

Sensory receptors

Sweat gland

Apocrine gland

Artery

Vein

Hair follicle

Figure 2-4. Skin comprises the superficial epidermal layer, internal dermal layer, and underlying hypodermal layer. The hair, nails, and glands of the skin are extensions of the epidermis and penetrate deep into the dermal layer.

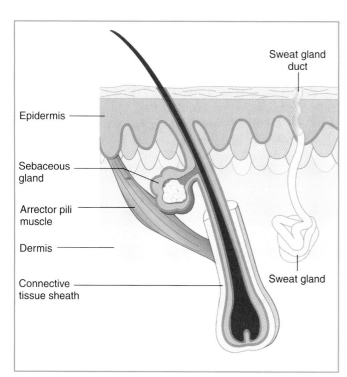

Sweat gland duct

Epidermis

Sebaceous gland

Arrector pili muscle

Dermis

Connective tissue sheath

Sweat gland

Figure 2-5. Hair and sebaceous gland secretions exit the epidermis at the hair follicle, whereas sweat glands exit by way of independent ducts.

HISTOLOGY

Hair Follicles

Hair follicles usually occur with sebaceous glands, and together they form a pilosebaceous unit. Sebaceous glands secrete fluid and lipids into the hair follicle ducts, which act as waterproofing. Sebaceous gland secretion is enhanced by androgen secretion at puberty Arrector pili muscles of the dermis attach to hair follicles and elevate the hairs when body temperature falls, producing "goose bumps."

form (straight or curly) depends on the shape of the hair in cross-section. Straight hair has a round cross-section; curly hair has an oval or ribbon-like cross-section. Curved follicles also affect the curliness of hair. Melanocytes in the bulb determine hair color.

Epidermal Glands

Three different types of glands are located on the epidermis. These glands are also composed of epithelial tissue; the glands themselves are secretory epithelia, and the ducts leading to the surface of the skin have exchange epithelia.

Sebaceous glands are found throughout the skin and are most abundant on the face, scalp, upper back, and chest.

They are associated with hair follicles that open onto the skin surface, where sebum (a mixture of sebaceous gland–produced lipids and epidermal cell–derived lipids) is released. Sebum has a lubricating function and bactericidal activity. Androgen is responsible for sebaceous gland development. In utero androgen causes neonatal acne; after puberty, increased androgen production again stimulates sebum production, often leading to acne in adolescents.

Eccrine sweat glands play an important role in thermoregulation. They are found within most areas of the skin, but are particularly numerous on the palms, soles, forehead, and axillae. Sweat is a dilute secretion derived from plasma. Eccrine gland secretion is stimulated by heat as well as by exercise and emotional stress.

Apocrine glands secrete cholesterol and triglycerides and occur primarily in the axillae, breast areola, anogenital area, ear canals, and eyelids. Sympathetic nerves stimulate apocrine secretion of a milky substance that becomes odoriferous when altered by skin surface bacteria. Apocrine glands do not function until puberty, and they require high levels of sex steroids in order to function. In lower order animals, apocrine secretions function as sexual attractants (pheromones), and the apocrine secretion musk is used as a perfume base. The role, if any, in humans is not established.

Dermis

The dermis is a connective tissue layer that gives the skin most of its substance and structure. The dermoepithelial junction contains numerous interdigitations that help anchor the dermis to the overlying epidermal layer. The papillary layer has loose connective tissue, mast cells, leukocytes, and macrophages. The reticular dermis has denser connective tissue and fewer cells than does the papillary layer. The dermis has a rich layer of blood and lymphatic vessels, including the arteriovenous anastomoses important in thermoregulation. The dermis also contains numerous nerve endings, including a wide variety of the cutaneous sensory nerve receptors.

Hypodermis

The subcutaneous hypodermis layer is a specialized layer of connective tissue containing adipocytes. This layer is absent in some sites such as the eyelids, scrotum, and areola. The depth of the subcutaneous fat layer varies between body regions and is based on the age, sex, and nutritional status of the individual. Hypodermal adipose functions as insulation from extremes of hot and cold, as a cushion to trauma, and as a source of energy and hormone metabolism.

●●● ROLE OF SKIN IN THERMOREGULATION

Body temperature is maintained at 37°C as a result of balance between heat generation and heat loss processes. This balance involves autonomic nervous system, metabolism, and behavioral responses. Even at rest, basal body metabolism generates an excess heat load that must be dissipated to an environment that is usually cooler than 37°C. Heat loss across the skin can be controlled, and consequently the skin plays a major role in the regulation of body temperature. Cutaneous participation in short-term thermoregulation involves blood flow and sweat production, part of complex process described in Chapter 1.

The dermal layer of the skin contains an extensive subcutaneous vascular plexus to assist in the regulation of body temperature (Fig. 2-6). This plexus has an extensive sympathetic innervation, and an increase in cutaneous sympathetic activity constricts the blood vessels, decreases cutaneous blood flow, and consequently diminished heat transfer to the environment. The hypothalamus is partly responsible for regulating adrenergic activity to the skin and therefore skin blood flow, particularly to the extremities, the face, ears, and the tip of the nose. Generally, the vessels dilate during warm temperatures and constrict during cold. Thermoregulation is assisted by countercurrent heat exchange between arterial and venous blood flow in extremities.

Under severe heat stress, increased cutaneous blood flow is inadequate to dissipate the thermal load. Eccrine glands produce sweat, and cooling is enhanced by fluid evaporation from the skin. Eccrine gland innervation is unique in that these sympathetic cholinergic nerves use acetylcholine (rather than norepinephrine) as the neurotransmitter. Sweating significantly enhances the body's capacity for thermoregulation.

Sweat elaborated from eccrine sweat glands is modified while passing through the sweat gland duct. There is some NaCl absorption that is enhanced in low flow states. Consequently, fast flow rates can increase the amount of NaCl lost from the body in the sweat. Sweat glands release an enzyme that causes formation of the vasodilator bradykinin, which acts in a local, paracrine fashion to increase cutaneous blood flow.

Heat production can also be regulated. Basal metabolic rate is increased by thyroid hormone and by dietary protein ingestion. Output of motor cortex controls skeletal muscle activity, allowing behavioral responses, such as movement, to assist thermoregulation. In addition, the hypothalamus regulates involuntary muscle activity, such as shivering.

Sensory Reception

The skin contains a wide variety of specialized receptors and nerves responding to pressure, vibration, pain, and temperature. In the dermal layer, touch (flutter) is sensed by Meissner corpuscles; pressure, by Merkel cells and Ruffini endings; vibration, by pacinian corpuscles; and hair movement, by hair follicle endings. The density of receptors determines the sensitivity of the skin. For example, two-point discrimination is most acute on the skin of the fingers and face, where the highest density of touch receptors occurs. In contrast, the skin on the back has a low density of touch receptors and the ability to localize touch is therefore reduced.

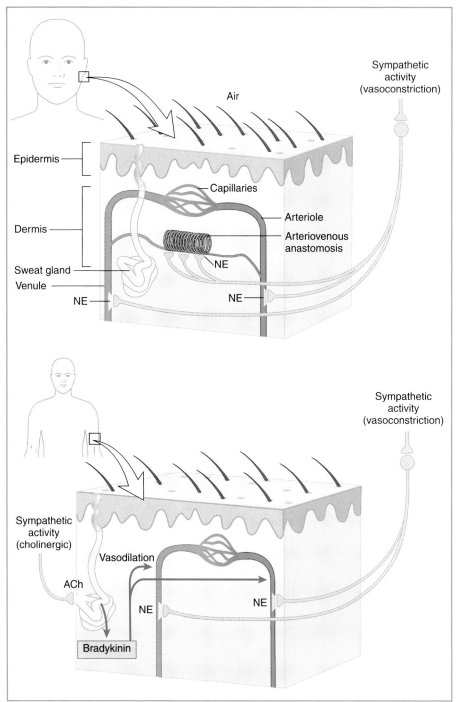

Figure 2-6. Blood flow to the true capillaries of the skin provides nutrition, and blood flow to the arteriovenous anastomoses assists in thermoregulation. The anterior hypothalamus regulates body temperature and controls the activity of the sympathetic nerves that innervate the cutaneous arteriovenous anastomoses. Skin temperature is directly proportionate to blood flow to the skin. Sweat gland activity is controlled by a unique branch of the sympathetic nervous system that uses acetylcholine as its neurotransmitter. A strong increase in sympathetic activity decreases cutaneous blood flow and increases sweat gland production, leading to skin that is cold and clammy (diaphoretic).

Temperature is sensed by specific thermoreceptors in the epidermis, and pain is sensed by free nerve endings throughout the epidermal, dermal, and hypodermal layers. The speed of axonal conduction of pain information to the cortex results in a functional division. "Fast" pain is transmitted by myelinated axons, is localized, but has a short latency. "Slow" pain is transmitted by unmyelinated C fibers, is more diffuse, and has a longer latency. Afferent axons transmit impulses arising from these cutaneous receptors to the somatosensory cortex, where the information is integrated into a somatotopic map.

●●● CUTANEOUS GROWTH AND REGENERATION

The thickness of the cutaneous layers varies based on remodeling, the endocrine environment, and the metabolic state. The dermal layer on the soles of the feet and palms of the hand thickens in response to continuing abrasive stress. Testosterone and estrogens both increase connective tissue growth, and consequently skin thickness, particularly during puberty. Excess cortisol secretion decreases collagen synthesis and consequently decreases skin thickness.

ANATOMY

Cardiovascular System

The arteries and veins are anatomically arranged in parallel, particularly for the circulation to the extremities. Blood flowing in these vessels is traveling in opposite directions, allowing a countercurrent exchange of heat. This anatomic arrangement permits cooling of arterial blood flowing from the warm body core toward the extremities, and warming of venous blood returning from the cool extremities to the body core. Countercurrent exchange assists the conservation of heat in the body core while maintaining blood flow to the cool extremities.

Epithelial cells are among the most rapidly growing cell population in the body. Epithelia of skin and GI tract are normally lost from abrasion, and the rate of epidermal cell growth and replacement has to match that loss. Epithelial cells respond to numerous growth agents, including epithelial growth factor. In addition, many hormones are tropic agents for epithelia, especially for the GI tract. Epithelial cells are the most rapidly dividing cells of the body, and consequently are often damaged or killed as a side effect of chemotherapy. Patients on chemotherapy often experience the loss of hair, and damage to the GI epithelia can impair nutrient absorption.

VITAMIN D PRODUCTION

The epidermis is involved in synthesis of vitamin D. In the presence of sunlight or ultraviolet radiation, a sterol found on the malpighian cells is converted to form cholecalciferol (vitamin D_3). Vitamin D_3 assists in the absorption of Ca^{++} from ingested foods.

IMMUNE FUNCTION

Immune cells in both the epidermis and dermis of the skin are important in the cell-mediated immune responses of the skin through antigen presentation. Langerhans cells of the epidermis are part of the cell-mediated immune response. Langerhans cells recognize antigens and process the antigen for recognition by T cells in the lymph nodes. Other lymphocytes are also located in the dermal layer. Any antigen entering immunologically competent skin is likely to encounter a coordinated response of Langerhans and T cells to neutralize its effect. An antigen entering diseased skin can induce and elicit cell- and antibody-mediated immune responses.

PHARMACOLOGY

Chemotherapy

Chemotherapy for cancer utilizes drugs that target rapidly dividing cells. Current chemotherapeutic agents include those that block the replication of DNA (alkylating agents, antitumor antibiotics, mitotic inhibitors), drugs that impede the repair of DNA (nitrosoureas), and drugs that block the metabolism of these rapidly dividing cells. Angiogenesis inhibitors can restrict the growth of new blood vessels, limiting the delivery of nutrients to tumors. Current chemotherapy often uses combinations of drugs to increase their effectiveness and limit side effects.

IMMUNOLOGY

Antigen Presentation

Langerhans cells are a type of antigen-presenting cell found in the skin. Antigens that enter the skin are recognized, phagocytized, and digested in lysosomes. Fragments of the antigen are bound to the extracellular surface of membrane proteins—the major histocompatibility complex proteins—and the Langerhans cells migrate to the lymph nodes, where they present these antigen fragments to antigen-specific T cells, resulting in T-cell activation.

TOP 5 TAKE-HOME POINTS

1. Epithelial cells are arranged in sheets joined by tight junctions, and they provide a barrier between the interior of the body and the external environment.
2. Epithelial cells have polarity, with an apical surface facing the outside the body and a basolateral surface facing the interior of the body.
3. The skin is the largest and most visible organ of the body, consisting of an epithelial epidermis, the dermis, and the hypodermis.
4. Skin maintains body temperature, prevents water loss, and has sensory receptors that are activated by touch, temperature, and pain.
5. Skin regulation is mediated by sympathetic adrenergic control of blood flow to arteriovenous anastomoses and by sympathetic cholinergic control of sweat glands.

Body Fluid Distribution 3

CONTENTS

●●● BARRIERS BETWEEN COMPARTMENTS

Body water accounts for about 60% of the total body weight. Selective barriers allow fluid compartments to differ in composition of electrolytes and other solutes. Consequently, these barriers help define anatomic and functional spaces. About two thirds of the body water is within the cells, called "intracellular fluid." The remaining third is outside the cells. This extracellular fluid includes plasma, cerebrospinal fluid, and the interstitial fluid that occupies the space between the cells (Fig. 3-1).

Most cells of the body have aquaporin water channels, and consequently water can be exchanged between the intracellular and extracellular fluid compartments in response to osmotic gradients. The exchange between plasma and interstitial fluid is quite rapid, as is the exchange between cellular and extracellular fluid. Some extracellular fluid compartments, however, have a very slow exchange rate. This includes the aqueous humor of the eye, cerebrospinal fluid, synovial fluid of the joints, and extracellular fluid in bone and cartilage.

The barriers can also restrict solute movement. The lipid bilayer of the cell membrane is impermeable to charged molecules but will allow movement of gases and other lipid-soluble molecules. Consequently, the ionic composition of the extracellular fluid can and does differ markedly from the intracellular fluid. The capillary endothelial cells separate the plasma volume from the remainder of the interstitial fluid. This barrier permits the exchange of ions and other small molecules, and it restricts the movement of only the high-molecular-weight proteins such as albumin.

●●● MEASUREMENT OF BODY FLUID COMPARTMENTS

Body fluid compartments can be measured by dilution of a compound that distributes only in the space of interest. The indicator dilution principle is based on the definition of a concentration. If the amount of the substance is known and the resulting concentration is measured, the volume can be calculated:

$$\text{Concentration} = \text{Amount/volume}$$
$$\text{Volume} = \text{Amount added/change in concentration}$$

This approach assumes that the compound distributes only in the space that you are interested in measuring and that the concentration measured represents the average concentration throughout the entire volume.

Blood volume represents a unique case in that it contains both intracellular water (within the erythrocytes and leukocytes) and plasma, an extracellular fluid. Blood volume represents approximately 8% of total body water, or about 5 L.

●●● MOVEMENT ACROSS BARRIERS

Movement of a compound, either solute or solvent, requires energy, and the barrier (cell membrane) provides a resistance to the movement. The energy can be in the form of ATP, or it can be stored in a concentration, electrical, or osmotic gradient.

Diffusion

Diffusion is described by Fick's law:

$$J = -DA\,\frac{\Delta \text{ concentration}}{\Delta \text{ distance}}$$

where J is the net flux (movement) of the compound; – indicates that the movement is from an area of higher concentration to an area of lower concentration; D is the

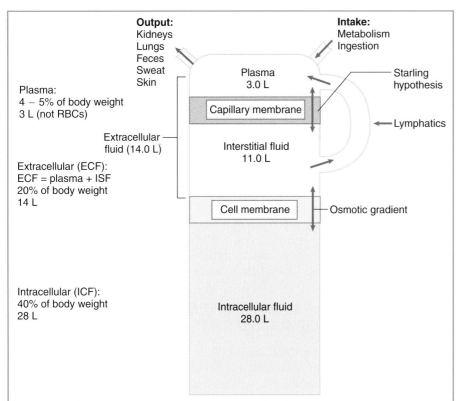

Figure 3-1. Barriers separate body fluid compartments. Changes in total body water first affect the plasma volume. If the change in plasma volume causes a change in plasma capillary pressure or plasma protein concentration, the interstitial fluid volume will change. If the change in extracellular fluid composition causes a change in extracellular fluid osmolality, there will be an osmotic equilibration with the cell water volume.

diffusion (permeability) coefficient, specific for the compound and for the barrier; A is the surface area involved; Δ concentration is the concentration gradient; and Δ distance is the distance over which the compound must travel. The diffusional movement of a compound is increased by increasing the surface area for exchange, by increasing the concentration gradient, or by decreasing the distance across which the compound has to move.

Transport across the cell membrane can occur by diffusion for lipid-soluble compounds. The movement of compounds with limited lipid solubility is facilitated by transport proteins embedded in the cell membrane. Some of these proteins provide a route to enable the compound to move down its concentration gradient, a process called *facilitated diffusion*. Other proteins are capable of moving compounds against a concentration gradient. This process requires energy, usually in the form of hydrolysis of ATP (*primary active transport*), or coupled to the diffusional movement of a second compound, such as the influx of Na^+ (*secondary active transport*).

Osmosis

Water movement between body fluid compartments occurs in response to osmotic gradients and in response to hydrostatic pressure gradients.

The osmotic pressure (π) of any solution is calculated as

$$\pi = RT\,(\tau ic)$$

where R is a constant, T is temperature, τ is an ionic dissociation coefficient, i is the number of ionic particles, and c is the concentration of the compound. For NaCl, $\tau = 0.93$ and $i = 2$ particles. A solution made with 0.9 g NaCl per 100 mL water (0.9%) has a molarity of 154 mmol/L, has an osmotic pressure of 286 mOsm/L and is isosmotic with normal body osmolarity. Consequently, 154 mmol/L NaCl is called "normal saline" or "isotonic saline."

Osmotic movement of water requires (1) a semipermeable barrier that permits movement of water but not the solute and (2) a difference in the solute concentration across the barrier. For cells, the cell membrane represents the semipermeable barrier. Water can freely cross the cell membrane, but ions such as Na^+, K^+, and Cl^- and larger compounds such as proteins cannot. Consequently, a difference in the total ionic concentration across the cell membrane will cause the osmotic movement of water. Water movement will persist until the ionic concentration inside the cell equals the ionic concentration outside the cell.

In the body, changes in extracellular fluid osmolarity (primarily due to changes in extracellular Na^+) determine the exchange between extracellular and intracellular water. The erythrocyte provides a model for studying the osmotic movement of water. Normal erythrocyte intracellular osmolarity is 290 mOsm. Placing the erythrocyte in a solution with an osmolarity of greater than 290 mOsm will cause water to exit the cell, and the cell will shrink (crenate). Placing the erythrocyte in a solution with an osmolarity less than 290 will cause the osmotic movement of water into the cell. The red blood cell will swell. There is a limit to the volume of fluid that the erythrocyte can contain. Placing an erythrocyte in a solution with an osmolality of less than 199 mOsm will cause the cell to swell and rupture (lyse) (Fig. 3-2).

BIOCHEMISTRY

Cell Membrane Permeability

The cell membrane is a phospholipid bilayer with a hydrophobic interior. Lipid-insoluble compounds can cross the membrane only by means of embedded protein channels or transport proteins.

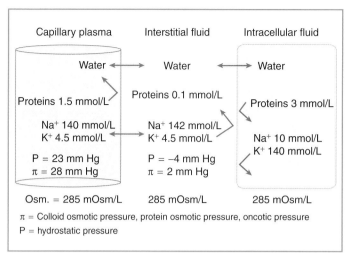

π = Colloid osmotic pressure, protein osmotic pressure, oncotic pressure
P = hydrostatic pressure

Figure 3-3. Water and solute permeability across body fluid compartment barriers. Both plasma and interstitial fluid are extracellular volumes. The major difference between plasma and interstitial fluid is the much higher protein concentration in plasma. This high protein concentration causes plasma to have a much higher oncotic pressure. Intracellular fluid has a much higher [K^+] and much lower [Na^+] than does extracellular fluid. In spite of these differences, the osmolality of all three fluids is equivalent. A change in the osmolality of any one fluid will result in redistribution of water until all three spaces come back into an osmotic equilibrium.

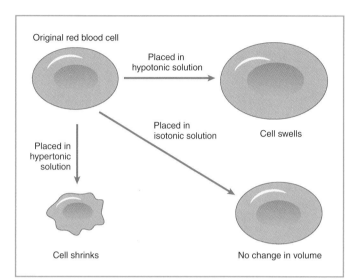

Figure 3-2. Changes in plasma osmolarity cause osmotic movement of water between the plasma and the cell water of the erythrocytes. A difference in intracellular and extracellular fluid osmolality causes an osmotic shift of water. Placing an erythrocyte in a hypotonic solution results in an osmotic shift of water into the cell, expanding its volume. Placing an erythrocyte in an isotonic solution does not cause a change in the cell volume. Placing an erythrocyte in a hypertonic solution causes an osmotic shift of water out of the cell.

Capillary Filtration

Osmotic pressure also contributes to the transcapillary movement of fluid in the cardiovascular system. The net movement across the capillary is called filtration, described by the Starling hypothesis:

$$Q = K\,[(P_c + \pi_i) - (P_i + \pi_c)]$$

In this case, Na^+ and Cl^- are not osmotically active particles, since both can freely cross the capillary endothelium. High-molecular-weight proteins, such as albumin, cannot cross the capillary endothelium. Consequently, osmotic pressure at the capillary barrier is determined by the concentration of the large plasma proteins and is called "colloid osmotic pressure" or "oncotic pressure." The balance of oncotic and hydrostatic forces determines exchange at the capillaries between plasma and interstitial fluid and is described in more detail in Chapters 8 and 9 (Fig. 3-3).

Volume and Osmotic Disturbances

Body fluid volume disturbances involve an imbalance of intake and loss. This imbalance is first reflected in a change in the volume or osmolarity of the plasma space, as shown at the top of Figure 3-1. Within the body, water will redistribute between the compartments only if there is a gradient. A change in oncotic or hydrostatic pressure will cause fluid movement between the plasma and interstitial fluid. A change in osmotic pressure will cause fluid movement between the extracellular and intracellular compartments.

If the volume disturbance does not alter extracellular osmolarity, then the fluid change is restricted to the extracellular space and intracellular volume is unchanged. Only body fluid volume disturbances that alter extracellular osmolarity will change the intracellular volume.

Volume Depletion

Renal and GI elimination are the major sources of body fluid loss. Under extreme heat load, sweat can also account for a significant fluid loss. The consequences of isotonic, hypotonic, and hypertonic fluid losses are described below. The letters correspond to those in Table 3-1 and Figure 3-4.

  A Diarrhea results in a loss of isotonic fluid from the GI tract. The lack of change in extracellular fluid osmolality means that the loss is restricted to the extracellular volume. The extracellular fluid volume includes both the plasma and the interstitial fluid volumes; consequently, prolonged diarrhea can lead to marked decreases in blood volume and blood pressure.

TABLE 3-1. Independent Changes in Extracellular Fluid (ECF) Osmolality and Body Fluid Volume

Body Volume*	ECF Osmolality		
	Low	Normal	High
High	Ingest water (F)	Infuse 0.9% (normal) saline (D)	Infuse 7.5% (hypertonic) saline (E)
Normal	Sweat, then drink same volume of water	Normal	Ingest salt tablets
Low	Incomplete compensation, dehydration (C)	Hemorrhage, diarrhea (A)	Dehydration (sweat) (B)

*Body fluid volume can increase both by ingestion of fluid and intravenous infusion. Body fluid volume will decrease when fluid loss exceeds fluid intake. The ECF osmolality becomes dilute when a dilute fluid is ingested or when there is loss of hypertonic solution. The ECF osmolality becomes concentrated when there is an ingestion or infusion of a hypertonic fluid or loss of a dilute fluid.

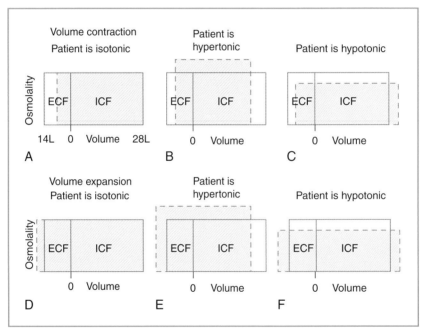

Figure 3-4. The six Darrow-Yannet diagrams show the relative changes in volume (x-axis) and osmolarity (y-axis) of the extracellular fluid (ECF) and intracellular fluid (ICF). Zero for the x-axis is on the line separating the ICF and the ECF. An increase in ECF volume expands the figure along the x-axis to the left, and an increase in ICF volume expands the figure to the right. **A,** There is a loss of an isotonic fluid, and only the extracellular volume is changed. **B,** There is a loss of a hypotonic fluid, and the original decrease in extracellular fluid volume is attenuated by movement of water from the intracellular volume to the extracellular volume. **C,** There is a loss of a hypertonic fluid, and the original decrease in extracellular fluid volume is augmented by a shift of fluid from the extracellular space into the cells. **D,** There is a gain of an isotonic fluid, and only the extracellular volume is changed. **E,** There is an addition of a hypertonic fluid, and any extracellular volume increase is a result both of the additional fluid and the movement of fluid from the cell volume to the extracellular fluid volume. **F,** There is a gain of a hypotonic fluid, and the expansion of the extracellular fluid volume space is attenuated by the movement of some of the new fluid into the intracellular fluid volume.

A Hemorrhage is a special case of isotonic fluid loss in that it involves loss of both the extracellular plasma volume and the cellular volume of the red blood cells. The loss is isotonic, so there is no osmotic change, and the remaining cellular volume is unaffected. The decrease in blood (capillary) pressure causes the reabsorption of interstitial fluid at capillaries. This reabsorbed fluid lacks red blood cells and albumin; consequently, hema-tocrit drops and plasma albumin concentration drops. The drop in plasma albumin causes a drop in plasma oncotic pressure. When blood pressure is restored, the drop in plasma oncotic pressure may cause a proportionately greater shift of the extracellular fluid from the plasma space to the interstitial fluid volume space.

B Sweat is an example of a hypotonic fluid volume loss. Fluid volume depletion caused by excessive sweating

PATHOPHYSIOLOGY

Hemorrhagic Shock

The decrease in blood pressure caused by hemorrhage is proportionate to the volume of the hemorrhage. During the recovery phase following hemorrhage, the combination of the low arterial pressure and the sympathetic nerve–mediated arteriolar constriction causes a drop in capillary pressure. The low capillary pressure favors the reabsorption of interstitial fluid, which is similar to plasma but lacks red blood cells and plasma proteins, including the clotting factors. Consequently, there is a drop in blood O_2 carrying capacity and clotting ability during recovery from hemorrhage. This deficit can be compounded by resuscitation with fluids such as isotonic saline that lack red blood cells and clotting factors.

TABLE 3-2. Daily Water Balance*

Water Gain	
Food and drink	2.2 L
Metabolism	0.3 L
Water Loss	
Insensible	0.9 L
Urine	1.4 L
Feces	0.1 L
Sweat	0.1 L

*Ingestion of food and drink is a major source of water gain to the body, with a smaller volume coming from metabolism of carbohydrates and fats. Urinary excretion represents the major source of water loss from the body, with a significant insensible volume also lost through respiration and transpiration. Smaller volumes of water are lost in the feces and in sweat. Changes in fluid ingestion and urinary excretion represent the major physiologic regulation of body water balance.

results in increased plasma osmolality. The increased osmolality causes an osmotic movement of water from the cellular space into the extracellular space. Consequently, the total body fluid deficit is larger than would be predicted from the increase in extracellular fluid osmolarity. During resuscitation, the volume of fluid needed to restore fluid volume and osmolarity to normal is greater than that calculated based solely on the extracellular fluid volume deficit. The loss of water from the cell space also causes the cells to shrink and increases the concentration of all water-soluble cellular components.

C Excessive antidiuretic hormone (ADH) secretion results in the renal excretion of hypertonic urine. Hypertonic fluid depletion causes a decrease in plasma osmolarity. Consequently, there is an osmotic shift of water into the cellular space, causing cell swelling and dilution of intracellular solutes. Cerebral edema in SIADH can lead to nausea and headache.

Volume Expansion

Dietary ingestion and intravenous infusion represent the most common routes for fluid gain. The consequences of hypotonic, isotonic, and hypertonic fluid expansion are contrasted below. Again, the letters correspond to those in Table 3-1 and Figure 3-4.

D Intravenous infusion of isotonic saline (0.9% NaCl) dilutes plasma albumin, does not change plasma osmolarity, but slightly increases plasma Na^+ and to a greater extent plasma $[Cl^-]$. The lack of an osmotic change means that the added fluid will expand only extracellular (plasma and interstitial fluid) spaces. Plasma albumin is diluted, resulting in a tendency for fluid to accumulate in the interstitial space.

E Hypertonic saline infusion increases plasma osmolarity. The increased osmolarity causes an osmotic movement of water from the cellular space to the extracellular space. Consequently, the extracellular volume expansion is larger than the volume of saline that was infused.

Again, the volume expansion causes a dilution of plasma albumin, and consequently some of the expanded plasma volume is lost to the interstitial fluid space.

F Intravenous H_2O infusion dilutes both plasma ions and plasma albumin. The decrease in osmolarity causes the osmotic movement of water into cells, including red blood cells. The dilution of albumin causes movement of water from the plasma into the interstitial fluid at the capillaries. Consequently, water infusion expands the plasma space, interstitial fluid space, and cell water space. Red blood cells exposed to an osmolarity of less than 200 mOsm will swell and rupture. Consequently, an effect equivalent to water infusion is achieved by infusing a 5% dextrose solution. The dextrose is gradually transported into the cells, and the water distributes as described above. Alternatively, a half-normal NaCl solution (0.045%, 77 mmol/L) can also be used to expand both the cellular and the extracellular volumes.

● ● ● BODY FLUID AND ELECTROLYTE BALANCE

Long-term fluid and electrolyte homeostasis requires balancing the accumulation of a compound (ingestion + production) against the elimination of the compound (excretion + metabolism). Intake of water and electrolytes is primarily from diet, with a small portion of water being generated from metabolism. There is a regulated loss of both water and electrolytes from the kidneys. For most compounds, there is a storage pool in the body to help buffer the body against interruptions in ingestion or elimination (Table 3-2).

Importantly, it is the plasma concentration of compounds, rather than the size of the body store, that is the regulated variable. Any deficit in plasma electrolyte concentration causes the release of a hormone that releases the compound from storage or reduces the excretion of that electrolyte, or both. Table 3-3 summarizes the acute and chronic regulation of Na^+, K^+, and volume by the kidneys and lists compounds and events that alter renal excretion.

Body Fluid Balance

Fluid intake is controlled by the thirst center in the hypothalamus. Thirst is stimulated by increases in plasma osmolality and by hypotension. This stimulation is augmented by antidiuretic hormone and angiotensin II.

Fluid loss occurs from variety of sites (Fig. 3-5). Urinary loss is heavily regulated, acutely by antidiuretic hormone (ADH, vasopressin) and chronically by renal perfusion

pressure. The water content of feces is poorly regulated. Finally, there is an "insensible" fluid loss from sweat and respiratory systems that is not regulated by volume control systems. Sweat loss is regulated, but by the thermoregulatory system.

In a 70-kg adult, a 2.5 L/day turnover of body fluid represents only 6% of the body water. Infants have a much higher percentage of their total body weight as water and also a much higher proportional turnover of that water. In a 3-kg infant, approximately 77% of the body weight is water, or about 2.3 L. The daily turnover of water in infants this size is approximately 0.375 L/day, or about 16% of the total body water. Consequently, infants are much higher risk than adults for dehydration and other body fluid disturbances.

Acutely, urine volume is controlled by antidiuretic hormone. Chronically, the major controller of urine volume is renal perfusion pressure. For this reason, hypertension is often viewed as a renal disease.

Sodium Balance

Sodium is an essential nutrient. In historic times, salt was used for exchange, and our word "salary" originates from the Roman use of salt as payment for services. Sodium enters the body by ingestion, partially regulated by a sodium appetite, or "taste." The body has multiple redundant mechanisms to assist renal sodium conservation.

Body Na^+ balance (Fig. 3-6) involves the hormonal adjustment of urinary Na^+ excretion to match dietary Na^+ intake. Cellular Na^+ stores are somewhat limited and play only a small role in the regulation of extracellular sodium concentration.

Urinary Na^+ excretion represents the primary route of loss. Short-term urinary loss is regulated by control of glomerular filtration rate (GFR) and of tubular Na^+ reabsorption. Angiotensin II, aldosterone, and renal sympathetic nerves enhance Na retention. Tubuloglomerular feedback also promotes sodium retention. Urinary excretion is enhanced by atrial natriuretic peptide (see Table 3-3).

Long-term Na^+ balance is regulated by a negative feedback control using antidiuretic hormone or, to a lesser extent, aldosterone. Sodium is the major extracellular ion and a primary determinant of plasma osmolarity. The hypothalamus

TABLE 3-3. Acute and Chronic Regulation of Fluid and Ion Balance

	Acute*	Chronic
Sodium†		
Conserve	Aldosterone Angiotensin II Sympathetic nervous system Blood pressure	Aldosterone
Excrete	Atrial natriuretic peptide (ANP)/urodilatin	Antidiuretic hormone (ADH) (dilutional)
Potassium		
Excrete	Filtered load Aldosterone	Aldosterone Filtered load
Volume		
Conserve	ADH	↓ Renal perfusion pressure
Excrete		↑ Renal perfusion pressure

*Measured in minutes, except for aldosterone, which is measured in hours.
†Multiple redundant factors control Na^+ balance. The acute sodium-conserving mechanisms act to reduce urinary Na^+ loss and are much more powerful than the hormones that increase Na^+ excretion. Chronic changes in plasma Na^+ result from endocrine diseases involving ADH or aldosterone. Plasma K^+ excretion is regulated by the filtered K^+ load and the aldosterone. Urinary volume excretion is acutely regulated by ADH. The long-term regulation of volume in the body is tied most closely to changes in renal perfusion pressure.

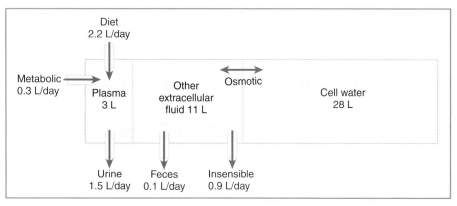

Figure 3-5. Body water balance requires the regulation of intake (thirst) and renal excretion to compensate for the unregulated loss of water through respiration and sweating.

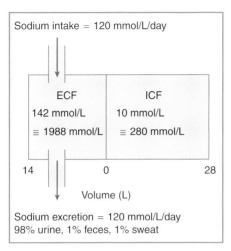

Figure 3-6. Body Na^+ balance is achieved primarily through control of renal Na loss. The amount of Na^+ ingested each day is equal to about 5% of the total body Na^+ stores. Urinary Na^+ excretion is regulated by numerous redundant hormonal control systems, and urinary Na^+ loss is adjusted to match dietary Na^+ intake.

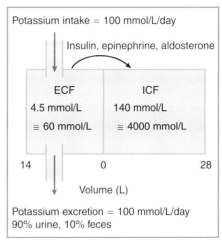

Figure 3-7. Cellular stores represent the vast majority of body K^+. Acute changes in extracellular fluid K^+ levels most commonly represent shifts between extracellular and intracellular K^+. The hormones insulin, epinephrine, and aldosterone all stimulate the movement of K^+ from the extracellular space into the cells and cause a decrease in plasma K^+ levels.

contains osmoreceptors that respond to changes in plasma osmolarity by adjusting ADH release. ADH acts on the kidney to promote water retention, causing osmolarity (and Na concentration) to decrease.

Hypernatremic Na disorders result from either a deficit in extracellular fluid volume or an excessive retention of Na. ADH normally promotes water retention. In the absence of functional ADH, there is an excess loss of water in the urine that can be offset only by enhanced fluid ingestion. Diabetes insipidus is due to an ADH defect. "Insipidus" refers to the fact that the excessive urine production is not characterized by the presence of glucose in the urine and consequently the urine is insipid, or "tasteless." Central diabetes insipidus results from impaired production or release of ADH. Nephrogenic diabetes insipidus results when kidneys do not respond to ADH, usually owing to impairment of the ADH (vasopressin) receptor. Another hormone imbalance, hyper-aldosteronism, can also cause hypernatremia, since excessive aldosterone production causes excessive Na retention and consequently increases plasma Na.

Hyponatremic Na disorders reflect the other side of impaired Na control. Hyponatremia can result from excessive water retention, characteristic of SIADH, the syndrome of inappropriate (excessive) ADH secretion. Hyponatremia can also be due to a loss of body Na stores, such as occurs when aldosterone secretion is impaired in Addison's disease. Finally, hyponatremia can result from excessive water ingestion.

Increased activity of the renal sympathetic nerves causes an increase in Na^+ reabsorption, as described in Chapter 11. The renal sympathetic nerves directly contract the afferent arterioles, thereby decreasing glomerular filtration rate. Activation of the renal sympathetic nerves also causes the release of renin, ultimately leading to the formation of angiotensin II. Norepinephrine and angiotensin II both increase Na^+ reabsorption at the proximal tubule cells.

Atrial natriuretic peptide (ANP) is a peptide hormone synthesized and released from the cardiac atria in response to stretch. An increase in circulating blood volume stretches the cardiac atria, releasing ANP and causing increased renal excretion of Na^+. The renal loss of Na^+ and water decreases circulating blood volume and removes the excessive stretch on the cardiac atria. ANP is a naturally occurring diuretic that was discovered only in the 1980s. Currently, pharmaceutical companies are examining ANP and its analogs for clinical management of hypertension and heart failure. One analog, urodilatin, differs from ANP by the addition of four amino acids. Urodilatin is secreted by the distal tubule in response to an increase in blood volume. Urodilatin is the active form of the ANP/urodilatin family within the kidney.

Potassium Balance

The vast majority of K^+ in the body is stored within the cells. The total amount of K^+ in the extracellular fluid represents less than 2% of the K^+ in the body. Movement of K^+ into and out of the cells represents a major mechanism for regulation of plasma K^+ levels (Fig. 3-7). Urinary K^+ loss is regulated, primarily by aldosterone. Dietary K^+ intake is poorly regulated and plays at best a minor role in K^+ balance.

Three endocrine agents cause the movement of K^+ from the extracellular fluid into the cells. Insulin, aldosterone, and β-adrenergic stimulation (epinephrine) all promote the uptake of K^+ by cells and consequently a decrease in plasma K^+ concentration. Aldosterone also lowers plasma K^+ by stimulating renal K^+ excretion and by increasing K^+ loss in the feces.

Plasma H^+ also impacts the transcellular movement of K^+. An increase in plasma H^+ (acidosis) causes an increase in H^+ entry into cells and an increase in K^+ movement out of cells. Acidosis is often associated with hyperkalemia.

Urinary K^+ excretion is determined in the short term by tubular load, by luminal pH, and by aldosterone (see Chapter 11). The long-term control of K^+ balance also relies on tubular load and on aldosterone. Hypokalemia can be caused by hyperaldosteronism, and hyperkalemia by impaired aldosterone secretion in Addison's disease. Hyperkalemia can result from significant cellular death and the movement of what was cellular K^+ into the extracellular fluid.

Calcium Balance

Plasma Ca^{++} (5 mEq/L) reflects dietary intake, excretion, and movement between body storage pools. Forty percent of plasma Ca^{++} is bound to plasma proteins, and 50% of plasma Ca^{++} is ionized (free). The remaining 10% is complexed to nonprotein anions.

Parathyroid hormone is the dominant regulator of plasma Ca^{++} (Fig. 3-8). A decrease in plasma Ca^{++} stimulates the release of parathyroid hormone. Parathyroid hormone then acts to stimulate Ca^{++} reabsorption by the loop of Henle and distal tubule by increasing dietary Ca^{++} absorption and by stimulating bone resorption. Together, these actions of parathyroid hormone help increase plasma Ca^{++} back toward normal levels.

●●● TOP 5 TAKE-HOME POINTS

1. Movement of water between the intracellular and the extracellular compartments is controlled by an osmotic gradient created by a difference in concentration of electrolytes.

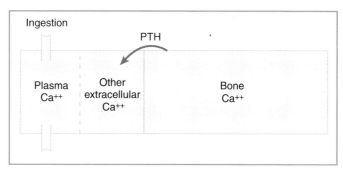

Figure 3-8. Body Ca^{++} balance represents the parathyroid hormone regulation of renal Ca^{++} loss and exchange with the large Ca^{++} storage pool in bone.

2. Movement of extracellular water between the plasma and the interstitial fluid is controlled by the hydrostatic pressures and the oncotic pressures in these two compartments.
3. Body fluid volume represents a balance between the gain of water from both ingestion and metabolism, and the loss of water through renal and GI elimination, as well as sweat and insensible water losses.
4. Body sodium, potassium, and calcium balance reflects the balance between ingestion and renal elimination, with buffering by extracellular and cellular body stores.
5. Acute and chronic regulation of water and electrolyte balance depend on the specific action of a variety of hormones and to a small extent the autonomic nervous system.

Cellular Function

4

◌◌●● CELL STRUCTURE AND FUNCTION

The cell is the basic unit of structure and function in biologic systems. Eukaryotic cells consist of a membrane-bound nucleus embedded in an aqueous cytoplasmic matrix surrounded by a phospholipid plasma membrane. Scattered within the cytoplasm are organelles, membrane-limited structures with a complex infrastructure. Organelle structure allows multistage metabolic and physiologic events to occur simultaneously while keeping one function separate from another. Cytoskeleton proteins provide the scaffolding on which the cellular components are organized (Fig. 4-1).

Cells perform the basic functions of life. Cells transfer energy, take up and assimilate materials from outside the cell, metabolize macromolecules, maintain a homeostatic environment, and reproduce as required.

Physiologic function requires interaction of many cellular components. Aerobic production of ATP occurs in the mitochondria but requires proper function of the cell membrane to regulate the cellular influx of carbohydrate or fat substrates, as well as O_2. Protein synthesis requires the coordinated function of the nucleus, endoplasmic reticulum, Golgi apparatus, ribosomes, and microtubules. Lipid synthesis requires the smooth endoplasmic reticulum, and cell replication requires the nucleus, centrioles, and the components involved in protein synthesis. A functional map of cellular processes is shown in Figure 4-2.

The Nucleus

The nucleus is the most prominent organelle in the eukaryotic cell. The nucleus contains DNA in the form of chromatin threads surrounded by a porous double phospholipid membrane, the nuclear envelope. Each cell, except the reproductive cells, contains an individual's entire genome located on 46 chromosomes.

The genome is the genetic blueprint for the body. Although each cell contains the entire genetic blueprint, an individual cell normally utilizes only a portion of the total DNA. The portion of the DNA that is available for transcription for each cell is determined as cells differentiate. Transcription is a highly controlled process, regulated by multiple factors, including hormones and other cell-signaling molecules (Fig. 4-3).

Transcription is the creation of messenger RNA from an "unzipped" portion of the DNA. The messenger RNA exits the nucleus and enters the cytoplasm for translation. During translation, the combination of a ribosome and the messenger RNA is used to create a protein. Translation is the reading of the nucleotide triplet code that determines the specific sequence of amino acids incorporated into a protein.

Cell Growth: Hypertrophy and Hyperplasia

Cell growth involves one of two processes—hypertrophy and hyperplasia. Although both processes will increase the size of a tissue, they are fundamentally and functionally different.

Hypertrophy is an increase in the size of a cell. Hypertrophy represents the remodeling of a cell, often in response to an increased workload. Muscle cells rarely divide. Consequently, most of the growth of a muscle is due to hypertrophy of existing muscle cells. For example, hypertension (an increase in arterial blood pressure) increases the workload on the left ventricle of the heart. The muscle cells of the left ventricle hypertrophy in order to handle the additional work. Another example is the increased size of the biceps muscle in individuals engaged in strenuous physical activity.

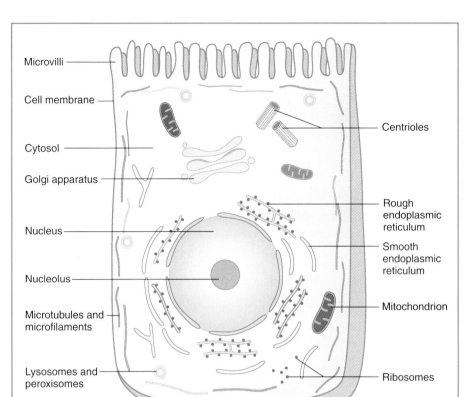

Figure 4-1. Organelles present in an epithelial cell.

Microvilli

Cell membrane

Cytosol

Golgi apparatus

Nucleus

Nucleolus

Microtubules and microfilaments

Lysosomes and peroxisomes

Centrioles

Rough endoplasmic reticulum

Smooth endoplasmic reticulum

Mitochondrion

Ribosomes

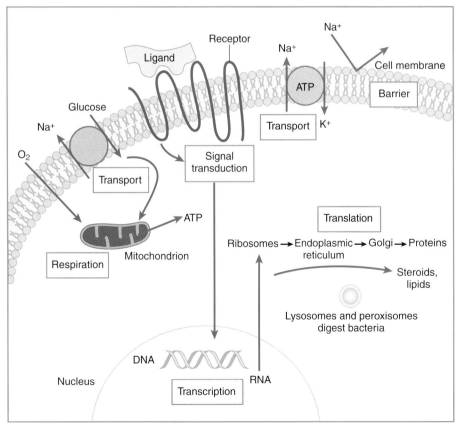

Figure 4-2. Cellular organelles assist the cellular life processes.

Na+

Receptor

Ligand

Na+

Cell membrane

Glucose

ATP

Barrier

Na+

Transport

K+

O₂

Signal transduction

Transport

ATP

Translation

Mitochondrion

Ribosomes → Endoplasmic → Golgi → Proteins
reticulum

Respiration

Steroids, lipids

Lysosomes and peroxisomes digest bacteria

DNA

Nucleus

RNA

Transcription

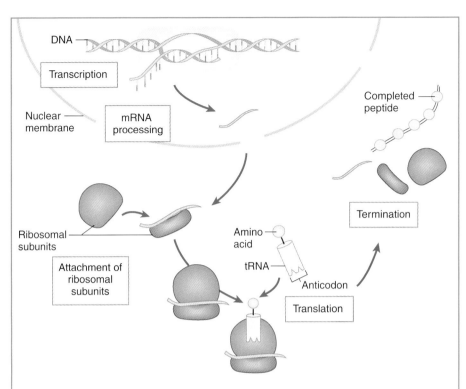

Figure 4-3. Protein synthesis results from transcription of the DNA code in the nucleus and translation of the RNA code in the ribosomes. The unzipping of the DNA helix by RNA polymerase allows for the construction of a complementary RNA sequence. This messenger RNA exits the nucleus and is attached to ribosomes, where the protein is synthesized one amino acid at a time. Each transfer RNA (tRNA) has an amino acid specific to the anticodon. Peptide synthesis is stopped when one of the three termination codons is read.

BIOCHEMISTRY

DNA Codons

DNA is composed of two nucleotide chains linked by the H^+ bonds between the purines and the pyrimidines to form a double helix. RNA polymerase binds to a section of DNA and uncouples the H^+ bonds, allowing a messenger RNA to be created that complements the DNA base sequence. The messenger RNA nucleotide sequence is "read" as triplets by the ribosome to create proteins.

Hyperplasia is an increase in cell number through mitosis. Most cells in the body replicate, although at varying rates. Epithelial cells, hematopoietic cells, and sperm replicate at a high constant rate. At the other extreme, following infancy, muscle cells and neurons replicate infrequently if at all. This inability to replicate means that the body has a limited capacity to repair damage resulting from the death of neurons.

Mitosis requires replication of the genetic information. The complementary DNA strands separate, and each strand serves as a template. Once the DNA has duplicated, somatic cells divide and produce two daughter cells with genetic content identical to that of the parent cell (unless altered by mutation). Gametogenesis occurs by meiosis and produces progeny cells, each having half the genetic content of the starting cell (23 rather than 46 chromosomes).

Following mitosis, cells can proceed along one of two paths. Stem cells enter G_1 phase and continue through another mitotic cycle. Alternatively, the cells may differentiate and enter G_0 phase (Fig. 4-4).

Mitosis can be divided into four phases: prophase, metaphase, anaphase, and telophase. In prophase, two centrioles move toward opposite poles of the cell, the nucleolus disappears, and the chromatin threads of DNA become visible as structures called chromosomes. By metaphase, the nuclear envelope has completely disappeared and the chromosomes are attached to their centromeres. At the end of this stage, the chromatin divides into separate strands of chromosomes. Anaphase further divides the cell, with evidence of pinching of the cell membrane. In telophase, the cell divides into two identical daughter cells having the same genetic content as the parent cell.

Successful replication requires the maintenance of the original DNA sequence. Mutations result when an error occurs in the DNA replication process. Mutations in somatic cells have unpredictable consequences—possibly benign, possibly fatal—but the change is limited to that individual. Mutations in gametes can be passed on to the offspring, altering the DNA in every cell of that offspring.

CELL DEVELOPMENT

Human life begins as a fertilized ovum, a single undifferentiated cell derived from the fusion of a sperm and an ovum. Within 1 week, the original cell has undergone multiple cycles of mitotic replication. The progeny cells begin to differentiate into cells that can be distinguished on the basis of both form and function. Differentiation is determined by a

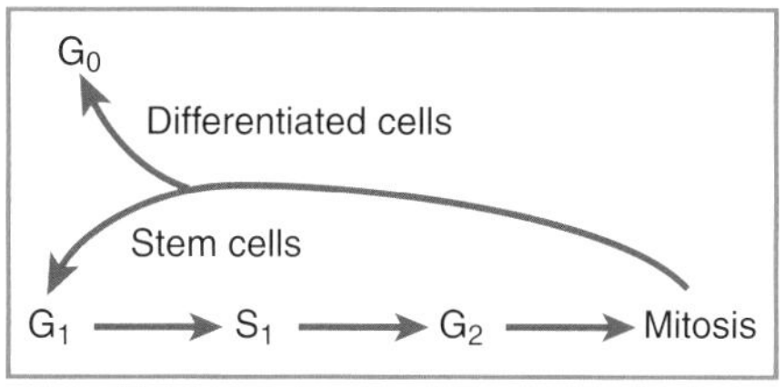

G₀
Differentiated cells
Stem cells
$G_1 \longrightarrow S_1 \longrightarrow G_2 \longrightarrow$ Mitosis

Figure 4-4. Cells participating in mitotic replication exit the G_0 phase and enter the cell cycle. Cell organelle growth occurs during the G_1 phase, followed by DNA synthesis in the S phase, followed by a second gap (G_2 phase). The mitotic process results in two identical progeny cells.

BIOCHEMISTRY

Replication Errors

Mitosis requires creation of an exact copy of the DNA that is distributed to each of the daughter cells. Mutations occur when there is an error in replicating the base pair sequence. Deletion of a single base pair results in a frame-shift error that affects all subsequent triplet codons. Deletion of three base pairs would result in the loss of only a single amino acid in the protein sequence.

combination of genetic programming and the influence of surrounding cells.

Eventually, the rate of cell reproduction begins to slow and finally stop. The tissues attain a steady-state level, in which replication is limited to replacement. The arrestment of growth is due to contact or density-dependent inhibition, and it is regulated by physical contact and the chemical microenvironment.

●●● CELL-TO-CELL COMMUNICATION

Normally the cell membrane isolates a cell from the adjacent tissue. As a consequence, any cell-to-cell message must first transit the cell membrane. One exception to that arrangement is a feature found in cardiac and smooth muscle cells: the gap junction. A gap junction is a direct pathway that joins the cytoplasm of adjacent cells formed by connexin proteins. When open, this pathway provides a direct electrical connection between the cells. An action potential generated in one cell will spread through all adjacent cells that are connected by an open gap junction. This arrangement allows a group of cells to function as a syncitium, a single unit.

Autocrine, paracrine, endocrine, and neurotransmitter signaling all involve the release of an agent from one cell into the extracellular space and the subsequent binding of the agent to a receptor on a target cell. For autocrine actions, the receptor is on the same cell that released the signal. For paracrine signaling, the receptor is on a cell in close proximity to the signaling cell. The distance is increased even further with endocrine signaling, which requires that the signal molecule be transported by the blood to reach the target

HISTOLOGY

Gap Junctions

Gap junctions are direct cytoplasmic connections between adjacent cells. The six transmembrane-spanning connexon monomers create a potential channel through the cell membrane. Connexons can bind to a similar channel located in the cell membrane of an adjacent cell. The connexon channel creates a pathway permitting movement of ions and small molecules up to 1200 Da, such as cAMP.

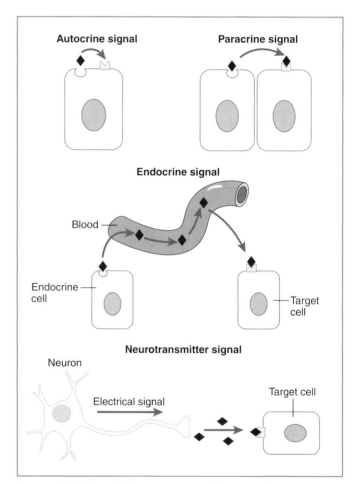

Figure 4-5. Extracellular messengers interact with receptors on the target cell. The distance between the cell secreting the messenger and the target cell containing the receptor is the basis for classifying the action as an autocrine, a paracrine, a neurotransmitter, or an endocrine event.

tissue. Neurotransmitter signaling is a special case in which agents released from the axon terminal diffuse over a short distance to the postsynaptic target cell (Fig. 4-5).

Characterization of a signaling molecule as an endocrine, autocrine, or paracrine agent is difficult, since one molecule can serve each of these purposes in the same system. Norepinephrine released at a sympathetic nerve terminal will bind to an α_2-adrenergic receptor on the presynaptic axon terminal (autocrine), bind to the postsynaptic cell receptor (neurotransmitter), and diffuse away from the synaptic cleft, where it can bind to receptors on adjacent cells (paracrine) or diffuse into the circulation, where it can be carried to distant cells (endocrine) (Fig. 4-6).

CELL MEMBRANE

The cell membrane is a phospholipid bilayer into which proteins, glycoproteins, and glycolipids are embedded (Fig. 4-7). This structure separates the intracellular fluid from the extracellular fluid and regulates exchange and communication across the cell membrane. Membranes also surround intracellular

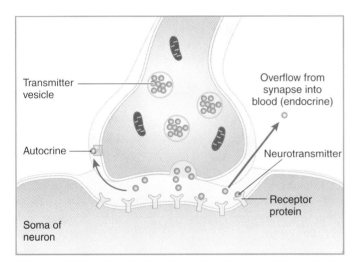

Figure 4-6. Norepinephrine released at the synaptic terminal interacts with multiple receptors. The norepinephrine that diffuses across the synaptic cleft to the postsynaptic membrane acts as a neurotransmitter. The norepinephrine that diffuses away from the synapse can act in an autocrine fashion on the presynaptic nerve terminal, a paracrine fashion on nearby cells, or an endocrine fashion when the overflow from the synaptic cleft enters the circulation.

organelles, such as vacuoles, mitochondria, the Golgi apparatus, and the nucleus, where they perform an equivalent role.

The phospholipid bilayer provides a barrier to diffusion. The lipid retards movement of ions and other charged molecules. In contrast, lipid-soluble substances easily diffuse across the membrane but have difficulty traveling through the aqueous extracellular and intracellular fluid. Lipophilic molecules can accumulate in the interior of cell membranes. Small polar molecules, such as water and urea, easily diffuse across the membrane, facilitated by selective channels that span the lipid bilayer. Diffusion of glucose and other large polar molecules is impeded by the plasma membrane, and cellular uptake of glucose requires specific transport proteins.

Proteins in the cell membrane selectively regulate the cellular entry and exit of water-soluble, but not lipid-soluble, materials. Movement across the membrane can occur passively down a concentration gradient (from high to low concentration) or by active transport against the concentration gradient (from low to high). Active transport processes require energy. The basic transport mechanisms are summarized in Figure 4-8.

Diffusion occurs down a concentration gradient. The effectiveness of diffusion is increased by increasing the concentration gradient, increasing the permeability, increasing

BIOCHEMISTRY

Fluid Mosaic Model of Cell Membrane

The cell membrane consists of a phospholipid bilayer oriented with the hydrophobic fatty acid tails facing the middle of the bilayer, and the hydrophilic polar heads facing interior and exterior surfaces. Proteins, glycoproteins, and glycolipids are embedded in the membrane, and cholesterol is inserted into the lipophilic interior. Proteins either can be partially inserted into the membrane and exposed on only one surface, or they can span the entire membrane. Channels and transport proteins are membrane-spanning structures.

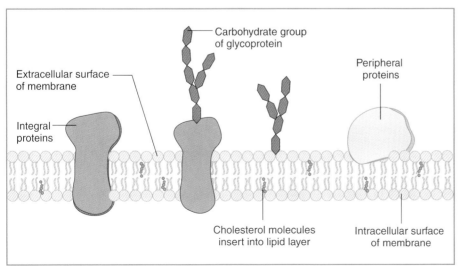

Figure 4-7. The cell membrane consists of proteins embedded in a phospholipid bilayer. Some proteins extend across the lipid bilayer and are exposed to both the intracellular and extracellular surfaces. Other proteins are more loosely attached to the cell membrane.

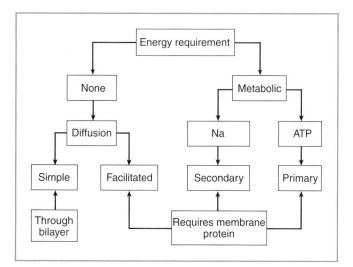

Figure 4-8. Transport across the cell membrane can be classified by energy requirements or by the involvement of membrane proteins. Processes requiring metabolic energy allow movement against a concentration gradient. Processes requiring membrane proteins exhibit the characteristic of saturation kinetics, in which the number of proteins sets a limit on the maximum rate of transport.

the surface area, or decreasing the distance over which the compound must travel (see Chapter 1).

$$J = -DA \frac{\Delta \text{ concentration}}{\Delta \text{ distance}}$$

Cell membranes exhibit a special case of facilitated diffusion. This transport process allows the transmembrane movement of compounds that are poorly soluble in the phospholipid bilayer. Glucose absorption across the intestinal epithelia illustrates both secondary active transport and facilitated diffusion. On the apical surface, glucose enters the cell by a secondary active transport process, coupled to Na^+ entry. This process allows glucose uptake even when the extracellular luminal glucose concentration is lower than the intracellular glucose concentration. Glucose exits the cell on the basolateral surface by facilitated diffusion. No energy is expended, and the glucose moves down the concentration gradient. The net effect is that glucose is absorbed from the lumen of the intestine into the body. Movement across the basolateral surface occurs by transport proteins, but no energy (other than the glucose concentration gradient) is involved. The reliance on transport proteins, however, means that compounds moving by facilitated diffusion show saturation kinetics, in which the number of transport proteins can limit the maximum rate of the compound.

In a completely random world, diffusion would ensure the even distribution of all substances. Life, however, depends on the development, maintenance, and utilization of concentration gradients. The development of concentration gradients cannot occur by diffusion. The energy required to move solutes against their concentration gradient comes from hydrolysis of ATP in primary active transport or from energy derived from a preexisting concentration gradient in secondary active transport.

Active Transport

Primary active transport uses energy obtained from ATP hydrolysis to move ions against a concentration gradient. Examples of this process include Na^+/K^+-ATPase on the membranes of all cells, Ca^{++}-ATPase on the sarcoplasmic and endoplasmic reticulum, and H^+-ATPase in the stomach and renal distal tubule.

Alternatively, a transcellular ion gradient can provide energy for secondary active transport. Examples include the Na^+ gradient–driven amino acid and glucose transport in the intestine and renal proximal tubule and the Na^+ gradient–driven $Na^+/K^+/2$ Cl^- transport in the loop of Henle in the kidney.

The Na^+/K^+-ATPase is particularly important to cellular function. The Na^+/K^+-ATPase pumps 3 Na^+ out of the cell and 2 K^+ into the cell for each ATP hydrolyzed. This pump plays two important roles in establishing the resting membrane potential. First, the pump is electrogenic in that it transports three positively charged ions out of the cell for every two positively charged ions that enter (Fig. 4-9). Consequently, pump activity creates a negative intracellular (about 5 to 10 mV) environment. Second, this pump activity establishes and maintains the transcellular ionic gradients for Na^+ and K^+. As explained below, the differences in intracellular and extracellular ion concentrations, along with permeabilities, generate the cell membrane potential. Decreased ATP production slows pump activity and acutely depolarizes the cell membrane by 5 to 10 mV. Chronic poisoning of the pump disrupts the ion concentration gradients, and if complete, will kill the cell.

Membrane proteins are also categorized by the number of compounds transported and by the direction of transport. Uniports carry only one agent across the membrane. Symports or co-transporters carry two agents in the same direction. Antiports or exchangers carry two agents in opposite directions.

Carrier-mediated transport requires binding a compound to a receptor site. Consequently, the process is characterized by specificity, saturation kinetics, and competitive inhibition. The rate of transport can reach a maximum and thereafter become independent of substrate concentration. The maximum rate of transport is proportionate to the number of carrier proteins (see Fig. 11-11 for an example). In contrast, diffusion-driven flux does not show saturation kinetics and continues to increase as the concentration difference increases.

Electrochemical Gradient

Cellular function depends on the close regulation of intracellular concentrations of K^+, Na^+, Cl^-, and Ca^{++}. Diffusion down the concentration gradient favors the efflux of K^+ and the influx of Na^+, Ca^{++}, and Cl^- (Table 4-1). Because ions are charged entities, an electrostatic attraction can be used to induce ion movement. For example, negatively charged Cl^- would be repelled from the inside of a cell whose inside was

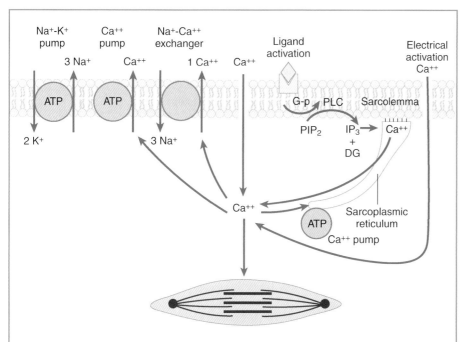

Figure 4-9. Na$^+$/K$^+$-ATPase on myocardial cells helps maintain low intracellular Na$^+$. The low intracellular Na$^+$ is then used in the secondary active transport to transport Ca^{++} out of the cell. Drugs such as digitalis will slow the activity of the Na$^+$/K$^+$-ATPase. The increase in intracellular Na$^+$ decreases the efficiency of the Na/Ca exchange, resulting in an increase in intracellular Ca^{++} and an increase in myocardial contractility. An increase in extracellular K$^+$ is one of the hallmarks of digitalis toxicity.

PHARMACOLOGY

Cardiac Glycosides

Digoxin and similar cardiac glycosides increase myocardial contractility and are used to treat congestive heart failure. Digoxin inhibits the activity of the Na$^+$/K$^+$-ATPase, resulting in an increase in intracellular Na$^+$ and a decrease in intracellular K$^+$. The increased cardiac contractility is tied to the increase in intracellular Na$^+$ and subsequent reduction in activity of the Na/Ca exchanger, the net result of which is an increase in resting Ca$^+$ levels.

TABLE 4-1. Typical Nernst Equilibrium Potentials for an Axon

	Extracellular	Intracellular	Nernst Equilibrium Potential
Na$^+$	144 mEq/L	15 mEq/L	+60 mV
K$^+$	4.5 mEq/L	120 mEq/L	−88 mV
Ca^{++}	5 mEq/L	0.0001 mEq/L	+144 mV
Cl$^-$	110 mEq/L	20 mEq/L	−46 mV

BIOCHEMISTRY

Similarities Between Hormone-Receptor Interactions and Enzyme Kinetics

Hormone-receptor interactions share many common characteristics of enzymatic reactions. Binding of the ligand (or substrate) is stereospecific, is reversible, and shows saturation kinetics. Binding is competitive in that ligand binding can be displaced by compounds having a similar structure.

negatively charged compared with the outside. In contrast, positively charged K$^+$ would be attracted toward the inside of a cell whose inside was negatively charged compared with the outside.

Two separate gradients affect K$^+$ movement: the chemical driving force from diffusion and an electrostatic driving force from the electrical charge. There can be a balance between these driving forces, so that the outward diffusional tendency

for K$^+$ is offset by the inward electrostatic attraction. This is a condition of steady state. When these forces are completely balanced, there will be no net movement between intracellular and extracellular K$^+$ pools. The Nernst equation describes the equilibrium potential for an ion, the electrical force that would balance the observed ion concentration gradient, based on the ratio of intracellular to extracellular ion concentrations:

$$E_M = -61.5/\text{valence} \, \log [\text{ion}]_{in}/[\text{ion}]_{out}$$

Using cardiac muscle cells as an example (Fig. 4-10), the calculated equilibrium potential for K$^+$ is −94 mV and for Na$^+$ is +73 mV. Importantly, a change in the intracellular or extracellular ion concentration will cause a shift in the Nernst equilibrium potential for that ion. For example, an increase in extracellular K$^+$ from 4.2 mEq/L to 8.0 mEq/L will cause the equilibrium potential to shift from −94 mV to −76 mV.

The Nernst equilibrium values have two important implications for the cardiac muscle cell shown in Figure 4-10:

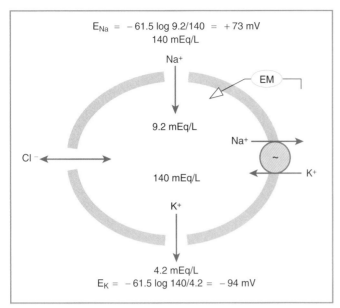

$$E_{Na} = -61.5 \log 9.2/140 = +73 \text{ mV}$$
140 mEq/L

Na+

EM

9.2 mEq/L

Na+

~

140 mEq/L

K+

K+

4.2 mEq/L

$$E_K = -61.5 \log 140/4.2 = -94 \text{ mV}$$

Cl⁻

Figure 4-10. Differential distribution of ions creates a chemical gradient that can be offset by an electrical charge. An equilibrium potential of +73 mV would be required to balance the diffusional movement of Na⁺. An equilibrium potential of −94 mV would be required to balance the diffusional movement of K⁺. The Nernst equation calculates the equilibrium potential based on the intracellular and extracellular concentrations of that ion.

TABLE 4-2. Ion Channel Classes

Class	Description
Na⁺	Voltage-gated Na⁺ channels Non-voltage-gated Na⁺ channels

K⁺	Voltage-gated K⁺ channels
	  Inward rectifier K⁺ channels
	  Delayed rectifier K⁺ channels
	Ca⁺⁺-sensitive K⁺ channels
	ATP-sensitive K⁺ channels
	Na⁺-activated K⁺ channels
	Cell volume–sensitive K⁺ channels
	Type A K⁺ channels
	Receptor-coupled K⁺ channels

Cl⁻	Extracellular ligand-gated Cl⁻ channels Cystic fibrosis transmembrane conductance regulator Voltage-gated chloride channels Nucleotide-sensitive chloride channels Calcium-activated chloride channels
Ca⁺⁺	Voltage-gated (N, P, Q, R, T subtypes) Ca⁺⁺ channels Ligand-gated Ca⁺⁺ channels Capacitive Ca⁺⁺ channels

(1) if K⁺ was the only ion that determined the membrane potential, the inside of the cell would be −94 mV when compared with the outside of the cell, and (2) for a cell with a resting membrane potential of −94 mV, K⁺ will not cross the membrane (again, no net movement).

Another cell, with slightly different internal and external ion concentrations, yields slightly different calculated Nernst equilibrium potentials (see Table 4-1). Extracellular Na⁺ and K⁺ rarely vary by more than 10%, and the calculated Nernst values for each of the ions is in a general range close to the values shown in Table 4-1.

The preceding discussion assumes that the cell membrane is freely permeable to the ions under consideration. Cell membrane ionic permeability, then, is an essential determinant of cell electrophysiology. Cell membrane permeability can change on the basis of the activity of ion selective channels. Some of the channels leak continuously, and others are gated (opened by stimuli). A ligand-gated channel changes shape (opens) when an agent binds to a specific receptor coupled to the channel. These channels are seen in cells that respond to hormones, drugs, or neurotransmitters. A voltage-gated channel opens or closes when there are changes in the electrical voltage across the membrane. A mechanically gated channel opens in response to deforming forces, such as pressure or friction.

Of the many ion channels found in the body, those listed in Table 4-2 play a particularly important role in multiple tissues. Other channels will be introduced in the discussion of a tissue in which they have a specific function.

Membrane Potential

The membrane potential results from the separation of an electrical charge across a membrane. By convention, it is expressed as the inside of the membrane compared with the outside of the membrane. A cell membrane potential of −90 mV means that the inside surface of the cell membrane is 90 mV more negative than the outside surface of the cell membrane. Polarization is based on a charge separation, so any movement away from 0 mV is a hyperpolarizing change and any movement toward 0 mV is a depolarizing change. Movement from −90 mV to −75 mV is therefore a 15 mV depolarization.

The membrane potential reflects the combined influence of all the ions and their permeability. The chord conductance equation provides a mathematical model of this relationship. Conductance is the electrical counterpart of ionic permeability, but for simplicity the term permeability is used in this text for both ionic events and electrical events. Qualitatively, the equation indicates that the most permeable ion will have the greatest effect on the cell membrane potential.

The chord conductance equation uses the term transference (T) to indicate the relative permeability for an ion. Transference for any ion is the conductance for that ion/ conductance for all ions in the system. Transference represents the percent of total ionic permeability that is due to one particular ion. In practice, Na⁺, K⁺, Cl⁻, and Ca⁺⁺ are the ions considered when looking at cell membrane events.

$$E_M = [(T_{Na})(E_{Na})] + [(T_K)(E_K)] + [(T_{Cl})(E_{Cl})] + [(T_{Ca})(E_{Ca})]$$

At rest, K$^+$ permeability is much higher than the permeability to any other ion. T for K$^+$ is greater than 95%, and T for the remaining ions is less than 5%. Consequently, the resting membrane potential (–90 mV) is close to the K$^+$ equilibrium potential. The membrane potential is not exactly equal to the –94 mV K$^+$ equilibrium potential, because even at rest there is some permeability to Na$^+$, which shifts the resting membrane potential slightly (but only slightly) toward the +73 mV Na$^+$ equilibrium potential.

Changing ion permeability causes a change in membrane potential. An increase in permeability to an ion shifts the membrane potential toward the Nernst equilibrium potential for that ion. A decrease in permeability to an ion shifts the membrane potential away from the Nernst equilibrium potential for that ion (Fig. 4-11).

CELL ELECTRICAL ACTIVITY

Cell membranes exhibit two distinct electrical behaviors based on the characteristics and the density of ion channels. Membrane areas that lack sufficient density of Na$^+$ channels generate only local currents. Areas with sufficient density of Na$^+$ channels are capable of generating an action potential. Figure 4-12 shows areas that exhibit these electrical behaviors.

Local Currents

Membrane potential is altered by the opening of ion selective channels. The magnitude of the electrical event is proportionate to the number of channels opened and the electrochemical driving force for the ion. Consequently, a region with many open channels has the greatest local potential.

Sites that exhibit local potentials include the end plate of the neuromuscular junction, the presynaptic nerve terminal, the postsynaptic dendrite, the neuron cell body, and many sensory receptors. These local potentials can be hyperpolarizing or depolarizing according to which ions are involved. For example, opening Na$^+$ channels would create a depolarizing local current. Opening K$^+$ channels would create a hyperpolarizing local current.

Local potentials are transmitted both along the cytosol and across the cell membrane. Increasing cytosolic resistance directs more current to flow along the membrane. Decreasing cytosolic resistance allows more current to flow through the cytosol and decreases the local potential across the membrane.

Transmission of the local potential along the membrane is called electrotonic conductance. The amplitude of local potentials that spread electronically decreases with distance.

The magnitude of the local potential is increased by temporal summation. A single, isolated local potential degenerates over time. A second stimulus, arriving before the first response has fully decayed, will add the new current to the existing current. The efficiency of temporal summation depends on the time constant.

The magnitude of the local potential also is increased by spatial summation. Each stimulus produces a local response. The simultaneous arrival of independent stimuli at the same region of the cell will produce a greater local potential than each alone. Inhibitory stimuli, which hyperpolarize the membrane, can also summate. The simultaneous arrival of an inhibitory and excitatory stimulus will decrease the normal local response to the excitatory stimulus.

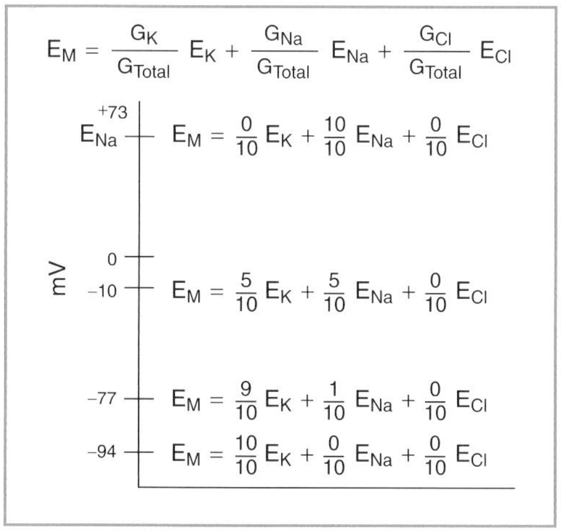

$$E_M = \frac{G_K}{G_{Total}} E_K + \frac{G_{Na}}{G_{Total}} E_{Na} + \frac{G_{Cl}}{G_{Total}} E_{Cl}$$

$$E_M = \frac{0}{10} E_K + \frac{10}{10} E_{Na} + \frac{0}{10} E_{Cl}$$

$$E_M = \frac{5}{10} E_K + \frac{5}{10} E_{Na} + \frac{0}{10} E_{Cl}$$

$$E_M = \frac{9}{10} E_K + \frac{1}{10} E_{Na} + \frac{0}{10} E_{Cl}$$

$$E_M = \frac{10}{10} E_K + \frac{0}{10} E_{Na} + \frac{0}{10} E_{Cl}$$

Figure 4-11. The chord conductance equation allows calculation of the membrane potential based on ion permeability. If Na$^+$ is the only permeant ion, the equilibrium potential for the membrane is the same as the Na$^+$ equilibrium potential. If both Na$^+$ and K$^+$ are equally permeable, the membrane potential will be halfway between the Na$^+$ and the K$^+$ equilibrium potentials.

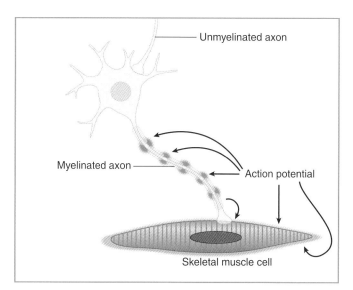

Figure 4-12. Both local potentials and action potentials occur in the neuromuscular system. Action potentials occur only when there is sufficient density of Na$^+$ channels, such as on unmyelinated axons, at the nodes of Ranvier on myelinated axons, and on the membrane of skeletal muscle cells. Local potentials occur in the neuron dendrites, neuron cell body, axon terminal, and end plate region of skeletal muscle cell.

Action Potential

Action potentials are the principal mechanism of nerve impulse propagation and transmission, and they allow depolarization at a single region of skeletal and cardiac muscle cells to spread across the entire cell. Action potentials require a stimulus that depolarizes the cell membrane potential to a threshold value, and then a sufficient density of voltage-gated channels to generate an electrical response. An action potential results from a sequential change in ion permeabilities. An action potential generated by a nerve axon is used to illustrate the characteristic changes in ion permeabilities and membrane potential (Figs. 4-13 and 4-14).

The fast Na^+ channel is a voltage-gated structure with two gates that can block the lumen of the channel (Fig. 4-15). The transition voltage for gate movement is around −70 mV, the threshold voltage. Both gates move whenever the membrane potential depolarizes or hyperpolarizes through this transition voltage value, but the gates move at different rates. The activation m-gate moves immediately, and the inactivation h-gate takes longer to get into position. At a resting membrane potential of −90 mV, the m-gate blocks the channel and the h-gate is open. As the membrane potential depolarizes past threshold, the gates move, with the m-gate opening the channel and the h-gate starting to close the channel. The channel remains open for a period of time until the h-gate is in the closed position. During repolarization through −70 mV, the gates again shift. The m-gate moves to block the channel, and the h-gate is still in place blocking the channel. Both gates block the channel until the h-gate moves to the open position. This gate dynamic results in a period of time during depolarization to threshold when both gates are open and Na^+ permeability is increased.

The resting membrane potential results from the high membrane permeability to K^+ relative to Cl^-, Na^+, and Ca^{++}. A stimulus generates a local potential that depolarizes a region of the membrane past the threshold value. The voltage-sensitive m-gate of the fast Na^+ channel opens, depolarizing the membrane. This depolarization opens more voltage-gated fast Na^+ channels, further increasing Na^+ permeability and further depolarizing the membrane in a positive feedback cycle. An action potential is generated if the density of functional fast Na^+ channels is sufficient to allow the progressive depolarization (see Fig. 4-15).

The Na^+ channels remain open for a limited period of time and then close as the h-gate inactivates the channel. Movement of the h-gate is also voltage dependent, and is initiated by the membrane depolarizing past threshold. One major difference is in the speed of movement. The h-gate closure is a slower event.

Even slower are the voltage-gated K^+ channels, which do not fully reach their open position until after the peak of the action potential. As the K^+ channels finally open, the membrane potential shifts toward the K^+ Nernst equilibrium value, possibly hyperpolarizing the membrane potential compared with the original resting membrane potential. The membrane potential returns toward the resting membrane potential as the voltage-gated K^+ channels close. As the membrane potential drops below −70 mV, the fast Na^+ channel gates reset. The m-gate quickly moves to block the channel, and the h-gate more slowly unblocks the channel. In contrast to the depolarizing event, the fast Na^+ channel is blocked by one or both gates during the repolarization phase.

The movement of the activation and inactivation gates of the voltage-gated Na^+ channel sets limits on the responsive-

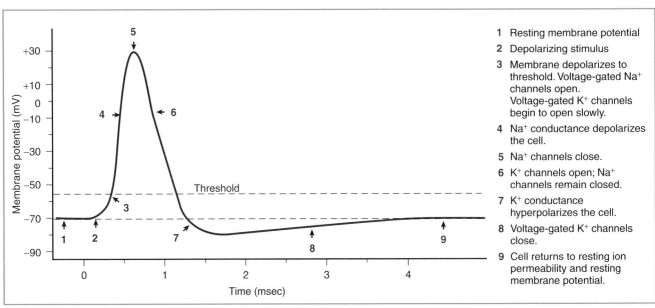

Figure 4-13. An action potential is an "all or nothing" response when the cell membrane is depolarized past the threshold value. The action potential consists of a rapid depolarization, a peak, a rapid repolarization, and a hyperpolarization period.

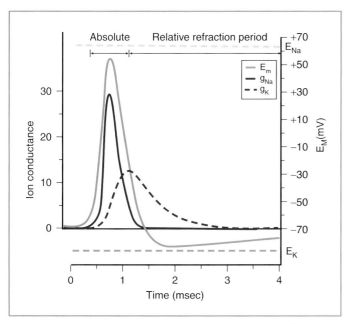

Figure 4-14. Changes in the ionic conductance to Na$^+$ and K$^+$ mediate the membrane electrical changes during an action potential. The depolarization is caused by a rapid increase in Na$^+$ permeability. The repolarization is caused by both a decrease in Na$^+$ permeability and an increase in K$^+$ permeability. The increase in K$^+$ permeability continues through the period of hyperpolarization, gradually returning to baseline values.

ness of the cell. The cell will not generate an action potential until after the fast Na$^+$ channel m-gate is reset. The period of time when the cell is unable to generate an action potential is called the absolute refractory period. A relative refractory period follows the absolute refractory period, and it persists until the voltage-gated K$^+$ channels close. During this time, the cell requires a greater than normal stimulus to reach threshold and generate an action potential. Action potentials of different tissues have characteristic forms and durations, based on the presence and density of fast Na$^+$ channels and the timing of the K$^+$ channel opening.

Threshold requires a critical density of open voltage-gated Na$^+$ channels so that the electrical depolarization becomes self-sustaining. A gradual depolarization allows some channels to open and inactivate without reaching critical

PHARMACOLOGY

Lidocaine and Other Local Anesthetics

Local anesthetics prevent both the generation and the transmission of an action potential by blocking Na channels. The differential ability to block a mixed nerve appears related to the diameter of the axon. Small-diameter neurons that transmit pain information are the first to be blocked, followed by temperature, touch, and finally deep pressure.

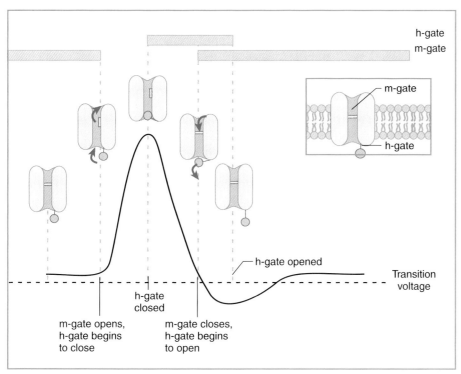

Figure 4-15. Movement of the activation m-gate and the inactivation h-gate on the fast Na$^+$ channel regulates neuronal Na$^+$ permeability.

current flow. Consequently, rapid depolarization more effectively generates an action potential than a more gradual depolarization does.

Changes in intracellular or extracellular ion concentrations will modify the action potential. The action potential is the result of changing ion permeabilities, driving the membrane potential toward that ion's Nernst potential. Increases in intracellular Na^+ or decreases in extracellular Na^+ will decrease the Na^+ Nernst potential and diminish the overshoot of the action potential. Decreases in intracellular K^+ or increases in extracellular K^+ will decrease the K^+ Nernst potential, and because of the high resting K^+ permeability, these changes will depolarize the resting membrane potential. Cl^- distributes passively based on the resting membrane potential, and changes in extracellular Cl^- will not greatly affect the action potential.

Maintained changes in ion permeabilities also will affect the resting membrane potential and the action potential. Maintained increases in Na^+ permeability will depolarize the cell, bringing the membrane potential closer to threshold. Maintained increases in K^+ permeability will hyperpolarize the cell and move the resting membrane potential farther from threshold. Maintained increases in Cl^- permeability have little effect on the resting membrane potential but will diminish the changes in membrane potential caused by alterations in the permeabilities of the other ions (see Fig. 4-11). This includes diminishing the Na^+-mediated overshoot and diminishing the K^+-mediated hyperpolarization.

Membrane Receptor Signal Transduction

Proteins, peptides, and charged molecules do not easily diffuse across the cell membrane. Consequently, the cell membrane can serve as a barrier to cell-to-cell communication when such agents are used as neurotransmitters and hormones. This communication barrier is overcome by use of proteins embedded in the cell membrane that function as receptors for signaling molecules. Agents that bind the active site of the receptor protein are called ligands. The ligand, which remains outside the cell, is considered the first messenger. The intracellular agents activated by the ligand are grouped as second messengers (Fig. 4-16).

Binding to Cell Membrane Receptors

Cell surface receptor proteins have active sites that recognize the three-dimensional structure of the ligand. Binding of the ligand to the receptor protein then activates a series of membrane or intracellular events. These may include activation of a G protein, activation of a kinase or other enzyme, or direct activation of an ion channel. Ultimately, intracellular second messengers will be formed or released, and can include cAMP, cGMP, diacylglycerol (DAG), and Ca^{++} released from the endoplasmic reticulum.

Ligands that bind the receptor and activate it are agonists or activators. Ligands that bind the receptor but do not activate it are called antagonists or blockers. Antagonists are named because the normal agonist cannot bind the receptor

and activate it so long as the antagonist is occupying the active site.

Some receptors are physically independent of the ion channel protein. Activation of the receptor activates a G protein. The G protein may directly open the ion channel, or the G protein may activate phospholipase C (PLC), guanylate cyclase, or adenylate cyclase to modify the activity of an ion channel (Table 4-3).

Activation of PLC splits phosphatidylinositol 4,5-bisphosphate (PIP_2) into diacylglycerol (DAG), which stays in plasma membrane, and inositol 1,4,5-trisphosphate (IP_3), which enters the cytosol (Fig. 4-17). IP_3 acts as second messenger to release Ca^{++} from the endoplasmic reticulum. Calcium often activates protein kinase C. Calcium actions may be further controlled by activity of protein calmodulin. DAG activates protein kinase C. Alternatively, hydrolysis of diacylglycerol may produce arachidonic acid, a precursor to prostaglandins and thromboxanes.

Other signal transduction pathways directly activate protein kinases. These kinases, through the phosphorylation of other intracellular proteins, cause protein activation or inactivation. These transduction pathways and the protein G–coupled receptor pathways described above are not exclusive, as cAMP can also activate protein kinases.

The biological advantage of a signal transduction cascade is the amplification of the response during each step of the cascade. The diversity and overlap of second messenger systems also provide multiple opportunities for potentiation and inhibition of signal transduction events.

Although most signal transductions produce immediate effects, the receptor tyrosine kinase mediates the chronic effects of peptides such as growth hormone, insulin-like growth factor I, and numerous other growth factors. Proteins activated by these kinases alter transcription and translation, accounting for chronic growth-related actions (Fig. 4-18).

Recent experiments have shown that steroid hormones and other lipophilic hormones also can activate membrane receptors to produce acute (within minutes) effects. Previously, steroid hormones were thought to work only on nuclear and perinuclear receptors to produce changes that took hours to become evident.

Lipid-Soluble Signal Transduction

The cell membrane is not a barrier to the entry of steroid hormones, thyroid hormone, and the gases nitric oxide (NO) and carbon monoxide (CO). Both NO and CO activate a soluble guanylyl cyclase in the cytosol, leading to the formation of cGMP. NO and CO work mostly as paracrine agents but play a significant role in the regulation of vascular smooth muscle relaxation.

The steroid hormones and thyroid hormone bind to intracellular receptors located within or adjacent to the cell nucleus (Fig. 4-19). The steroid hormone–receptor complex enters the nucleus and acts as a transcription factor, promoting the transcription of specific genes. The transcription/translation process requires hours or days to exert an effect.

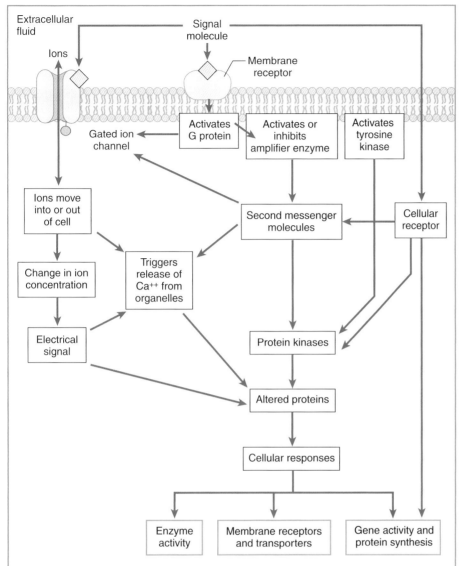

Figure 4-16. Overview of signal transduction pathways showing multiple mechanisms where an extracellular signal can alter cellular function. Hydrophilic ligands bind membrane receptors to directly alter membrane ionic permeability or to generate a second messenger by activating G proteins, amplifier enzymes, or tyrosine kinases. Lipophilic molecules bind intracellular or perinuclear receptors before altering gene transcription or other second messenger systems.

PHARMACOLOGY

Agonists and Antagonists

Agonists bind to a receptor and activate it to produce a response. Agonists usually share a common structure with the binding component of the natural ligand. Competitive antagonists inhibit the interaction of the ligand and the receptor by binding to the active site of the receptor. Consequently, some competitive antagonists have partial agonist properties. The maximal response of a partial agonist is by definition less than that of a full agonist. Noncompetitive antagonists alter the conformation of the receptor so that it can no longer elicit a response. This is done via an allosteric mechanism or through irreversible inhibition of the receptor, such as might be seen with an alkylating agent.

TABLE 4-3. Heterometric G Protein Target Kinases

Protein	Action
G_s	Stimulates adenylate cyclase—increases cAMP, targets PKA
G_i	Inhibits adenylate cyclase—decreases cAMP, targets PKA
G_q	Through phospholipase C, releases IP_3 and DAG, targets PKC
G_t	Decreases cGMP, targets PKG

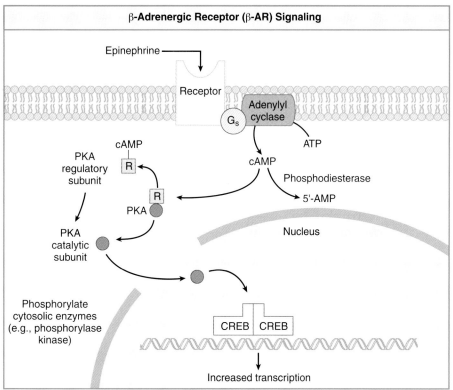

A

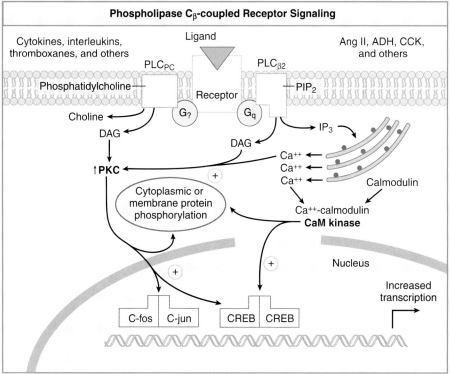

B

Figure 4-17. A, β-Adrenergic receptor signaling illustrates the steps involved in G protein–coupled second messenger systems. Binding to the β-adrenergic receptor activates a G_s protein and increases adenylyl cyclase activity, forming the second messenger cAMP. cAMP has multiple intracellular targets, including intracellular proteins, Ca^{++} released from sarcoplasm reticulum, and nuclear transcription. **B**, Phospholipase C receptor activation proceeds by one of two second messenger pathways, both of which involve diacylglycerol. The G_q pathway hydrolyzes PIP_2 to DAG and IP_3, with the IP_3 causing Ca^{++} release. An alternative G pathway hydrolyzes phosphatidylcholine to choline and DAG without generating IP_3 production and Ca^{++} release.

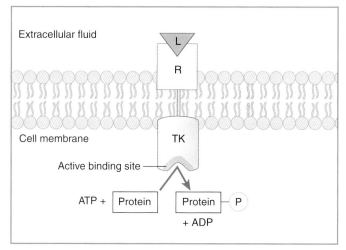

Figure 4-18. Tyrosine kinase second messenger systems can be directly coupled to the cell membrane receptor or can be more loosely coupled.

●●●● MODULATION OF TISSUE RESPONSE TO LIGAND

The biological response to a ligand results from a complex series of events, each of which is subject to modulation. First, the production, release, and concentration of the ligand can vary. In addition, the number of functional receptors on the cell can be increased (up-regulated) or decreased (down-regulated). The binding of the ligand to the receptor can be diminished by antagonists or enhanced by cooperativity. The coupling of the receptor to a second messenger system can be enhanced or diminished. Finally, the responsiveness of the effector within the cell can be modulated (Fig. 4-20).

Ligand production, particularly for hormones and neurotransmitter release, is under negative feedback control (described for each hormone in Chapter 13). For ligands that circulate in the plasma complexed to binding proteins, the total amount in the plasma will differ from the free amount in the plasma. The amount of free ligand is the biologically significant number, and bound versus free is an important concept in evaluating the biological concentrations of thyroid and steroid hormones.

The number of functional receptors is regulated. Over-production of thyroid hormone, for example, leads to an increase in the expression of adrenergic receptors and consequently an enhanced response to circulating norepinephrine. Hormone receptor expression also is often under negative feedback control based on the hormone levels. When circulating hormone levels are chronically high, the number of functional receptors is down-regulated. With fewer receptors, the tissue shows an attenuated sensitivity to the hormone. Conversely, when circulating hormone levels are chronically depressed, there is an up-regulation of receptors, leading to an increase in tissue sensitivity to the hormone.

The active site of the receptor has specificity for the three-dimensional structure of a specific ligand. Agonists are agents

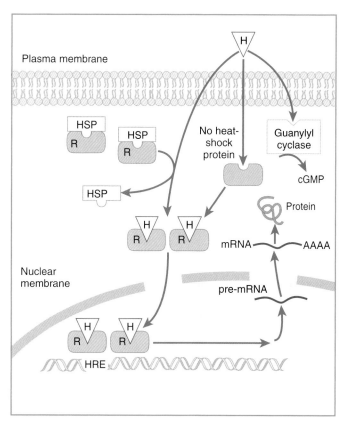

Figure 4-19. Lipophilic signaling molecules (H) bind to intracellular receptors (R). About half of the steroid receptors are coupled to heat-shock proteins (HSPs), which dissociate when the steroid binds the receptor. NO and CO bind to soluble guanylyl cyclase, generating cGMP and from that point following the normal G protein–coupled second messenger pathway.

BIOCHEMISTRY

Hormone Response Elements

Hormone response elements are sequences of DNA that recognize and bind a specific hormone-receptor complex. For steroid hormones, binding specificity is achieved through the TATA box of the hormone response element of the promoter area of the gene and the zinc fingers on the receptor. The specificity of hormone response elements results in the capacity of a steroid hormone to stimulate the synthesis of only a few proteins from the entire genome.

that have a similar structure to a ligand and their binding to the receptor activates it much in the same way as that ligand does. Antagonists interfere with the correct binding of the ligand to the receptor.

There can be more than one biological ligand for a receptor. The catecholamines norepinephrine, epinephrine, and dopamine each bind the cellular α-adrenergic receptors but with different affinities. Peptides and proteins that share

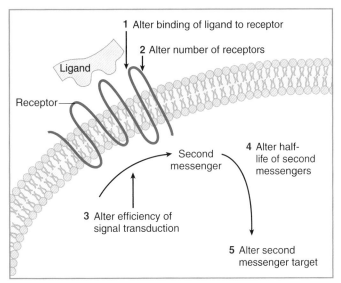

Figure 4-20. Modulation of hormone signaling pathways can occur at any step in the signaling cascade.

a common amino acid sequence, such as the secretin family, can bind and activate the same receptor.

There can also be more than one receptor for a given ligand. Epinephrine binds to the multiple α- and β-adrenergic receptors. Consequently, epinephrine works through a variety of second messenger systems. The exact response, and the second messenger system involved, are characteristic of the individual target tissues.

The robustness of second messenger cascades is modulated, particularly by protein kinases. This allows interaction of ligands, both synergistic and antagonistic, to occur at the second messenger level. For example, insulin works through a tyrosine kinase to activate protein kinase B, stimulating the translocation of GLUT4 transporters into the skeletal muscle cell membrane and enhancing glucose uptake by skeletal muscle. Growth hormone, working through the JAK/STAT second messenger system, blocks the activation of protein kinase B. Consequently, an increase in insulin, in the presence of growth hormone, does not stimulate skeletal muscle glucose uptake.

●●● TOP 5 TAKE-HOME POINTS

1. Like organisms, individual cells perform all the functions of life, including replication, but on a smaller scale.
2. Cells differentiate in order to express the specialized proteins to facilitate their function.
3. The nervous system, endocrine system, and numerous paracrine agents coordinate cellular function by means of cell-to-cell communication.
4. Signaling ligands bind receptors on the target tissue and generally exert an effect by activating cell-signaling pathways.
5. Modulation of cellular signaling can occur at the level of the ligand or receptor or within the signal transduction pathway.

Musculoskeletal System 5

CONTENTS

There are three general types of muscle in the body: skeletal, cardiac, and smooth. The muscle types are distinguished based on the presence of striations, source of innervation, and mechanism of contraction (Table 5-1).

The musculoskeletal system consists of skeletal muscle attached to the bony skeleton. Physiologically, the musculoskeletal system enables changes in movement and position. The rigid bony skeleton provides support, protection, and a movable frame. The connective tissue of joints and ligaments allows adjacent bones to articulate smoothly as they move. Skeletal muscle attaches to the bones of the skeleton. Skeletal muscle contraction shortens the length of the muscle and generates movement of this frame.

Skeletal muscle is the effector organ for movement (Fig. 5-1). Movement is initiated in the upper motor neurons of the central nervous system (CNS) motor cortex. Efferent motor cortex axons synapse on the spinal cord and generate an action potential in the α-motor neuron. The action potential travels to the axon terminal, releasing acetylcholine into the synaptic cleft. Acetylcholine binds a receptor on the skeletal muscle cell and generates an action potential, increasing Ca^{++} release from the sarcoplasmic reticulum. Ca^{++} initiates contraction, resulting in shortening of the muscle cell and, consequently, movement.

The musculoskeletal system contributes to electrolyte and metabolic balance. The skeleton is a storage pool for Ca^{++} and other ions. Skeletal muscle cells, which account for 40% to 50% of body weight, are a major storage pool for body K^+. Skeletal muscle also plays a major role in metabolism and in temperature regulation.

Cardiac and smooth muscle support the activities of the cardiovascular, respiratory, GI, and renal systems. Cardiac muscle generates the pressure that propels blood through the body (see Chapter 7). Smooth muscle also regulates movement of numerous substances, including blood, within the body. GI smooth muscle controls gastric motility (see Chapter 12). Respiratory airway smooth muscle determines airway resistance to airflow (see Chapter 10). Vascular smooth muscle controls resistance to blood flow (see Chapters 8 and 9). This chapter describes the normal function of skeletal and smooth muscle as a tissue.

●●● STRUCTURE OF SKELETAL MUSCLE

Skeletal muscle is attached to the bones of the skeleton by very thin extensions of fascia or by tendons. *Tendons* (fibrous cords) make strong connections to bone. The contraction of skeletal muscle exerts force on bones or skin and moves them. Most skeletal muscles are under voluntary control of the nervous system.

Skeletal muscle is composed of successively smaller structures: the muscle fascicle, muscle fiber, and finally myofibrils. Skeletal muscle has a regular arrangement of actin (I band) and myosin (A band) filaments, giving it a striated appearance. Myofibrils are attached to each other within the I band at the Z disk. *Actin* filaments are composed of actin, tropomyosin, and troponin proteins. *Myosin* filaments are composed of myosin proteins. *Titin* is a structural protein that provides an elastic connection between the opposing ends of the actin and myosin filaments (Fig. 5-2).

Muscle cells can be functionally classified into smaller segments called sarcomeres, delineated by Z bands. The *sarcomere* is the structure in the muscle where the actual contraction occurs. Two primary myofilaments are present in the sarcomere: thick myosin filaments and thin actin filaments. The filaments are proteins that briefly attach and

TABLE 5-1.   Comparison of the Three Muscle Types

Characteristic	Skeletal Muscle	Cardiac Muscle	Smooth Muscle
Histologic appearance	Striated	Striated	Smooth
Contraction speed	Fastest	Intermediate	Slowest
Fiber proteins	Actin, myosin, troponin, and tropomyosin	Actin, myosin, troponin, and tropomyosin	Actin, myosin, and tropomyosin

Control	Voluntary
	  Ca^{++} and troponin
	  Fibers are independent
		Involuntary
		  Ca^{++} and troponin
		  Gap junctions join fibers
			Involuntary
			  Ca^{++} and calmodulin
			  Gap junctions join fibers

Nervous control	α-Motor neuron	Autonomic neurons	Autonomic neurons
Morphology	Multinucleate; large, cylindrical fibers	Uninucleate; shorter branching fibers	Uninucleate; small spindle-shaped fibers
Key internal structures	T tubule and SR	T tubule and SR	No T tubules; SR reduced or absent
Activation	Troponin	Troponin	Calmodulin MLCK
Calcium source	Intracellular (SR)	Extracellular and SR	Extracellular and SR
Calcium mobilization	T-tubule depolarization DHPR/RyR coupling	ΔE_M/DHPR trigger Ca^{++}	IP_3 ΔE_M-gated channels Ligand-gated channels
Regulation of force	Recruitment	Δ Contractility	MLC20 latch

DHPR, dihydropyridine receptor; MLC20, myosin light chain of 20 kDa; MLCK, myosin light-chain kinase; RyR, ryanodine receptor; SR, sarcoplasmic reticulum.

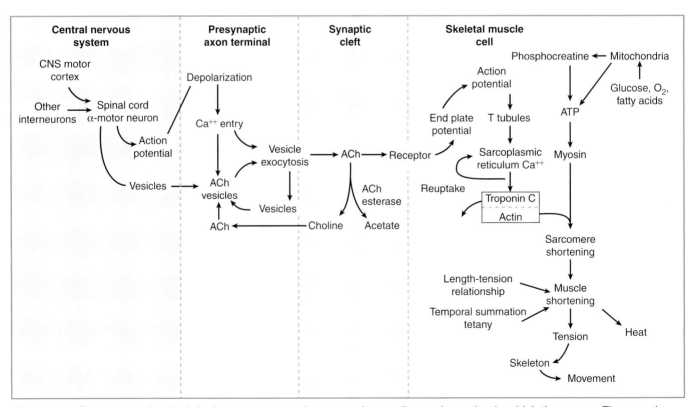

Figure 5-1. Skeletal muscle physiologic processes can be grouped according to the region in which they occur. The neural signal for voluntary movement originates in the CNS and passes along the motor neurons to the neuromuscular junction. Acetylcholine, released from the presynaptic neuron, depolarizes the muscle cell and initiates muscle contraction.

Skeletal Muscle

Skeletal muscles are named according to the following properties: (1) action (e.g., flexor, extensor), (2) shape (e.g., quadrilateral, pennate), (3) origin (i.e., stationary attachment of muscle to skeleton), (4) insertion (i.e., movable attachment of the muscle), (5) number of divisions, (6) location, or (7) direction of fibers (i.e., transverse).

ratchet or slide across one another causing the muscle to generate force or movement.

●●● SKELETAL MUSCLE TYPES

Skeletal muscle consists of two different types of fibers. *Fast twitch fibers* have a myosin ATPase that rapidly hydrolyzes ATP. Consequently, fast twitch fibers have a relatively rapid rate of tension development. Fast twitch fibers generally are large and depend on glycolysis for energy. Fast fibers are white in appearance because of the relatively low amount of myoglobin and the low number of mitochondria. These muscles respond and fatigue rapidly and consequently are adapted for short bursts of activity.

Slow twitch fibers have a myosin ATPase that more slowly hydrolyzes ATP. Slow twitch fibers generally are smaller than fast twitch fibers and depend on oxidative phosphorylation for energy. Slow fibers respond more slowly than fast fibers but are resistant to fatigue. The high concentration of the oxygen-binding protein myoglobin gives the slow twitch muscles a red appearance. These muscles are adapted for maintained activity, such as standing.

Human muscles are mixtures of fast and slow twitch fibers. The relative proportion of fast versus slow twitch is characteristic of individual muscles. Extensive aerobic training can cause some fibers in fast twitch muscles to perform in a more oxidative fashion, functionally mimicking slow twitch fibers (Table 5-2).

Neuromuscular Transmission

Neuromuscular transmission represents a prototype for synaptic transmission. At the neuromuscular junction, an action potential carried along the axon of an α-motor neuron releases acetylcholine (ACh) into the synaptic cleft. ACh diffuses across the synaptic cleft and binds to nicotinic receptors on the end plate region of the skeletal muscle cell. An action potential is initiated in the skeletal muscle cell, which is transduced to an intracellular Ca^{++} signal that triggers muscle contraction.

α-Motor neurons are large, myelinated fibers that originate in the anterior horns of the spinal cord. An axon can branch at its terminal and innervate multiple muscle cells. A muscle cell, however, receives only one synapse. This means that a muscle cell is dependent on a single motor neuron for

activation, providing great specificity for muscle control. In contrast, a given motor neuron can innervate multiple muscle cells, allowing a coordinated response of larger muscles. The motor unit consists of the motor neuron and all the muscles that it innervates.

The number of muscle fibers making up each motor unit determines the degree of control of contraction that is possible. Small motor units allow fine control, such as the muscles of the hand involved in writing. Large motor units coordinate the response of large muscles, such as the muscles of the leg used for lifting.

The neuromuscular junction, or motor end plate, consists of a nerve terminal that rests in a trough on the muscle cell surface called the synaptic trough. The membranes of the two cells are separated by a 20 to 30 nm space called the synaptic cleft. The neuron is considered to be the presynaptic cell, and the muscle cell is the postsynaptic cell (Fig. 5-3).

The presynaptic nerve terminal contains approximately 300,000 synaptic vesicles that contain the neurotransmitter acetylcholine. The sides of the presynaptic membrane contain voltage-activated Ca^{++} channels. The synaptic region of the presynaptic membrane is called the active zone because it is the site where ACh is released.

The synaptic gap spans the distance between the presynaptic and postsynaptic membranes. Acetylcholinesterase, which degrades ACh into acetate and choline, is found in the synaptic cleft. The postsynaptic membrane is part of the muscle cell end plate region and contains numerous ACh receptors.

Figure 5-3 illustrates the steps in synaptic transmission:

1. Vesicles arrive at the axon terminal and are loaded with acetylcholine.
2. An action potential in the presynaptic neuron depolarizes the nerve terminal.
3. Depolarization activates voltage-sensitive Ca^{++} channels in the active zone, and Ca^{++} enters the axon terminal.
4. The influx of Ca^{++} activates calcium/calmodulin–dependent kinase and leads to translocation of vesicles to the presynaptic membrane, where they dock.
5. After docking, fusion proteins bind Ca^{++} and prime the vesicles, and the vesicle contents are released by exocytosis.
6. The ACh diffuses across the cleft and binds to ACh receptors on the muscle membrane. The ACh receptor channels open, and ion movement creates a depolarizing end plate potential.
7. ACh dissociates from the receptor, and the channel closes. ACh is broken down to choline and acetate in the cleft. Choline is transported into the terminal in an Na^+-dependent secondary active transport process.
8. Membrane that was added to the terminal membrane during exocytosis is taken up and reused to form new vesicles.

Approximately 200 vesicles fuse with the membrane at the active zone and release ACh into the cleft during excitation of the motor neuron. Each vesicle contains approximately 10,000 ACh molecules. These numbers become important in describing the both the efficiency of neuromuscular transmission and also the characteristics of neuromuscular diseases.

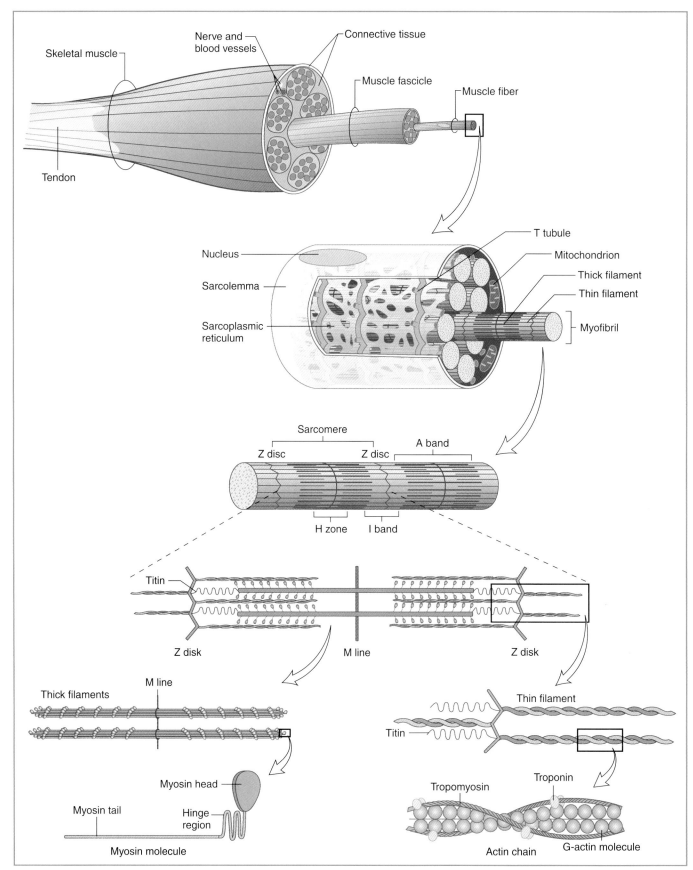

Figure 5-2. Skeletal muscle can be broken down into progressively smaller units, ending with the functional unit of the sarcomere. The histology of the sarcomere is based on the regular arrangement of thin and thick filaments, containing actin and myosin, respectively. Sarcomeres are the structural elements of the muscle fibers, and the muscle fascicle is a bundle of muscle fibers.

TABLE 5-2. Classification of Fiber Types in Skeletal Muscle

Characteristic	Slow Twitch Fiber	Fast Twitch Fiber
Other names	Type I	Type II
	Oxidative	Glycolytic
	Red	White
Myosin isoenzyme ATPase rate	Slow	Fast
Calcium-pumping capacity of sarcoplasmic reticulum	Moderate	High
Diameter	Moderate	Large
Glycolytic capacity	Moderate	High
Oxidative capacity (correlates with content of mitochondria, capillary density, myoglobin content)	High	Low

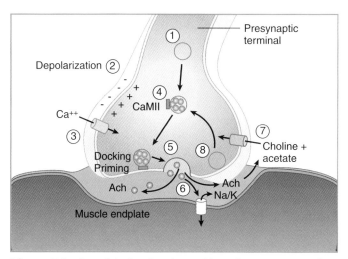

Figure 5-3. Acetylcholine is released into the neuromuscular cleft following depolarization of the α-motor neuron nerve terminal. Depolarization causes the entry of extracellular Ca^{++}, which causes translocation and binding of vesicles to the presynaptic membrane and stimulates exocytosis. CaMII, calmodulin-dependent kinase.

Presynaptic Event Details

Neurotransmitter vesicles are assembled in the cell body of the neuron and transported by kinesins along the axon microtubule system to the axon terminal. In the terminal, the vesicle is acidified by an H^+-ATPase. Acetylcholine is then transported into the vesicle in exchange for H^+. Drugs that disrupt microtubules, such as paclitaxel, can cause temporary paralysis owing to a reduction in the number of synaptic vesicles.

ACh vesicles in the axon terminal can be at the active zone, ready for exocytosis, or away from the active zone in

PHARMACOLOGY

Botulinum

Botulinum toxin produced by *Clostridium botulinum* bacteria depresses end plate potential amplitude. The toxin is extremely potent, with a lethal dose of 2 to 3 mg. The mechanism involves cleavage of proteins involved in vesicle priming (synaptobrevin, syntaxin, and SNAP-25) and subsequent inhibition of Ca^{++}-induced vesicle release from presynaptic terminals and degeneration of the terminals. Very dilute preparations of botulinum toxin can be used to treat disorders involving hyperactivity of neuromuscular junctions, such as would be seen in cases of prolonged muscle spasm, and to reduce facial muscle contractions that cause wrinkles.

the cytosol. Cytosolic vesicles must be translocated to the active zone, dock with the membrane, and be prepared for fusion (primed) when needed. The SNAP-SNARE mechanism mediates vesicle exocytosis. Synapsin 1, synaptobrevin, SNAP-25, syntaxin, synaptotagmin, and synaptophysin are proteins involved in vesicle translocation and exocytosis. Intracellular Ca^{++} enters during depolarization, and following repolarization Ca^{++} exits the cell. Repetitive depolarization causes an increase in intracellular Ca^{++} in the terminal, and thus facilitates vesicle release in response to subsequent excitation.

Prior to activation by depolarization, numerous vesicles are docked and primed, allowing for maximal release upon the arrival of an action potential. The quantity of ACh released is greater than what is required to generate an action potential in the skeletal muscle cell, thereby creating a "safety factor." The excess release of ACh normally ensures that nerve activation leads to muscle activation. The amount of ACh released with each action potential decreases as more action potentials invade the nerve terminal. The decrease is due to the time required for new vesicles to be positioned at the active zone and fully primed. Consequently, the safety factor decreases with high-frequency stimulation, but in normal individuals no loss of function is observed.

Postsynaptic Event Details

The skeletal muscle end plate region has a high density of nicotinic ACh receptors. This ACh receptor is an integral membrane protein consisting of five subunits that form a cation-selective ion channel. Simultaneous binding of 2 ACh molecules to the receptor protein opens the channel, allowing Na^+ and K^+ to diffuse across the membrane. The same protein functions both as the ACh receptor and the channel—no signal transduction is required.

The ACh receptor channel conducts Na^+ and K^+ with equal ease. Normally, a channel that conducts only one ion shifts the membrane potential toward the Nernst potential for that ion. Opening a K^+ channel shifts the membrane potential toward −90 mV, and opening an Na^+ channel shifts the membrane potential toward +60 mV (Fig. 5-4). The skeletal muscle ACh receptor conducts both ions equally, and opening

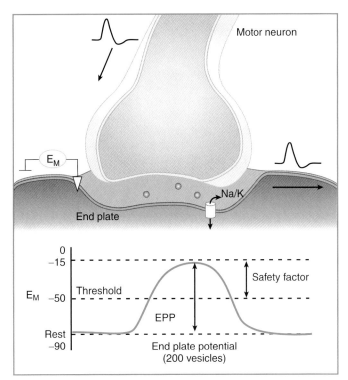
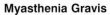

Figure 5-4. Release of acetylcholine causes depolarization of the end plate region of the postsynaptic membrane on the skeletal muscle cell. The 200 vesicles of acetylcholine released during neuromuscular transmission is sufficient to depolarize the end plate to –15 mV (end plate potential), well past the threshold required to initiate an action potential in the skeletal muscle cell. This excess depolarizing ability creates a safety factor, ensuring that neuromuscular transmission causes the depolarization and contraction of the muscle cell.

the channel shifts membrane potential at the end plate region of the skeletal muscle toward the arithmetic average of the Na$^+$ and K$^+$ Nernst values, about –15 mV.

The binding of ACh to the muscle cell ACh receptors causes depolarization. The amplitude of the depolarization is dependent on the number of functional receptors and the percentage of the functional receptors bound by ACh. ACh is released from the axon terminal in packets of 10,000 molecules, the amount in one vesicle. Release of one vesicle causes a 0.4 mV depolarization of the skeletal muscle end plate region, called a miniature end plate potential (MEPP). MEPPs occur spontaneously at neuromuscular junctions and are thought to be due to unstimulated exocytosis of single ACh vesicles.

Normal neuromuscular transmission causes the release of up to 200 vesicles, and that amount of ACh causes a 75 mV depolarization, from the resting membrane potential of –90 mV to –15 mV. This depolarization is an end plate potential (EPP). Depolarization of the muscle end plate to –50 mV is sufficient to activate voltage-sensitive Na$^+$ channels in the muscle cell membrane and induce an action potential, so the normal 75 mV depolarization provides a safety factor ensuring that each neuromuscular transmission causes depolarization and contraction of the target skeletal muscle.

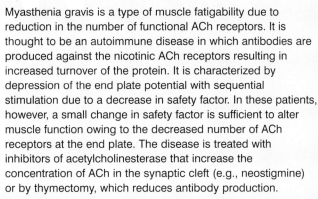

PATHOLOGY

Myasthenia Gravis

Myasthenia gravis is a type of muscle fatigability due to reduction in the number of functional ACh receptors. It is thought to be an autoimmune disease in which antibodies are produced against the nicotinic ACh receptors resulting in increased turnover of the protein. It is characterized by depression of the end plate potential with sequential stimulation due to a decrease in safety factor. In these patients, however, a small change in safety factor is sufficient to alter muscle function owing to the decreased number of ACh receptors at the end plate. The disease is treated with inhibitors of acetylcholinesterase that increase the concentration of ACh in the synaptic cleft (e.g., neostigmine) or by thymectomy, which reduces antibody production.

ACh is rapidly cleared from the synaptic cleft by acetylcholinesterase. This process ensures that continuing ACh receptor stimulation depends on continuing release of ACh from the motor neuron. Sustained contraction, or tetany, depends on sustained activity of the motor neuron. EPP amplitude is not constant but is dependent on the amount of ACh in the cleft and number of functional nicotinic receptors in the postsynaptic membrane. Action potentials that are close together in time increase EPP amplitude through a process known as facilitation. *Facilitation* is enhanced ACh release due to increased priming of vesicles by Ca^{++} in the presynaptic terminal. Increased ACh concentration in the cleft leads to a larger than normal EPP. Facilitation plays a role in normal activation of muscle but is most noticeable in patients with decreased numbers of functional nicotinic ACh receptors. In these patients, initial attempts to activate a muscle lead to weak contractions. Continued use facilitates the release of ACh, which partially compensates for the decreased numbers of receptors, and contraction strength improves.

The size of the EPP increases as motor neuron action potential frequency increases. A high-frequency stimulation that yields a maximal EPP is called a tetanic stimulation. During a normal contraction, muscle cells are stimulated by the innervating motor neuron at a tetanic frequency.

The extended series of motor neuron action potentials leads to posttetanic potentiation. Following high-frequency stimulation, a subsequent action potential in the motor neuron evokes an EPP that is larger than normal owing to enhanced release of ACh.

At the other extreme, high-frequency stimulation for prolonged periods can lead to transient depletion of primed ACh vesicles near the membrane and depression of neuromuscular transmission, or synaptic fatigue. Depression is rarely observed in normal individuals under voluntary control. However, it is routinely observed in some diseases of the neuromuscular junction, such as myasthenia gravis.

A number of toxins and drugs affect the ACh receptors at the neuromuscular junction and induce flaccid paralysis.

Curare, d-tubocurarine, and gallamine block the nicotinic channels from opening and induce flaccid paralysis. These agents are used for relaxing skeletal muscle during surgical procedures. Succinylcholine is an agonist of the nicotinic ACh receptor, but it is not degraded by AChE. Therefore, it causes prolonged depolarization of the muscle end plate and inactivation of the fast Na^+ channels, leading to elevation of threshold in the muscle cell and relaxation. Elapid snake venoms (krait and cobra) contain α-bungarotoxin, a curare-like drug with high affinity for the ACh receptor.

The skeletal muscle action potential is similar to the motor neuron action potential except that it is longer in duration and does not exhibit a hyperpolarizing afterpotential. The long duration of the muscle action potential allows time for mobilization of Ca^{++} and activation of actomyosin ATPase.

Excitation-Contraction Coupling

The action potential generated at the motor end plate region spreads along the membrane of skeletal muscle cell and into the T tubules. The T tubules contain dihydropyridine receptors that connect to the Ca^{++} channels of sarcoplasmic reticulum. Depolarization of T tubules opens the sarcoplasmic reticulum Ca^{++} channels. Calcium exits the sarcoplasmic reticulum and diffuses through the cytoplasm (Fig. 5-5).

Contraction results from the interaction of the actin and myosin filaments, a process described as the sliding filament mechanism. The sequence of the interaction of the actin and myosin proteins is shown in Figure 5-6. The troponin C component of the actin filament binds Ca^{++} and exposes the active sites of the actin protein. Actin now binds strongly to myosin (1), and the myosin filament heads pivot (2), using previously hydrolyzed ATP as an energy source. This pivoting generates a "power stroke," sliding the actin filaments along the myosin filaments toward the center of the sarcomere and causing the sarcomere to shorten. Pivoting also releases P_i and ADP (3, 4) and allows new ATP to bind the head of the myosin (5). The binding of new ATP detaches the myosin from the actin (6). The myosin hydrolyzes ATP, and the myosin head stores the energy until bound again by actin. The process

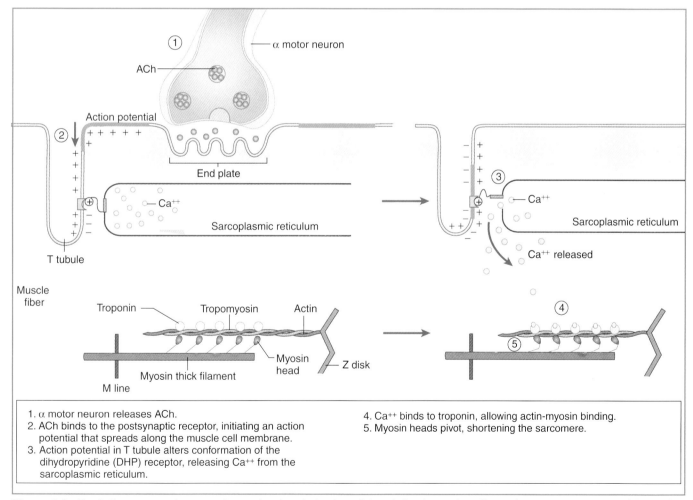

1. α motor neuron releases ACh.
2. ACh binds to the postsynaptic receptor, initiating an action potential that spreads along the muscle cell membrane.
3. Action potential in T tubule alters conformation of the dihydropyridine (DHP) receptor, releasing Ca^{++} from the sarcoplasmic reticulum.
4. Ca^{++} binds to troponin, allowing actin-myosin binding.
5. Myosin heads pivot, shortening the sarcomere.

Figure 5-5. Excitation-contraction transduces the depolarization of the skeletal muscle cell membrane to movement of the actin and myosin filaments. An action potential generated at the neuromuscular junction (2) spreads through the cell membrane and T tubule system of the skeletal muscle cell. Dihydropyridine receptors on the T tubule (3) stimulate the release of Ca^{++} from the sarcoplasmic reticulum. Ca^{++} exposes the binding surface of the actin protein (4), allowing it to bind to myosin and initiate the contraction process (5).

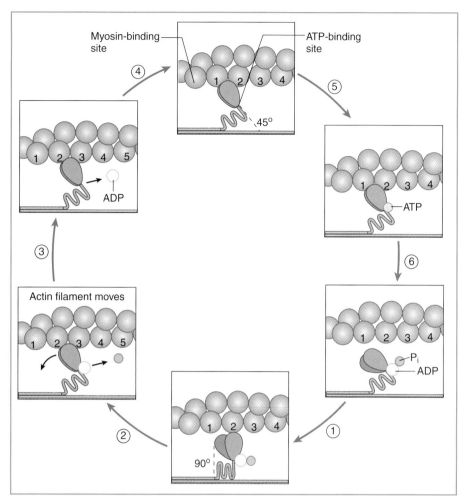

Myosin-binding site

ATP-binding site

45°

ADP

Actin filament moves

90°

ATP

Pᵢ
ADP

Figure 5-6. Muscle movement is due to conformational of changes in the myosin motor protein. Ca^{++} entry exposes the actin-binding sites. The contraction process is initiated (1) by the binding of the myosin head to actin. Release of inorganic phosphate (P_i) (2) initiates the power stroke, moving the myosin heads to a 45-degree angle, and shortening the sarcomere. (3) Following the power stroke and dissociation of ADP, (4) myosin is tightly bound to actin at a 45-degree angle in a rigor complex. (5) Binding of ATP to myosin breaks the actin-myosin bond. Hydrolysis of ATP moves the myosin head to a 90-degree angle, where it can again bind to actin, returning to (1). Following the power stroke, the process repeats provided that there are sufficient stores of ATP and that Ca^{++} keeps the actin-binding sites exposed.

repeats until Ca^{++} is resequestered or ATP stores are depleted.

ATP used for muscle contraction and active transport of ions comes from phosphocreatinine, glycolysis, and oxidative phosphorylation. Phosphocreatinine is the first energy store accessed and provides up to 10 seconds of energy. The high-energy phosphate on the creatinine is hydrolyzed during the resynthesis of ATP from ADP and P_i. Skeletal muscle stores of glycogen provide the next pool of energy, as anaerobic glycogenolysis allows the replenishment of ATP. The final— and most abundant—energy source is the mitochondrial oxidative phosphorylation. This process depends on the number of mitochondria and the availability of O_2.

The excitation contraction process stops when Ca^{++} is resequestered in the sarcoplasmic reticulum. The SERCA (*s*arcoplasmic and *e*ndoplasmic *r*eticulum *c*alcium *A*TPase) moves Ca^{++} from the cytosol back into the sarcoplasmic reticulum against a significant concentration gradient, thus requiring ATP for function. Free [Ca^{++}] within the sarcoplasmic reticulum is buffered by Ca^{++} binding to the proteins calsequestrin and calreticulin.

BIOCHEMISTRY

Oxidative Phosphorylation

Oxidative phosphorylation is the process by which ATP is formed by the mitochondrial transfer of electrons from the electron donors NADH and $FADH_2$ to O_2. Complete oxidation of a molecule of glucose to CO_2 and H_2O consumes up to 2 ATP and generates up to 38 ATP. This includes 26 ATP generated from NADH, 4 from FADH, and 6 from substrate-level phosphorylation. The net maximum energy production is 36 molecules of ATP from each molecule of glucose.

Skeletal Muscle Mechanics

A skeletal muscle is composed of numerous muscle fibers and motor units. Contraction of the intact muscle is the result of the contraction of a portion of the muscle fibers in the muscle.

Tension developed by the muscle contraction is increased by temporal summation and by recruitment. Temporal summation results from an increase in the rate of individual motor unit activity. This produces tetanization, or sustained contraction of skeletal muscle. Recruitment increases the number of motor units activated, increasing the tension developed by the contracting muscle. Tension developed in the contracting muscle is transmitted to the skeleton by tendons.

The mechanics of contraction are best modeled at the sarcomere level. The muscle striations are due to the regular arrangement of the thin actin and thick myosin filaments. Sarcomere contraction results from the sliding of the overlapping actin and myosin filaments, rather than from shortening of the actual proteins themselves. Consequently, the A-band length does not change, but the adjacent Z lines are brought closer together (Fig. 5-7).

The sarcomere model also illustrates the length-tension relationship. The tension developed by a contracting muscle depends on the number of points of attachment between actin and myosin during the myosin power stroke. The maximum amount of tension developed by the sarcomere is at the middle of the length-tension curve, where every myosin head is across from an actin molecule. At lengths longer than the optimal, some myosin heads are not across from an actin. These heads cannot participate in the power stroke, and consequently the tension developed by the contracting sarcomere is diminished. At sarcomere lengths shorter than optimal, the myosin filaments are already approaching the

point of attachment for the actin filaments, and consequently shortening is impeded (Fig. 5-8).

This effect carries over to the intact muscle, since both overstretch and understretch of resting muscle diminishes developed tension. The resting length of the muscle (before contraction is initiated) helps determine the maximal amount of tension that can be developed during contraction. For skeletal muscle, the optimal length is close to the normal resting length of the muscle. For cardiac muscle, the amount of stretch on the muscle before a contraction has special significance and is called preload.

Normal muscle activity is a combination of isometric and isotonic contractions. An isometric contraction involves the development of tension without any change in length. An isotonic contraction involves a change in length without any change in tension. The apparatus in Figure 5-9 illustrates the tension and length changes developed by a contracting muscle.

The bar on the right side can be adjusted to set the resting length. The muscle is attached to a tension gauge and an immovable plate at the top. The muscle is attached to a spring and finally to a weight at the bottom. Stimulation of the muscle by an electrode induces contraction.

Stage 1 shows the length and tension of the muscle at rest. Any tension is the result of stretch of the muscle connective tissue, caused by altering the resting length. Following stimulation, there is an increase in tension as the sarcomeres shorten and develop force during the isometric phase of contraction (stage 2). The weight remains on the platform because the tension developed in the muscle is not sufficient to lift the weight. The sarcomere shortening only stretches the elastic tissue within the muscle. Stage 3 occurs when the tension developed by the muscle equals 10 kg, the same as the weight. At this point, there is no further increase in tension, and contraction of the sarcomere now results in shortening of the muscle. This is the isotonic portion of the contraction. When the stimulus is removed, the muscle ceases its contraction, passing through stage 4, an isotonic period in which the muscle is lengthening, and as the weight returns to the platform, stage 5, in which the tension in the muscle is diminished and the elastic tissue returns to the starting condition.

The load to be lifted determines both the maximum tension that is developed and the velocity of shortening. In the contracting muscle, tension develops until it is sufficient to lift the load, at which point the muscle shortens. The tension does not change further; consequently, the load sets the maximum tension. In contrast, velocity of shortening is decreased as the load increases. At zero load, the muscle contracts with a maximal velocity of shortening. A heavy load that cannot be lifted does not allow shortening of the muscle, producing an isometric (same length) contraction.

Strength of muscle contraction is also increased by previous activity, called a staircase, or treppe, effect. This effect is probably due to enhanced intracellular Ca^{++} levels in

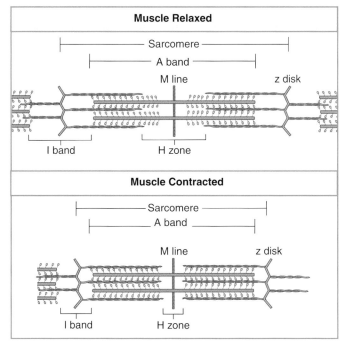

Figure 5-7. Contraction of the sarcomere involves the sliding of thick and thin filaments past each other. During contraction, the adjacent Z lines move toward each other, and the length of the A band does not change.

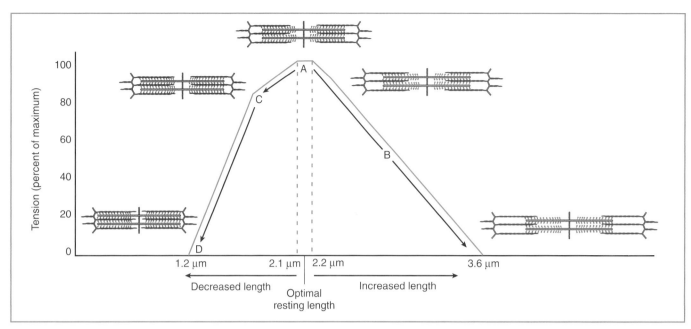

Figure 5-8. The optimal sarcomere length of 2.2 μm reflects the point at which there is a maximal overlap of the heads of the myosin filaments with the binding sites of the actin filaments. Any overstretching or understretching of the sarcomere decreases the maximum amount of tension that can be developed during contraction.

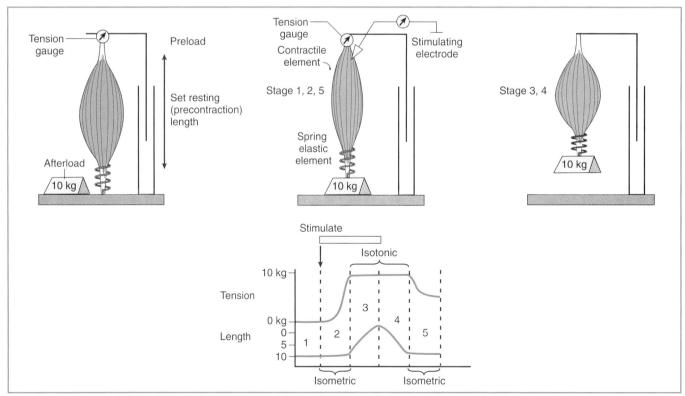

Figure 5-9. Contraction of the skeletal muscle causes a combination of an increase in tension and a shortening. The resting stretch on the skeletal muscle (preload) determines the overlap of the actin and myosin filaments and determines the peak tension that can be achieved during contraction. As contraction develops, tension in the muscle is increased until it is sufficient to move the weight (afterload). The afterload determines what portion of the total energy available during contraction will be used to develop tension, and what portion of the total energy available will be used to shorten the muscle.

the muscle. This is a muscle effect and should not be confused with facilitation of the presynaptic nerve terminal ACh release.

Skeletal muscle remodels based on the workload. Repetitive strong contractions increase muscle mass, which is called hypertrophy. Lack of muscle use decreases muscle mass, called atrophy. These changes reflect a change in the size of individual muscle cells and not a change in the number of muscle cells in the tissue.

● ● ● SMOOTH MUSCLE

Smooth muscle is so named because it has no visible striations. Its contraction is involuntary. It is found in the walls of hollow organs (e.g., digestive tract, blood vessels, urinary bladder) and other areas (e.g., the iris). Smooth muscle is controlled by the autonomic nervous system, hormones, and intrinsic factors in the organ.

Smooth muscle fibers are smaller and shorter than skeletal muscle fibers. Multiunit smooth muscle is primarily under neural control. This is characteristic of vascular smooth muscle and ciliary muscles and iris of the eye. Single-unit smooth muscle is usually made up of cells that are coupled by gap junctions, allowing ions and action potentials to pass between adjacent cells. This arrangement allows the entire sheet of smooth muscle to function as a unit, or a syncytium, and is characteristic of GI smooth muscle.

Contraction

Smooth muscle uses actin and myosin filaments for contraction. The mechanism, illustrated in Figure 5-10, differs from that in skeletal muscle. Smooth muscle has tropomyosin but lacks troponin C. Calcium acts through calmodulin to activate myosin light-chain kinase to phosphorylate the myosin heads. This increases myosin ATPase activity. The calcium/calmodulin complex also uncovers the actin-binding site by binding to and phosphorylating calponin. Myosin hydrolyzes ATP, and the released energy causes the myosin head to pivot. Contraction develops more slowly but lasts longer than skeletal muscle. The actual rate varies greatly between groups of smooth muscle. ATP usage is much less than for a similar contraction of skeletal muscle.

Calcium flux is the primary ionic event, and sodium plays a smaller role in smooth muscle action potentials. Extracellular Ca^{++} directly activates smooth muscle actin, whereas the sarcoplasmic reticulum is the primary source of Ca^{++} in skeletal muscle. Some smooth muscle uses sarcoplasmic reticulum to enhance the contraction from extracellular Ca^{++}. Contraction ends when Ca^{++} is pumped out of the cell or back into the sarcoplasmic reticulum. Some smooth muscle shows spontaneous depolarization of the membrane potential, called a slow wave. Slow-wave depolarization can reach threshold and initiate an action potential. The rate of depolarization determines the frequency of action potentials. In regions such as the stomach, slow-wave generation can act as a pacemaker, setting the rate of contraction for the organ.

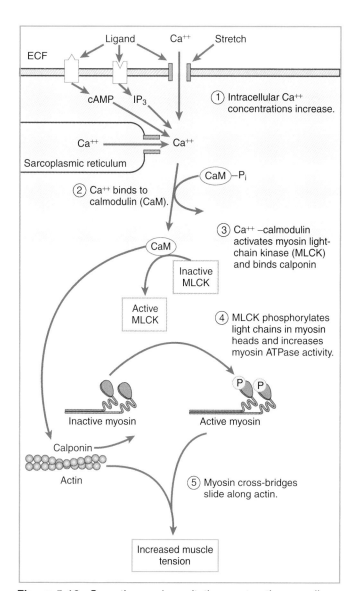

Figure 5-10. Smooth muscle excitation-contraction coupling depends on the calcium/calmodulin activation of kinases. The myosin light-chain kinase increases the activity of the myosin ATPase and moves calponin to expose the binding site on the actin protein.

Excitation

Multiple interacting mechanisms mediate the excitation-contraction coupling for smooth muscle. Stretch opens stretch-sensitive channels, depolarizes smooth muscle, and can initiate contraction. Cell membrane receptors respond to a variety of ligands, and working through inositol-1,4,5-trisphosphate (IP_3), stimulate sarcoplasmic Ca^{++} release and smooth muscle contraction. Hormones that increase cAMP can release Ca^{++} from intracellular stores and cause contraction without causing an action potential. Alternatively, some ligands promote the entry of extracellular Ca^{++}, directly stimulating contraction. The calcium/calmodulin contractile mechanism depends on protein phosphorylation and consequently is sensitive to modulation by multiple kinases.

In contrast to skeletal muscle, nerve activity can initiate smooth muscle contraction without causing action potentials. Neuromuscular junctions are more difficult to identify than in skeletal muscle. Neurotransmitters are released from axons and diffuse to the smooth muscle cell. The ability of nerves to initiate an action potential depends on the amount of neurotransmitter released and the amount of depolarization required to reach threshold. Acetylcholine stimulates contraction in some smooth muscle and relaxation in other smooth muscle types through the release of nitric oxide. Acetylcholine-mediated parasympathetic activity and norepinephrine-mediated sympathetic activity often have opposing effects on smooth muscle.

●●● CARDIAC MUSCLE

The myocardium is a type of involuntary muscle that is found only in the heart. It is composed of branched, striated muscle cells connected by gap junctions. Cardiac muscle is controlled by intrinsic factors (e.g., the amount of venous return to the right atrium), hormones, and signals from the autonomic nervous system. Cardiac muscle is discussed in more detail in Chapter 7.

●●● SKELETON

The adult body contains 206 bones, which together represent a tissue that is capable of growth, adaptation, and repair. Bone consists of an organic framework of proteins in collagen fibers. Hydroxyapatite crystals are embedded in this framework and provide a significant store that helps regulate plasma Ca^{++} levels (see Chapter 13).

Joints are articulations at the place of contact between two or more bones. Most of the joints in the body are synovial. They are freely movable, permitting position and motion changes. Ligaments and tendons reinforce the joint and help limit motion. Articular disks are located between the bones in some synovial joints and act to buffer forceful impact. Fibrous joints are articulations in which bones are held together by fibrous connective tissue. Cartilaginous joints are held together by cartilage, such as the ribs.

Bone marrow is the source of pluripotent blood cells (see Chapter 6). In adults, blood cells form in marrow cavities in the skull, vertebrae, ribs, sternum, shoulder, and pelvis. There are two types of bone marrow: yellow and red. Yellow marrow is composed mostly of fat cells and is found in the shafts of long bones. Yellow marrow does not normally produce blood cells. Red marrow has a hematopoietic function, manufacturing both red and white blood cells. It is located in the cancellous spaces of flat bones.

Bone contains three types of cells. Osteoblasts form bone by catalyzing the crystal formation of Ca^{++} and PO_4^- in a collagen meshwork. Osteocytes are osteoblasts that are encased in the bone matrix. Osteoclasts resorb damaged or old bone cells during periods of growth or repair. They are also crucial in returning Ca^{++} from bone to the bloodstream.

ANATOMY

Epiphyseal Plate

In children and young adults, the epiphyses are separated from the diaphysis by *epiphyseal cartilage* or plates, where bone grows in length. Estrogen and testosterone release at puberty initiates closure of the epiphyseal plates. When bone growth is complete, the epiphyseal cartilage is replaced with bone, which joins it to the diaphysis. Fractures of the epiphyseal plates in children can lead to slow bone growth or limb shortening.

The coordinated activity of these bone cells allows bone to grow, repair itself, and change shape. Even mature bone constantly changes, with new cells being formed and old cells being destroyed. The process of bone turnover is called remodeling, and it is one of the major mechanisms for maintaining Ca^{++} balance in the body. As much as 15% of the total bone mass normally turns over each year. Rebuilding of bone requires normal plasma concentrations of Ca^{++} and PO_4^- and is dependent on vitamin D.

Movement

Skeletal muscle contraction occurs when an α-motor neuron excites an individual muscle fiber. Outflow from the CNS motor cortex descends to the anterior horn of the spinal cord, where a synapse leads to activation of an α-motor neuron. The axon from the α-motor neuron transmits the action potential to the neuromuscular junction. ACh released at the neuromuscular junction binds to receptors on the muscle end plate, initiating an action potential in the muscle cell. The action potential spreads through the T tubules, causing release of Ca^{++} from the sarcoplasmic reticulum and contraction of the muscle.

Movement requires a shift of the position of the bones as they articulate across a joint. Skeletal muscle is attached to two different bones by fibrous tendons. Shortening of the skeletal muscle causes angles connecting the bones to decrease (for flexor muscles, i.e., biceps) or to increase (for extensor muscles, i.e., triceps). The musculoskeletal system functions as a unit to allow movement of the body.

Heat Production

The activity of skeletal muscle produces heat as a metabolic byproduct, which usually must be transmitted to the environment. Some of this heat can be used to maintain body temperature, as described in Chapter 1.

●●● TOP 5 TAKE-HOME POINTS

1. Skeletal, cardiac, and smooth muscle all use the motor protein myosin, the structural protein actin, ATP, and Ca^{++}

for contraction. Muscle types differ in the source of Ca^{++}, arrangement of actin and myosin, excitation contraction coupling, and regulation of contraction.

2. Skeletal muscle contraction is initiated by the release of the neurotransmitter ACh from the α-motor neuron synapse, binding to cholinergic receptors on the muscle cell end plate region.

3. Skeletal muscle depolarization causes release of Ca^{++} from the sarcoplasmic reticulum, the binding of myosin to actin, and contraction of muscle.

4. The force developed during contraction is determined by the resting length of the muscle, the weight to be lifted, and the availability of ATP.

5. Smooth muscle contraction is initiated by membrane events that allow the influx of extracellular Ca^{++}. Calcium binds with calmodulin to phosphorylate a series of proteins, leading to the development of actin-myosin binding and contraction.

Blood and Hematopoiesis   6

CONTENTS

Blood is a complex suspension of cells and formed elements in plasma. Blood flow serves multiple functions within the body, including the transport of O_2 and nutrients to the tissues for use and storage and the transport of metabolic wastes to the kidney, liver, and skin for elimination. Blood also transports hormones from the endocrine glands to the target tissues and transports heat to the skin for exchange.

The formed elements of blood originate in bone marrow from pluripotent bone marrow stem cells. This stem cell line differentiates into erythrocytes (red blood cells [RBCs]), leukocytes (white blood cells [WBCs]), and the megakaryocytes that produce platelets.

In an adult, blood makes up 8% of the total body weight, approximately 5 to 6 L in a young 70-kg male and 4 to 5 L in a young 60-kg female. Blood volume as a percentage of body weight decreases with age and also decreases as the body mass index (BMI) increases. Approximately 45% of the blood volume is RBCs (48% for males, 42% for females); less than 1% is WBCs, and the remainder is plasma.

Blood provides a barrier that protects the internal environment. Hemostasis and clotting seal any disruptions in the vascular system. Vascular injury initiates a sequence of responses that limit blood loss from the site of the injury. Injured vascular smooth muscle contracts, diminishing blood flow to the injured area. Bleeding causes extravascular swelling and consequently compression of the damaged vessels, further limiting future blood loss. Platelet adhesion and coagulation seal the site of injury (Fig. 6-1).

The barrier function is supplemented by the immune function of blood. Immunity can be innate or acquired. Innate immunity is a generic defense system. It includes barrier functions such as the skin, which prevents entry of pathogens. There is also nonspecific destruction of bacteria such as by acid in the stomach, or phagocytosis by tissue macrophages. Innate immunity is supplemented by complement and other plasma components. Acquired immunity requires exposure to a specific antigen. Acquired immunity uses the B (bursa, bone) leukocytes, such as the plasma cells and the memory B cells used to produce antibodies. Acquired immunity also makes use of the T (thymus) lymphocytes to mediate delayed allergic reactions and the rejection of foreign tissue, viruses, fungi, and some bacteria. Topics related to WBCs and immunity are discussed in more detail in the immunology book in this series.

⬤⬤⬤ HEMATOPOIESIS

Hematopoiesis is the synthesis of blood cells. Pluripotent hematopoietic stem cells in the bone marrow divide and differentiate into erythrocytes, leukocytes, or megakaryocytes. Replication and differentiation are regulated by hormones, cytokines, and growth factors (Fig. 6-2).

The aggregate weight of adult bone marrow is 3 kg, comparable in mass to the liver. Bone marrow is categorized by appearance as red or yellow. Red bone marrow consists of hematopoietic cells interspersed with sinusoidal capillaries. Yellow bone marrow has a limited number of hematopoietic cells, and the yellow appearance is from adipose. New cells synthesized in bone marrow enter the circulation by way of the marrow sinusoids.

In utero, active hematopoiesis occurs in the liver and spleen. At birth, all bone marrow is active in hematopoiesis. Following puberty, the red bone marrow in the shafts of the long bones is gradually replaced by yellow bone marrow. The femur and tibia have functional bone marrow up until about the age of 20 years. In adult life, erythropoiesis is found only at the ends of the long bones and in some flat bones, such as the vertebrae, sternum, and ribs.

Erythropoiesis is the synthesis of RBCs. RBCs arise from the hematopoietic stem cell line, and differentiation into a mature RBC occurs over 7 days. RBC production requires functional bone marrow, erythropoietin, thyroid hormone, and adequate supplies of iron, vitamin B_{12}, folic acid, pyridoxine, and protein and traces of copper. The absence of any of these components leads to either an impaired rate of RBC production or to the formation of atypical cells.

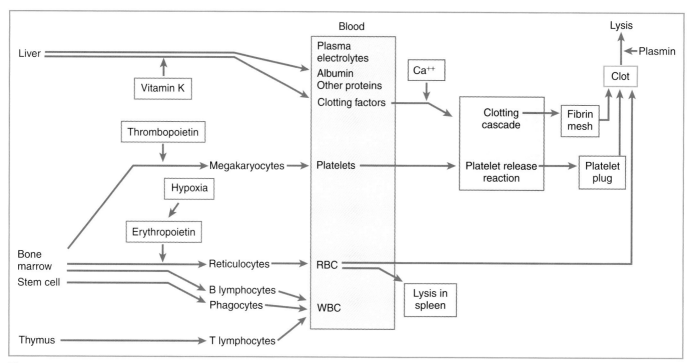

Figure 6-1. Blood and hemostasis map shows the convergence of clotting factors, platelets, and RBCs in forming a clot. Blood components are synthesized in the liver, bone marrow, and thymus. A major functional role for blood is the formation of a platelet plug or a clot in response to vascular injury.

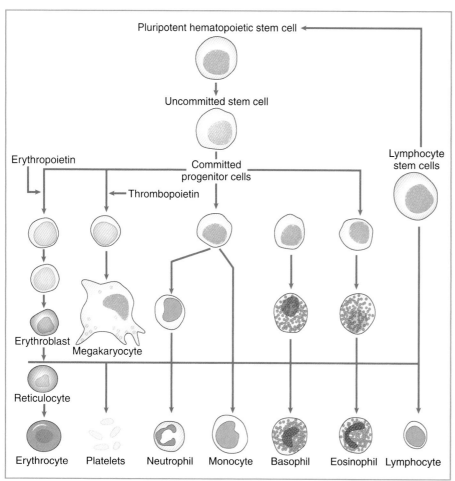

Figure 6-2. A single hematopoietic stem cell gives rise to RBCs, platelets, and WBCs. RBC production is regulated by the hormone erythropoietin, platelet production is regulated by the hormone thrombopoietin, and WBC production is regulated by various cytokines.

PATHOLOGY

Iron Deficiency Anemia

Iron deficiency is the most common cause of anemia. Iron deficiency can result from inadequate dietary iron consumption, poor absorption of iron from the diet, or hemorrhage, particularly associated with gastrointestinal ulcers. Blood analysis consistent with iron deficiency anemia shows abnormally small red blood cells, low serum ferritin, and low serum iron.

PHARMACOLOGY

Epoetin Alfa

Epoetin alfa is a synthetic version of the renal hormone erythropoietin used to stimulate bone marrow to produce red blood cells. Epoetin alfa is used to prevent or treat anemia caused by renal failure or anemia that occurs during chemotherapy for cancer. Because it is a protein, epoetin alfa is administered by injection or intravenous infusion.

Stem cells differentiate into RBCs and synthesize their major intracellular protein, hemoglobin. One molecule of hemoglobin is composed of four protein chains, each of which surrounds an iron atom core. Hemoglobin is specialized for transport of O_2 and CO_2 (see Chapter 10).

Iron is essential to hemoglobin production. Total body iron ranges between 2 and 6 g. Hemoglobin accounts for about two thirds of the total iron, and the remaining iron is in the bone marrow, spleen, liver, and muscle. As an iron deficiency develops, the latter iron stores are depleted first, followed by a gradual loss of the iron contained in hemoglobin.

Immature erythrocytes leave the bone marrow via veins in the marrow and enter the general circulation as nucleated reticulocytes. After their release from the marrow sites, the reticulocytes travel to the spleen, where they lose their nucleus and evolve into mature erythrocytes before being released back into the circulation.

The hormone erythropoietin controls the rate of RBC formation. Erythropoietin is synthesized primarily in the kidneys. Tissue oxygenation controls erythropoietin release. Anemia or prolonged exposure to altitude (hypoxia) increases RBC synthesis. Impaired cardiac or pulmonary function also increases RBC synthesis, as does pregnancy. It takes 5 days for erythropoietin to increase the rate of RBC formation.

Erythropoiesis can replace about 1% of the circulating RBC mass each day, or about 100 million cells. Under maximal stimulation, bone marrow can increase this rate of synthesis eightfold, forming up to 800 million new cells each day.

Anemia results from an imbalance between the rate of RBC synthesis and the rate of RBC loss. RBC synthesis may be decreased by deficiencies in iron, vitamin B_{12}, intrinsic factor, or folic acid. Anemia can also result from the RBC loss that accompanies hemorrhage and from the increased fragility characteristic of the sickle cell mutation (Box 6-1).

BLOOD COMPONENTS

Plasma

Plasma is one of the three body fluid compartments described in Chapter 3. Plasma is separated from blood by addition of an anticoagulant and subsequent centrifugation. Fresh plasma is a straw-colored fluid decanted from the top of the centrifuge tube, and it is 92% water. Serum is a cell-free fluid decanted from clotted blood. Serum lacks

BOX 6-1. CAUSES OF ANEMIA

Accelerated red blood cell loss

Blood loss: cells are normal in size and hemoglobin content but low in number
Hemolytic anemias: cells rupture at an abnormally high rate
Hereditary defects
Membrane defects (e.g., hereditary spherocytosis)
Enzyme defects
Abnormal hemoglobin (e.g., sickle cell anemia)
Parasitic infections (e.g., malaria)
Drugs
Autoimmune reactions

Decreased red blood cell production

Defective red blood cell or hemoglobin synthesis in the bone marrow
Aplastic anemia: can be caused by certain drugs or irradiation
Inadequate dietary intake of essential nutrients
Iron deficiency (iron is required for heme production)
Folic acid deficiency (folic acid is required for DNA synthesis)
Vitamin B_{12} deficiency: may be due to lack of intrinsic factor for B_{12} absorption (vitamin B_{12} is required for DNA synthesis)
Inadequate production of erythropoietin

the clotting proteins but otherwise is identical to plasma (Fig. 6-3).

Plasma consists of water, electrolytes, nutrients, wastes, and proteins. The protein components include albumin, α-, β-, and γ-globulins, clotting factors, complement, enzymes, precursors and their substrates, hormones, specific carrier proteins, and apolipoproteins. Table 6-1 lists the normal values for plasma.

Red Blood Cells

RBCs are the primary cellular component of blood. RBCs are shaped as biconcave disks with a depression in the center, a structure that provides the maximal ratio of cell surface area to cell volume. This specialized shape facilitates diffusion, allowing the hemoglobin in the RBC to equilibrate rapidly with O_2 dissolved in the plasma. RBCs also contain carbonic anhydrase, an enzyme that assists in the blood transport of

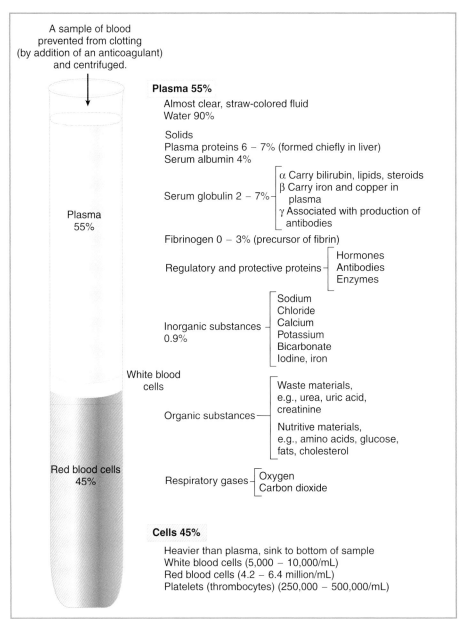

A sample of blood
prevented from clotting
(by addition of an anticoagulant)
and centrifuged.

Plasma
55%

White blood
cells

Red blood cells
45%

Plasma 55%

Almost clear, straw-colored fluid
Water 90%

Solids
Plasma proteins 6 – 7% (formed chiefly in liver)
Serum albumin 4%

Serum globulin 2 – 7%
- α Carry bilirubin, lipids, steroids
- β Carry iron and copper in plasma
- γ Associated with production of antibodies

Fibrinogen 0 – 3% (precursor of fibrin)

Regulatory and protective proteins
- Hormones
- Antibodies
- Enzymes

Inorganic substances 0.9%
- Sodium
- Chloride
- Calcium
- Potassium
- Bicarbonate
- Iodine, iron

Organic substances
- Waste materials, e.g., urea, uric acid, creatinine
- Nutritive materials, e.g., amino acids, glucose, fats, cholesterol

Respiratory gases
- Oxygen
- Carbon dioxide

Cells 45%

Heavier than plasma, sink to bottom of sample
White blood cells (5,000 – 10,000/mL)
Red blood cells (4.2 – 6.4 million/mL)
Platelets (thrombocytes) (250,000 – 500,000/mL)

Figure 6-3. Centrifugation separates blood into plasma, WBCs, and RBCs. RBCs are the most dense and collect at the bottom of the tube. A WBC layer sits atop the RBCs, and plasma accumulates at the top. Hematocrit is the percentage of blood that consists of RBCs and is calculated based on the centrifuged (packed) RBC volume.

CO_2. The functional importance of these proteins is described in Chapter 10.

The RBC nucleus is lost during the final stages of maturation (see Fig. 6-2). Consequently, mature RBCs cannot transcribe new proteins. Newly formed RBCs do retain their nucleus for the first 1 to 2 days following release from the bone marrow. These recently formed RBCs can be identified under a microscope and are called reticulocytes. The average life span of RBCs is 120 days, so approximately 1% of RBCs normally are removed from circulation each day, and the number of reticulocytes is normally less than 2% of the number of RBCs.

The average RBC count is 5,500,000 cells/mm^3 of blood. Hematocrit is the proportion of blood that is cells, normally 48% for men and 42% for women. Hematocrit is determined by centrifugation of heparinized blood (see Fig. 6-3). Alternatively, blood hemoglobin concentration provides

equivalent information, and normal hemoglobin values are 16 g/dL for men and 14 g/dL for women. Finally, RBCs are heavier than water, so the density of blood can be used as an estimation of hematocrit. Density and hematocrit can be influenced by osmotic changes in red cell water.

The liver, lung, and spleen sequester some of the peripheral blood erythrocytes, providing a reserve supply whenever the RBC count drops significantly. In humans, the liver is the primary organ that sequesters RBCs and releases them during times of enhanced sympathetic nervous system activity. This release of stored RBCs, along with changes in plasma volume, can produce changes in hematocrit that are unrelated to RBC synthesis or destruction.

RBC membranes are distensible, and their unique shape allows them to deform to pass through small-diameter capillaries and vascular sinuses. The normal RBC is 7 μm in diameter. The normal capillary diameter is 5 to 10 μm, so

TABLE 6-1. Laboratory Values for Arterial Blood

Component	Typical Value	Reference Range
Calcium, serum (Ca^{++})	9 mg/dL	8.4–10.2 mg/dL
Cholesterol, serum	200 mg/dL	140–250 mg/dL
Creatinine, serum	1 mg/dL	0.6–1.2 mg/dL
Sodium	140 mEq/L	135–147 mEq/L
Chloride	100 mEq/L	95–105 mEq/L
Potassium	4 mEq/L	3.5–5.0 mEq/L
Bicarbonate	24 mEq/L	22–28 mEq/L
pH	7.4	7.35–7.45
P$_{O_2}$	100 mm Hg	75–105 mm Hg
P$_{CO_2}$	40 mm Hg	33–45 mm Hg
Glucose, serum	100 mg/dL	Fasting: 70–110 mg/dL
Osmolality, serum	290 mOsmol/kg	275–295 mOsmol/kg
Proteins		
Total	7 g/dL	6.0–7.8 g/dL
Albumin	4 g/dL	3.5–5.5 g/dL
Globulins	3 g/dL	2.3–3.5 g/dL
Urea nitrogen, serum (BUN)	10 mg/dL	7–18 mg/dL
Uric acid, serum	6 mg/dL	3.0–8.2 mg/dL

RBCs can flow through the capillary. The sinuses of the spleen, however, are only about 3 μm in diameter, and RBCs have to deform to pass through the spleen. RBC membranes become more rigid as they age. This deformation of the membrane causes older RBCs to lyse (rupture), and the spleen and the liver are important sites for removal of older RBCs from circulation.

After RBCs lyse, the hemoglobin components are scavenged in the liver and spleen. Hemoglobin is scavenged by the protein haptoglobin. Heme is scavenged by hemopexin, and iron is scavenged by transferrin. These scavenging and transport proteins return the RBC components to the marrow, liver, and spleen for reuse. Any heme remaining in the circulation is excreted as bilirubin and biliverdin in the bile and lost in the feces.

Blood Groups and Blood Typing
RBCs express numerous membrane glycoproteins or glycolipids that can serve as antigens. Only three of these antigens, A, B, and Rh, are commonly used in blood compatibility testing. The ABO system blood type is inherited as an autosomal trait. The genotype and phenotype used for blood typing are shown in Table 6-2.

The four major blood types of the ABO system are A, B, AB, and O. Blood is typed according to the antigens found on the RBC and the antibodies found in the serum. The two major antigens within the blood group system are antigens A and B. Antibodies against the A and B antigens are formed shortly after birth because some proteins in the environment have sufficient homology with the A and B antigen and elicit an immune response. Individuals born with the A or B antigen do not mount an immune response and consequently lack antibodies against that antigen.

The Rh blood groups are nearly equal in clinical importance to the ABO groups. The D antigen is the most clinically significant of the more than Rh 20 antigens. The term *Rh-positive* indicates the presence of the D antigen, and *Rh-negative* indicates the absence of the D antigen.

In contrast to the spontaneous development of antibodies against the A or B antigen, an Rh-negative individual must first be exposed to the Rh antigen to develop anti-Rh antibodies. Exposure of an Rh-negative individual can occur through transfusion of Rh-positive blood or by exposure to Rh-positive fetal blood during pregnancy or delivery. Individuals with Rh-negative blood do not mount an immune response on first exposure because their blood does not yet contain anti-Rh antibodies (anti-D). Following exposure, about 50% of people develop sensitivity and form antibodies against the D antigen. If a sensitized individual receives a subsequent exposure to the D antigen, some degree of RBC destruction will occur. It is usually possible to prevent sensitization from occurring following the first exposure by administering a single dose of anti-Rh antibodies in the form of Rh$_0$(D) immune globulin (RhoGAM) immediately following exposure to the D antigen.

Platelets

Platelets are small, disk-shaped fragments of megakaryocytes. Platelet production is regulated by the hepatic hormone thrombopoietin. Platelets have two roles in hemostasis: occlusion of small openings in blood vessels and contribution of platelet factor III to the intrinsic clotting pathway.

Normal platelet count is 250,000 to 500,000/mL of blood. Platelets have a life span of 8 to 12 days, and the time required for the formation of human platelets is about 5 days. Cytoplasmic extensions from megakaryoblasts are extruded into the bone marrow sinusoids, and platelets are formed by fragmentation at the terminal ends of the filaments. Bone marrow may have up to 6 million megakaryocytes per kilogram of body weight, with each megakaryocyte being able to give rise to a thousand or more individual platelets.

●●● HEMOSTASIS

Hemostasis is the formation of the platelet plug and activation of the coagulation cascade. Normal hemostasis seals a break in the vascular system in order to limit blood loss. This repair process is attenuated by anticoagulants and fibrinolytic agents so that the clot is restricted to the damaged area of the circulation.

Damage to the endothelial cell lining initiates platelet plug formation and possibly clotting. Platelets adhere to the exposed subendothelial (collagen) surface. Formation of a platelet plug depends on the presence of fibrinogen and is

TABLE 6-2. Summary of ABO System

Blood Type	Genotype	Agglutinins in Plasma	Frequency in United States (%)	Plasma Agglutinates Red Cells of Type
O	OO	Anti-A, anti-B	45	A, B, AB
A	AA or AO	Anti-B	41	B, AB
B	BB or BO	Anti-A	10	A, AB
AB	AB	None	4	None

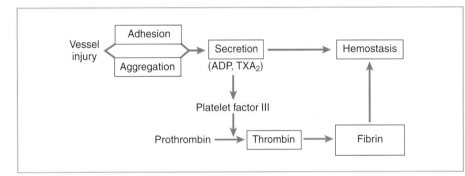

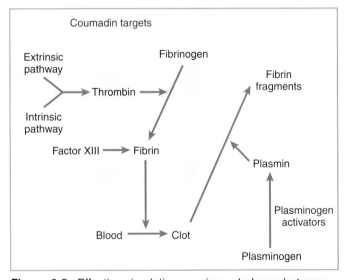

Figure 6-4. A platelet plug forms to seal a small injury to the vascular endothelium. Exposure to damaged endothelium initiates a platelet release reaction, promoting adhesion and aggregation of additional platelets to the site of injury. If the platelet plug is insufficient to repair the injury, platelets participate in the development of a blood clot.

enhanced by clotting factor VIII. Platelet granules containing ADP, serotonin, and thromboxane A are released by exocytosis. ADP attracts additional platelets, and serotonin and thromboxane A cause platelets to adhere and also cause vasoconstriction. Simultaneously, the clotting mechanism is activated, and thrombin promotes further platelet aggregation and release reactions. The fibrin mesh helps trap additional platelets and RBCs and completes the hemostatic plug (Fig. 6-4).

Platelets plugs alone control hemostasis when the damage involves a small area of the blood vessel. If the damage involves a large area, coagulation factors must join with platelets to form a permanent clot. Coagulation depends on the sequential activation of a number of clotting factor enzymes, most of which circulate in plasma in an inactive state.

The fibrin mesh is formed by the action of thrombin on fibrinogen. The extrinsic pathway for fibrin formation is triggered by the release of tissue thromboplastin. The intrinsic pathway for fibrin formation uses clotting factors that are normally present in the blood. Hemostasis is enhanced by emotional stress, strenuous physical activity, epinephrine, pyrogens, and vasopressin. All of these probably work through endothelial plasminogen activators (Fig. 6-5).

The clotting cascade is a series of enzymatic reactions leading to fibrin polymerization. Activation of either the extrinsic or intrinsic pathways leads to the formation of prothrombin activator. Prothrombin activator catalyzes thrombin formation. Thrombin catalyzes fibrin formation. Fibrin polymerizes into a network of strands that traps cells and forms a clot. The extrinsic pathway is activated by disruption of the vascular endothelium and contact of blood

Figure 6-5. Effective circulation requires a balance between the ability to form clots to repair vascular injury and the need to maintain blood flow through vessels. The clotting cascade results in the formation of a fibrin mesh, which traps platelets and RBCs to form a clot. Formation of the fibrin mesh is blocked by anticoagulants. Fibrinolytic agents, but not anticoagulants, can dissolve a clot after it is formed.

with thromboplastin in the tissue spaces. Intrinsic pathway activation occurs following blood stasis or contact with negatively charged surfaces such as glass or collagen (Table 6-3).

Clotting factors are synthesized primarily in liver except factor VIII, von Willebrand factor, which comes from

TABLE 6-3. System for Naming Blood-Clotting Factors

Clotting Factor*	Names
I	Fibrinogen
II	Prothrombin
III	Thromboplastin
IV	Calcium
V	Proaccelerin, labile factor, accelerator globulin
VII	Proconvertin, SPCA, stable factor
VIII	Antihemophilic factor (AHF), antihemophilic factor A, antihemophilic globulin (AHG)
IX	Plasma thromboplastic component (PTC)
X	Stuart-Prower factor
XI	Plasma thromboplastin antecedent (PTA), antihemophilic factor C
XII	Hageman factor, glass factor
XIII	Fibrin-stabilizing factor, Laki-Lorand factor
HMW-K	High-molecular-weight kininogen, Fitzgerald factor
Pre-K$_a$	Prekallikrein, Fletcher factor
Ka	Kallikrein
PL	Platelet phospholipid

*Factor VI is not a separate entity and has been dropped.

PATHOLOGY

Hemophilia A

The most common form of hemophilia in the United States is hemophilia A, which is deficiency of the blood-clotting protein factor VIII. Hemophilia is inherited as a sex-linked recessive pattern; females with the defective chromosome are carriers, and males exhibit the disease. The severity of the disease can vary markedly between individuals, but the symptoms are related to uncontrolled bleeding.

endothelial cells and megakaryocytes. Calcium is a necessary cofactor for many of the clotting enzymes. Hepatic synthesis of clotting factors requires vitamin K and can be blocked by dicumarol and warfarin. These agents diminish the tendency for a new clot to form.

●●●● FIBRINOLYSIS AND ANTICOAGULANTS

The ability to create clots to limit blood loss from sites of vascular injury is balanced by systems designed to limit clot formation and to dissolve existing clots. The blood contains natural anticoagulants that act continuously to inhibit clot formation. Fibrinolytic agents dissolve existing clots. In doing so, blood flow through the vascular system can be maintained.

Anticoagulants reduce the ability of clots to form and also prevent unrestricted clot growth. Clinically, heparin, warfarin, and aspirin are the most commonly used anticoagulants. Heparin acts immediately to potentiate antithrombin III action and prevent clot formation. Warfarin interferes with the vitamin K–dependent hepatic synthesis of clotting factors. Consequently, treatment with warfarin has little immediate effect but is useful for chronic suppression of clotting ability. Aspirin is classified as an anticoagulant, but it acts on platelets to reduce their clotting ability by blocking thromboxane production rather than acting on the clotting cascade. In vitro clot formation can be prevented by the Ca^{++} chelators citrate, EGTA, and EDTA. Protein C, which is activated by the clotting factor thrombin, can prevent further clot growth, and thus the normal clotting cascade produces an enzyme that helps stop the clotting process.

Fibrinolysis is the dissolution of clots, primarily due to action of the enzyme plasmin. The fibrinolytic mechanism is activated a few hours after clot formation. Plasmin is formed by the action of tissue plasminogen activator on the plasma protein plasminogen. Plasmin is a proteolytic enzyme that dissolves fibrin, fibrinogen, and factors V and VIII. Fibrin degradation products produced by clot lysis also act as anticoagulants. Plasmin additionally is formed from plasminogen by streptokinase, staphylokinase, and urokinase as well as intrinsic pathway components. Clinical trials contrasting the effectiveness of the different fibrinolytic agents in myocardial infarction are under way.

Disorders can occur due to insufficient or inappropriate clotting activity. Insufficient clotting activity can be due to thrombocytopenia, the lack of thrombocytes due to impaired production, enhanced breakdown, or enhanced use of thrombocytes. Thrombocytopenia leads to a prolonged bleeding time. In contrast, thrombocytosis is defined as a platelet count greater than 800,000, but it also is characterized by inappropriate bleeding.

Inappropriate clotting can cause thrombosis, the occurrence of a clot within a blood vessel. This can occur following endothelial damage, blood stasis, or enhanced coagulability. An embolus is a clot that breaks free of its attachment site and is carried within the circulation. Emboli are trapped by the branching pattern characteristic of the precapillary side of the circulation. Venous emboli are trapped in the lungs, which have enhanced clot lysis abilities. Left ventricular emboli become trapped in the systemic circulation and block blood flow to the areas distal to the occlusion. Emboli are often responsible for strokes and myocardial infarction.

Blood vessels break and are repaired continuously in the body. The multiple and complex interactions between clot formation, clot lysis, and anticoagulation allow normal vessel repair without precipitation of a massive clot throughout the vascular system. Functional tests of coagulation include bleeding time, clot retraction, and platelet aggregation (Table 6-4).

TABLE 6-4. Laboratory Values for Intrinsic Pathway Activation

Hematologic Parameter	Typical Value	Reference Range
Bleeding time	5 min	2–7 min
Erythrocyte count		
Male	5.0 million/mm^3	4.3–5.9 million/mm^3
Female	4.2 million/mm^3	3.5–5.5 million/mm^3
Hematocrit		
Male	48%	41–53%
Female	42%	36–46%
Hemoglobin, total		
Male	15 g/dL	13.5–17.5 g/dL
Female	14 g/dL	12.0–16.0 g/dL
Partial thromboplastin time (activated)	35 sec	28–40 sec
Platelet count	300,000 mm^3	150,000–400,000 mm^3
Prothrombin time	13 sec	11–15 sec
Reticulocyte count	1%	0.5–1.5% of red cells
Thrombin time		<2 sec deviation from control

Response to Injury

Trauma to blood vessels initiates compensatory and repair responses. Stretch of vascular smooth muscle causes vasoconstriction, which decreases the size of the opening. This response is more pronounced as trauma increases. Consequently, crushing injuries bleed less than cuts.

Clot retraction occurs following coagulation, using actin and myosin in platelets. The platelet plug also releases growth factors. Vascular smooth muscle and endothelial cells grow into the damaged area, and infiltration of fibroblasts initiates scar tissue formation. Tissue growth provides a permanent seal of the damaged area.

●●● TOP 5 TAKE-HOME POINTS

1. Blood is a complex suspension of plasma, solutes, and the formed elements RBCs, WBCs, and platelets.
2. The formed elements are synthesized from a stem cell population in the bone marrow under the control of cytokines and the hormones thrombopoietin (for platelets) and erythropoietin (for RBCs).
3. The four blood types are determined by the presence of an antigen (A or B) on the surface of the red blood cell.
4. Blood, through the formation of platelet plugs and the clotting cascade, seals vascular damage to limit hemorrhage. This clotting ability is balanced by the presence of anticoagulants, which act to restrict clot formation to the site of injury.
5. Vascular repair involves dissolution of the clot and repair of the damaged area by vascular growth.

The Heart

7

CONTENTS

The cardiovascular system (Fig. 7-1) consists of blood, a four-chambered heart, and a vast network of vessels through which blood circulates in the body. The heart is a dual pump contained within one organ. Each side of the pump has an atrium and a ventricle. The heart pumps blood from the low-pressure veins to the high-pressure arteries. The output of the right ventricle enters the pulmonary artery, and the output of the left ventricle enters the aorta. Pump output is under intrinsic control and can be extrinsically regulated by autonomic nerves and circulating hormones.

Two series of blood vessels distribute blood to the tissues and collect blood for return to the heart. The peripheral circulation transports blood from the aorta to most tissues of the body. The pulmonary circulation transports blood from the pulmonary artery to the lung for gas exchange. Diameter of the blood vessels can be altered by constriction of vascular smooth muscle. Local control of vascular smooth muscle contraction is supplemented by autonomic nerves and circulating hormones.

The cardiovascular system transports nutrients to tissues and removes metabolic wastes, including heat. Exchange of nutrients and wastes between the blood and the tissues occurs in the small blood vessels. Neural and hormonal regulatory systems maintain a constant arterial pressure, and the tissues control local blood flow by adjusting vascular resistance. Cardiovascular control systems must also adapt to stress, such as exercise.

● ● ● STRUCTURE OF THE HEART

The heart weighs about 300 g and is located within the mediastinum; it is cone-shaped and tilted forward and to the left. Because of rotation during fetal development, the apex of the heart (tip of the cone) is at its bottom and lies left of the midline. The base is at the top, where the great vessels enter the heart and lies posterior to the sternum (Fig. 7-2). The heart consists of four chambers: two smaller atria at the top (the base) and two larger ventricles at the apex. A band of fibrous tissue separates the atria from the ventricles and seats the four cardiac valves. A muscular septum separates the right from left atrium and the right from left ventricle.

In cross section, the wall of the heart contains the innermost endocardium, thick myocardial layer, and outer epicardium, all encased in a fibrous pouch, the pericardium. The innermost layer of the endocardium is a lining of endothelial cells. The thin endocardium also contains the nodal tissue, bundle of His, and bundle branches and provides a point of attachment for the cordae tendineae. The thick ventricular myocardium consists of striated muscle cells. The outer epicardial surface contains the major coronary blood vessels and is separated from the pericardium by a thin layer of fluid.

● ● ● CARDIAC ELECTROPHYSIOLOGY

Cardiac tissue has distinctive electrical characteristics. Intercalated disks allow action potentials to pass to adjacent cells. Myocardial cells can spontaneously depolarize, a process called automaticity. This spontaneous depolarization generates a pacemaker potential or prepotential and is caused by decreasing K^+ and increasing Ca^{++} and Na^+ permeability. This occurs at the fastest rate in sinoatrial (SA) node, so the SA node acts as the normal pacemaker for the heart. If cells other than SA node dominate rhythm, the pacemaker is called "ectopic."

The fibrous tissue that seats the cardiac valves provides a border between the atria and the ventricles. This tissue lacks gap junctions and consequently electrically isolates the atria from the ventricles. This electrical insulation allows the atria and ventricles each to function as an independent syncitium.

Ionic movements, or conductances across the myocardial membrane, occur in response to the electrochemical potential gradient and are controlled by selective ion permeability. For

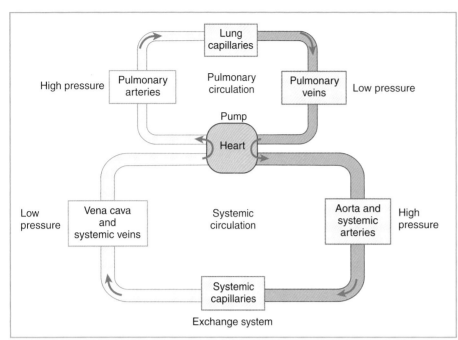

Figure 7-1. Blood flows sequentially through the right heart, pulmonary circulation, left heart, and systemic circulation. The four chambers of the heart function as two independent pumping systems. The right atrium and the right ventricle propel blood from the systemic veins into the pulmonary artery. The left atrium and the left ventricle propel blood from the pulmonary veins into the aorta.

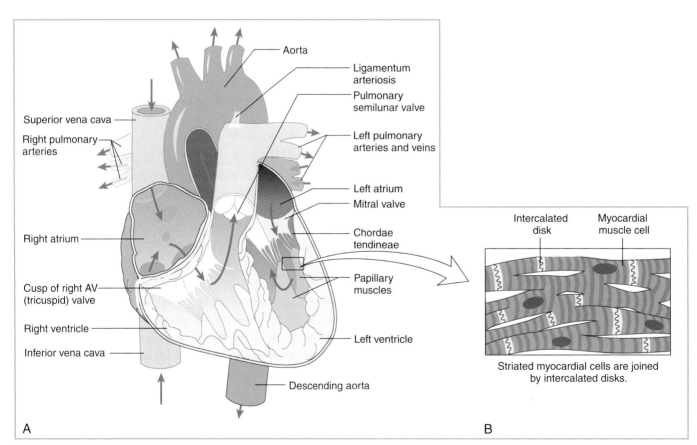

Figure 7-2. Gross and fine structures of the heart. **A**, The myocardium consists of the thin-walled atria and thicker walled ventricles. The atria and the ventricles are separated from each other by a band of connective tissue that also seats the four cardiac valves. **B**, The ventricular myocardium consists of striated muscle cells, connected to each other by gap junctions in the intercalated disks.

ventricular myocytes, the Nernst equilibrium value for Na$^+$ is +61 mV, for Ca^{++} is +132 mV, and for K$^+$ is −95 mV. Increasing the permeability of any ion will drive the membrane potential toward the Nernst equilibrium value for that ion, and conversely, decreasing the permeability of any ion will drive the membrane potential away from the Nernst equilibrium value for that ion.

Multiple types of Na$^+$ channels are found on myocardial cells. Voltage-gated Na$^+$ channels are blocked by local anesthetics such as lidocaine and by tetrodotoxin. L-type Na$^+$ channels also allow passage of Ca^{++} and can be blocked by verapamil. The presence of voltage-gated Na$^+$ channels results in a "fast" type of myocardial action potential, characterized by a rapid rate of transmission. This type of action potential is characteristic of ventricular muscle and ventricular conductive tissue. The absence of voltage-gated Na$^+$ channels results in a "slow" type of myocardial action potential, characterized by a slower rate of transmission. This type of action potential is characteristic of SA node and atrioventricular (AV) node tissue.

Ion permeability is altered to produce the five phases of the ventricular muscle action potential (Fig. 7-3). Phase 0 is rapid depolarization, caused by an increase in Na$^+$ permeability through the voltage-gated fast Na$^+$ channels. Phase 1 is a small recovery toward resting membrane potential, caused by an increase in Ca^{++} permeability while Na$^+$ permeability decreases. Phase 2 is a plateau, characterized by continuing Ca^{++} permeability. Phase 3 is repolarization, caused by an increase in K$^+$ permeability and a decrease in Ca^{++} permeability. During this phase, Ca^{++} is resequestered into the sarcoplasmic reticulum. Phase 4 is the resting membrane potential, characterized by high K$^+$ permeability.

Slow (SA nodal) action potential phases are not so sharply defined. Nodal cells have a less negative resting membrane potential that spontaneously depolarizes. This phase 4 depolarization is due to decreasing K$^+$ permeability or increasing slow Ca^{++}/Na$^+$ permeability, or both. The voltage-gated Na$^+$ channels, if present, are inoperative because the h-gate is closed (see Fig. 4-15 for gate movement of the fast Na channel).

Pacemaker activity is stimulated by sympathetic nerves and inhibited by parasympathetic nerves. The autonomic neurotransmitters act through altering membrane conduc-

tances (Fig. 7-4). The sympathetic neurotransmitter norepinephrine (Fig. 7-4A) acts through β$_1$-adrenergic receptors to increase Na$^+$ permeability and increase the heart rate. Acetylcholine (Fig. 7-4B) acts on muscarinic receptors to increase K$^+$ permeability, which hyperpolarizes the cell, decreases the slope of phase 4 depolarization, and consequently slows the heart rate. Parasympathetic nervous system activation also changes the threshold to a less negative value. This decreases the slope of the phase 4 depolarization and consequently decreases the heart rate.

Coordination of Cardiac Electrical Activity

The sequence in which the wave of depolarization spreads across the myocardium increases pumping efficiency of the heart. The SA node, at the junction of the vena cava and right atrium, normally initiates depolarization. The impulse spreads cell by cell through the intercalated disks through the atria. The contraction of the atria propels blood in the atria toward the AV valves.

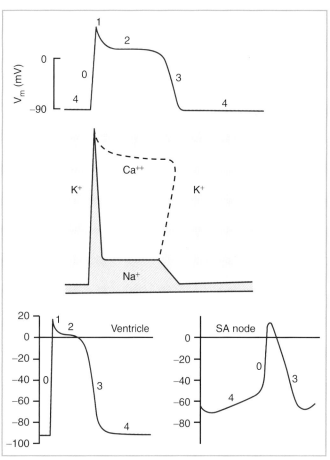

Figure 7-3. The ventricular muscle and the SA node represent two extremes of the type of action potential found in the heart. The rapid phase 0 depolarization of ventricular muscle is due to opening of voltage-gated Na$^+$ channels. The phase 4 diastolic depolarization of the SA node is due to a gradual decrease in K$^+$ permeability and to increases in Na$^+$ and Ca^{++} permeability.

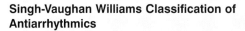

PHARMACOLOGY

Singh-Vaughan Williams Classification of Antiarrhythmics

Antiarrhythmic drugs work by altering Na$^+$, K$^+$, or Ca^{++} ion channels. Class I drugs block the Na channel and slow cardiac conduction. Class II drugs block the β-adrenergic receptors, slowing conduction and heart rate. Class III drugs delay repolarization by blocking potassium conductance and currently are the preferred agent. Class IV drugs block the L-type calcium channel, slowing both heart rate and AV node conduction.

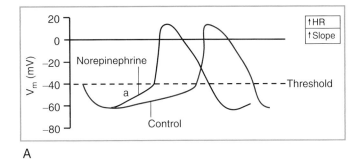

A

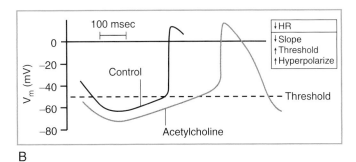

B

Figure 7-4. **A,** Sympathetic nervous system activation increases heart rate by increasing Na^+ and Ca^{++} permeability, which increases the slope of the phase 4 diastolic depolarization. **B,** Parasympathetic nervous system activation decreases heart rate by increasing K^+ permeability, which hyperpolarizes the cell and decreases the slope of the phase 4 diastolic depolarization.

AV nodal tissue has a slow conduction velocity and delays the passage of depolarization into the ventricles, allowing atrial contraction to complete before the onset of ventricular contraction. Once the wave of depolarization exits the AV node, it spreads through the common bundle of His on the surface of the right interventricular septum, through bundle branches, and into each ventricle. Finally, Purkinje fibers carry impulses from the endocardial surface into the ventricular wall, and the basal epicardial surface of the left ventricle is normally the last region of the heart to depolarize.

Electrocardiography

The electrocardiogram (ECG), an electrical potential recorded on the body surface, is a consequence of the flow of current from an area of depolarized myocardial tissue to polarized myocardium. The ECG provides a one-dimensional view of the current flow during the cardiac cycle recorded against time. Electrode placement markedly affects the measurement. Placement for humans was standardized by Einthoven as shown in Figure 7-5.

In this system, the right leg is used as the electrical ground. Three bipolar limb leads (I, II, and III) and three augmented unipolar limb leads (aVR, aVL, and aVF) view current movement in the frontal plane of the body. Augmented unipolar limb leads are 50% larger than bipolar leads. Chest leads (V_1 through V_6) provide information in the transverse plane of the body, based on six anatomically determined positions of exploring electrode (V) on the chest (Table 7-1).

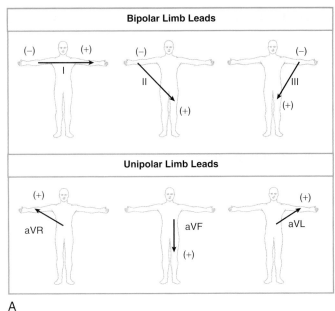

A

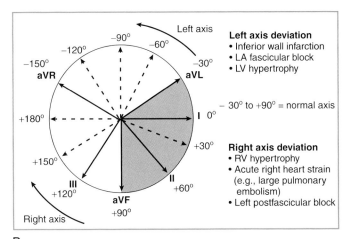

B

Figure 7-5. Einthoven standardized the electrode positions for recording ECG limb leads. **A,** The right arm, left arm, and left leg form a triangle, and leads I, II, and III are the sides of that triangle. The unipolar (augmented) leads are a variation of this triangle. **B,** The six limb leads can be drawn originating from a common center point. In this analysis, lead I provides a horizontal axis, and lead aVF provides a vertical axis. Deviation from −30 to +90 degrees, the normal range of the ventricular mean electrical axis, provides useful diagnostic information. aVR, aVL, aVF, three augmented unipolar limb leads; LA, left atrium; LV, left ventricle; RV, right ventricle.

The ECG is a record of the current flow caused by electrical activity in the heart. Cardiac depolarization originates in the SA node and then spreads through the cardiac chambers (Table 7-2 and Fig. 7-6). The numbers on the heart illustrate in milliseconds the interval between the origin of the depolarization at the SA node and the appearance of the depolarization in the different regions of the heart. The tracings on the right show the temporal relationship between the myocardial action potentials and the ECG. The P wave represents atrial depolarization, the QRS complex represents

TABLE 7-1. Locations for Electrocardiogram Leads

Lead	Positive Electrode	Negative Electrode
I	Left arm	Right arm
II	Left leg	Right arm
III	Left leg	Left arm
aVR	Right arm	(Left arm + left leg)
aVL	Left arm	(Right arm + left leg)
aVF	Left leg	(Right arm + left arm)
V_{1-6}	Six positions on chest	(Right arm + left arm + left leg)

TABLE 7-2. Electrocardiogram Events

Elapsed Time	Record	Cardiac Event	Duration
0.00 sec	P wave	Atrial depolarization	0.06 sec
	P-R interval	Delay of impulse at AV node	0.18 sec
0.18 sec	QRS complex ventricular depolarization		0.08 sec
	Q-T interval	Ventricular systole	40 sec
0.40 sec	T wave	Ventricular repolarization	0.15 sec

P-R interval is the time between atrial depolarizations, 0.83 sec = the inverse of heart rate.
Terminology: segments do not include a wave; intervals include at least one wave and one segment.

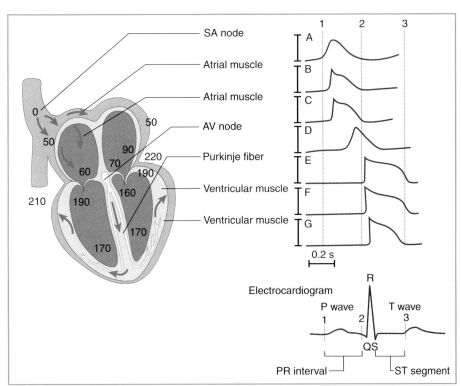

Figure 7-6. The SA node originates in an action potential that subsequently spreads through the cardiac chambers. The numbers on the heart illustrate in milliseconds the elapsed time interval between the origin of the depolarization at the SA node and the appearance of the depolarization in the different regions of the heart. The tracing on the right shows the temporal relationship between the myocardial action potentials and the ECG. The P wave represents atrial muscle depolarization, the QRS complex represents ventricular muscle depolarization, and the T wave represents ventricular muscle repolarization.

ventricular depolarization, and the T wave represents ventricular repolarization.

The mean electrical axis is a single vector representing the sum of current flow during ventricular depolarization. It is constructed from any two ECG leads by addition of vectors (dropping perpendicular lines). The mean electrical axis can be used to predict the magnitude of the QRS complex in any lead.

In the analysis of the ECG, the six limb leads can be drawn originating from a common center point. Lead I provides a horizontal axis, and lead aVF provides a vertical axis. Deviation from the normal range of the ventricular mean electrical axis provides useful diagnostic information.

●●● MYOCARDIAL PHYSIOLOGY

Myocardial cells have distinctive anatomic and physiologic characteristics. Under a microscope, striations are visible owing to the arrangement of actin and myosin as in skeletal muscle. T tubules increase the contact area of the cell membrane and extracellular fluid space.

At rest, cardiac muscle obtains 99% of its energy from aerobic metabolism. Myocardial cells have numerous mitochondria to support energy production. In addition, high capillary density ensures adequate blood delivery to support aerobic metabolism. Multiple substrates can provide energy for the heart. At rest, 60% of energy is derived from metabolism of fat, 35% from carbohydrates, and 5% from amino acids and ketones.

Myocardial Mechanics

Excitation-contraction coupling ties electrical depolarization to the mechanical shortening of myocardial cells (Fig. 7-7). Myocardial depolarization allows influx of extracellular Ca^{++} during phase 2 of myocardial action potential. This extracellular Ca^{++} "triggers" the release of Ca^{++} from sarcoplasmic reticulum (SR). Over 90% of the Ca^{++} involved in the contraction comes from the SR. By the end of systole, Ca^{++} is resequestered in SR, and extracellular Ca^{++} is removed by an electroneutral 2 Na^+/Ca^{++} exchange.

There is a time delay before Ca^{++} that is taken up by the SR is available for release by the next depolarization. A premature depolarization has diminished SR Ca^{++} release and consequently lower than normal force generation. In contrast, enhanced contractile strength characterizes a delayed depolarization because of the additional time for processing of SR Ca^{++} into the available pool.

Myocardial cell action potential precedes the contraction (Fig. 7-8). Contraction of the ventricular muscle cell (curve B in Fig. 7-8) requires the entry of Ca^{++} during phase 2 of the

ventricular muscle action potential (curve A), and relaxation begins during phase 3. During an action potential, the ventricular muscle cell cannot initiate a second action potential, since it is in the absolute refractory period. During the end of the action potential, there is a relative refractory period during which only a greater than normal stimulus can initiate a subsequent action potential. The ventricular muscle cell contraction is completed shortly after this relative refractory period. Consequently, ventricular muscle contraction is a series of twitch contractions, and the myocardium cannot enter tetany.

Contractile activity of the heart can be modeled by the activity of a contractile component and an elastic component in series. The contractile element reflects the action of actin and myosin. A parallel elastic element reflects the tendency of connective tissue to resist stretch, so stretch causes some tension in the muscle even without a contraction. The series elastic element has no anatomic counterpart, and it reflects the tendency of the muscle to develop tension before actual shortening occurs.

Developed force is inversely proportionate to velocity, and both are increased by elevations in intracellular Ca^{++}. The maximal velocity of contraction occurs when there is no load on the system. Peak force is developed during the isometric phase of the contraction.

Contractility is defined as the change in developed force at any given fiber length, independent of preload and afterload. Contractile force is altered by changing intracellular Ca^{++} levels. Digitalis (a cardiac glycoside) increases Ca^{++} by inhibiting Na^+/K^+-ATPase. The resultant high intracellular Na^+ acts to slow the electroneutral 2 Na^+/Ca^{++} exchange and increase intracellular Ca^{++}. Catecholamines increase influx of extracellular Ca^{++} during the action potential, and possibly

PATHOLOGY

Determination of Mean Electrical Axis

Mean electrical axis is estimated by finding a QRS complex with zero net voltage and identifying a lead perpendicular to it. The mean electrical axis will lie along the perpendicular lead.

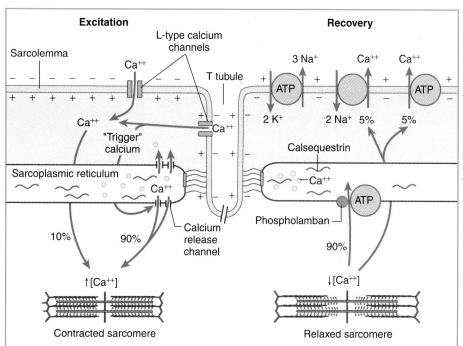

Figure 7-7. Calcium is released, then resequestered by myocardial depolarization. The events on the left side of the figure illustrate Ca^{++} release during the myocardial action potential, and the events on the right side of the figure illustrate the removal of intracellular Ca^{++} during the time between action potentials. Most of the Ca^{++} causing contraction of the myocardium is released from the sarcoplasmic reticulum following entry of trigger Ca^{++} from the extracellular stores.

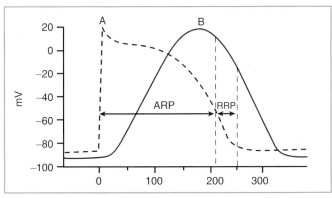

Figure 7-8. Depolarization of the ventricular muscle cell (curve A) precedes contraction (curve B). Contraction is initiated after entry of Ca^{++} during phase 2 of the ventricular muscle action potential. During an action potential, the ventricular muscle cell cannot initiate a second action potential and is in an absolute refractory period (ARP). At the end of the action potential, there is a relative refractory period (RRP), during which only a greater than normal stimulus can initiate a subsequent action potential. The ventricular muscle cell contraction is completed shortly after this relative refractory period. Consequently, ventricular muscle contraction is a series of twitch contractions, and the muscle cannot enter tetany.

PHARMACOLOGY

Congestive Heart Failure

Treatment for congestive heart failure is based on the severity of the disease and often involves an angiotensin-converting enzyme (ACE) inhibitor and a diuretic. The ACE inhibitor and diuretic both lower blood pressure, thereby reducing the workload on the ventricle. The benefit of ACE inhibitors appears tied to a reduction in remodeling of the myocardium. The excessive preload characteristic of heart failure is no longer enhancing pumping ability, and the diuretic helps reduce the volume load in the body.

through altering Ca^{++} transport by the SR. Tachycardia decreases the time for Ca^{++} to be resequestered into the SR, so free intracellular Ca^{++} levels rise. Any other agents that increase Ca^{++} will increase contractility, producing a positive inotropic effect.

CARDIAC MECHANICAL ACTIVITY

There are three major determinants of myocardial performance: preload, afterload, and contractility. Maximal force in a myocyte is developed at sarcomere lengths of 2 to 2.4 μm. The actual sarcomere length normally is shorter than 2 μm, since connective tissue prevents overstretching of heart muscle. For the left ventricle, preload is represented by left ventricular end-diastolic pressure, afterload is represented by aortic pressure, and Δ length/Δ time (slope of left ventricular pressure curve) is represented by contractility (Table 7-3).

TABLE 7-3. Correspondences of Cardiac Performance

Measure	Papillary Muscle	Ventricle	Measures
Preload	Resting length	End diastolic volume	Right atrial pressure, left ventricle end diastolic pressure, pulmonary capillary wedge pressure
Afterload	Weight	Aortic pressure	Mean arterial pressure
Contractility	$\frac{\Delta\ length}{\Delta\ time}$	$\frac{\Delta\ pressure}{\Delta\ time}$	Intracellular Ca^{++}

The active myocardial length-tension relationship (Frank-Starling relationship) shifts with changes in contractility. The active length-tension relationship is determined by overlapping of actin and myosin filaments. The passive length-tension relationship is due to stretching of cardiac tissue. An increase in preload provides a better overlapping of actin and myosin filaments, allowing the muscle cell to generate more contractile force. The afterload determines how much of this force is used to generate pressure and how much is used for shortening. Changes in contractility provide a preload-independent mechanism to increase contractile force.

Myocardial preload enhances myocardial performance. An increase in end-diastolic pressure causes an increase in ventricular pressure development. An increase in venous return will increase end-diastolic pressure and, consequently, increase the pumping ability of the heart. This means that within physiologic limits, the heart can pump all of the blood that is returned to it via the vena cava. Increasing the initial fiber length causes a more forceful contraction but does *not* affect contractility. Afterload affects Δ length/Δ time and the onset of shortening (Fig. 7-9).

The pericardium is a fibrous sac covering the heart. It contains fluid that acts as a lubricant to reduce friction during movements associated with contraction. The pericardium also helps prevent overstretching of ventricles during filling. Abnormal fluid accumulation (pericarditis) within the pericardium prevents expansion of ventricles during filling (pericardial tamponade) and therefore diminishes cardiac output.

Cardiac Cycle

The cardiac cycle integrates pressure, volume, and electrocardiographic and valvular movements during the systolic and diastolic periods (Fig. 7-10). The ECG illustrates the electrical events that drive the mechanical events of the cardiac cycle. The P wave of the ECG represents atrial depolarization, which is followed by contraction and an increase in pressure in the atria (atrial systole). The AV valves

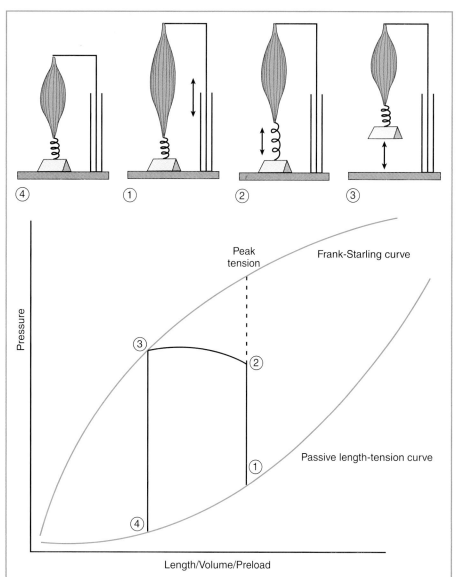

Figure 7-9. The active myocardial length-peak tension relationship (Frank-Starling relationship) shifts with changes in contractility. The passive length-tension relationship is due to stretching of the cardiac tissue. The active length-tension relationship is determined by overlapping of actin and myosin filaments. An increase in preload provides better overlapping of actin and myosin filaments, allowing the muscle cell to generate more contractile force. The afterload determines how much of this force is used to generate pressure, and how much is used for shortening. Changes in contractility provide a preload-independent mechanism to increase contractile force.

are open, and there is no valve between the atria and veins, so this small increase in pressure is also evident in the ventricle (a wave) and in the veins. Most ventricular filling occurs early in ventricular diastole, but atrial contraction at the end of ventricular diastole causes a small increase in ventricular volume. The QRS wave of the electrocardiogram represents ventricular depolarization, which is followed by contraction and an increase in pressure in the ventricles (ventricular systole). The T wave of the ECG represents ventricular repolarization and relaxation of the ventricular muscles (ventricular diastole).

Pressures on the left side of the heart are normally higher than pressures on the corresponding right side. Pressure range in the left atrium is 2 to 8 mm Hg, and in the right atrium is 0 to 5 mm Hg. Pressure in the left ventricle is 2 to 120 mm Hg, and in the right ventricle is 0 to 35 mm Hg. Pressure in the aorta is 80 to 120 mm Hg, and in the pulmonary artery is 10 to 25 mm Hg. The higher pressures on the left side mean that any disruption in the interatrial

septum or interventricular septum will result in blood flow from the left side of the heart to the right side of the heart.

Pressure waveforms characterize different areas of the circulation. For the atrial pressure waveform, the "a" wave is due to atrial contraction, the "c" wave is due to ventricular contraction, and the "v" wave is due to ventricular filling. The atrial waveforms are similar to jugular venous waveforms, because there is no valve between the right atrium and the vena cava.

The aortic (arterial) waveform has a systolic and a diastolic portion. The systolic portion consists of upstroke, peak, downstroke, and dicrotic notch (incisura). Diastole consists of a gradual decline in pressures.

The volume in the ventricles is greatest before the contraction occurs and lowest immediately following ejection. End-diastolic volume is the blood in the ventricle after closure of the AV valves, typically about 140 mL in an adult. End-systolic volume is the residual volume in the ventricle after closure of the aortic or pulmonic valve, about 70 mL in

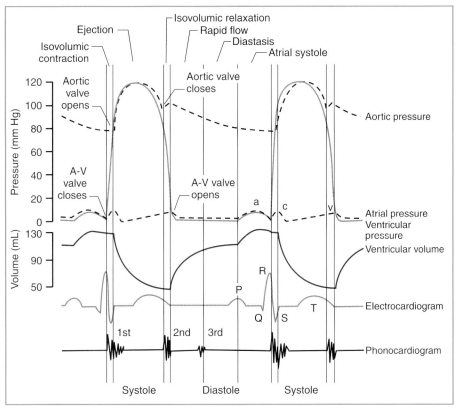

Figure 7-10. The cardiac cycle integrates pressure, volume, and electrocardiographic and valve movements during systole and diastole. Atrial depolarization is followed by contraction (atrial systole), an increase in pressure in the atria (a wave), and a small increase in ventricular volume. Ventricular depolarization is followed by contraction (ventricular systole) and an increase in pressure in the ventricles. Ventricular repolarization causes relaxation of ventricular muscles (ventricular diastole).

an adult. Stroke volume is the volume of blood ejected by ventricular contraction, also about 70 mL in an adult. Ejection fraction is the percentage of end-diastolic volume ejected during the contraction, typically about 50%.

The cardiac cycle is divided into a recurring series of intervals. The valve movement that ends the interval follows in parentheses.

- Atrial contraction (mitral valve closes)
- Ventricular isovolumetric contraction—occurs when both valves are closed (aortic valve opens)
- Rapid ventricular ejection
- Slow ventricular ejection (aortic valve closes)
- Ventricular isovolumetric relaxation occurs when both valves are closed (mitral valve opens)
- Ventricular filling
- Diastasis

Heart sounds are due to reverberation of blood when cardiac valves close or to the turbulent flow of blood. The first heart sound results from closure of the AV valves (mitral and tricuspid). The second heart sound results from closure of the aortic and pulmonary valves. The third heart sound is due to turbulent flow of blood into ventricles. Although rare, a fourth heart sound, if present, is due to turbulent flow during atrial contraction. The first and second sounds may "split" and be audible as distinct sounds because left and right ventricular systoles are unequal. The closing of the aortic valve before the pulmonic valve causes a splitting of the second heart sound and is often more prominent during inspiration.

PATHOLOGY

Cardiac Murmurs

Cardiac murmurs are primarily caused by turbulent flow of blood across a cardiac valve. Stenosis is narrowing of a valve; turbulence is audible during the portion of the cardiac cycle when the valve normally is open. Regurgitation is retrograde flow of blood through a normally closed valve; turbulence is audible during the portion of the cardiac cycle when the valve normally is closed. The timing and the position on the chest of the loudest sound allow identification of specific valve defects.

A murmur is an abnormal heart sound generated by the turbulent flow of blood. This often occurs as a result of an increased velocity as blood flows across a narrow opening, usually a cardiac valve. A bruit is an equivalent sound in a major blood vessel caused by turbulent flow, often caused by a narrowing of an artery.

The ventricular pressure-volume loop relates myocardial mechanics (see Fig. 7-9) to heart function (Fig. 7-11). The events of the ventricular pressure-volume loop are identical to those in the cardiac cycle of Figure 7-10. As the ventricles begin to contract, pressure in the ventricle exceeds that in the atrium, and the mitral valve closes (step 1 in Fig. 7-11). The ventricles continue to contract and generate pressure until the pressure in the ventricle is greater than that in the aorta, and the aortic valve opens (2). The ventricles continue to contract and now eject volume. As the ventricles begin to

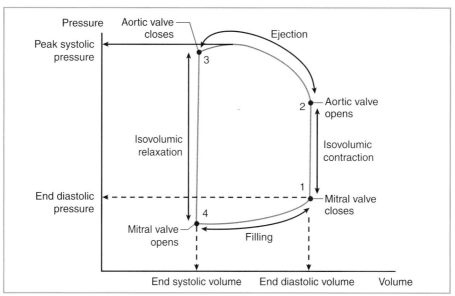

Figure 7-11. Events of the ventricular pressure-volume loop are identical to those in the cardiac cycle shown in Fig. 7-10, but the function of the valves is shown more clearly. Point 1 represents end-diastolic pressure and end-diastolic volume. During the early phase of ventricular systole, pressure in the ventricle exceeds that in the atrium and the mitral valve closes (1). The ventricles continue to contract and generate pressure (isovolumic contraction) until the pressure in the ventricle is greater than that in the aorta, and the aortic valve opens (2). The ventricles continue to contract and now eject volume. As the ventricles begin to relax, pressure in the ventricles drops below that in the aorta, and the aortic valve closes (3). The ventricles continue to relax (isovolumic relaxation) until pressure in the ventricles drops below the pressure in the atrium, and the mitral valve opens (4). The ventricles then fill until the cycle begins again.

relax, pressure in the ventricles drops below that in the aorta, and the aortic valve closes (3). The ventricles continue to relax, until pressure in the ventricles drops below the pressure in the atrium, and the mitral valve opens (4). The ventricles then fill, until the cycle begins again.

Cardiac Output

The cardiac output is the volume of blood pumped by the heart each minute. It can be calculated as stroke volume times heart rate. Factors that alter stroke volume or heart rate will change cardiac output. Normally it is about 5 L/min (70 mL/beat × 72 beats/min). Cardiac index is defined as cardiac output/body surface area, and it allows comparisons of cardiac function between individuals of different sizes.

Cardiac output measurements are direct or indirect. Direct determination uses a type of flowmeter. A Doppler flowmeter actually measures velocity, which is converted to an estimation of flow based on the vessel cross-sectional area. Indirect measurement often involves the Fick principle.

Cardiac output

$$= \frac{O_2 \text{ consumed per minute}}{\text{Pulmonary venous } O_2 - \text{pulmonary arterial } O_2}$$

An indicator dilution technique involves injection of a known amount of dye and measurement of the consequent concentration change downstream. However, dye can accumulate if multiple measurements are taken. Thermal dilution involves injection of cold saline and measurement of the resultant change in temperature downstream. This approach can be performed with a Swan-Ganz catheter and is suitable for multiple determinations.

Improved ventricular imaging techniques allow accurate measurement of ventricular end-diastolic and ventricular end-systolic volumes. Consequently, imaging combined with electrocardiographic measurement of heart rate allows non-invasive measurement of cardiac output and ejection fraction.

●●● NEURAL AND HORMONAL REGULATION OF THE HEART

The intrinsic spontaneous rate of the SA node depolarization is 90 to 100 beats/min and is modulated by autonomic nerve inputs. The parasympathetic nervous system (PNS) normally is dominant. The right vagus nerve, with acetylcholine as its neurotransmitter, innervates the SA node. Acetylcholine slows SA node depolarization and therefore lowers heart rate. The left vagus nerve innervates the AV node, at which the neurotransmitter acetylcholine decreases the velocity of impulse transmission. Nodal areas have high acetylcholinesterase activity, so they rapidly clear acetylcholine.

Cardiac sympathetic nerves (SNS) originate from spinal nerves C-7 to T-6, pass to the stellate ganglion, then to the epicardial plexus. The right epicardial plexus, with norepinephrine as the neurotransmitter, innervates the SA node. Norepinephrine increases heart rate. Elevated temperature and stretch also can act directly on the SA node to increase heart rate. The left epicardial plexus innervates the AV node, at which norepinephrine increases conduction velocity.

The external environment of the heart also influences myocardial performance. Endocrine agents with cardiac actions include the adrenal catecholamines epinephrine and norepinephrine, whose actions mimic those of the cardiac sympathetic nerve; thyroid hormone and growth hormone, which play a nutritive role and set the basal tone of the cardiovascular system; and insulin and glucagon, which both have a direct positive inotropic effect.

Blood gases can directly and indirectly alter cardiac function. Severe hypoxia directly depresses myocardial function. Very high CO_2 directly depresses myocardial function, and acidosis decreases Ca^{++} release from SR and consequently decreases contractility. Indirectly, moderate hypoxia causes activation of the sympathetic nervous system, and increases heart rate, contractility, and therefore cardiac output. Moderate hypercapnia also causes a sympathetic activation and increases heart rate, contractility, and therefore cardiac output.

●●● TOP 5 TAKE-HOME POINTS

1. The sinoatrial node of the right atrium serves as the cardiac pacemaker region by spontaneously generating a wave of depolarization that spreads sequentially through the atria and ventricles.
2. Myocardial depolarization allows the entry of Ca^{++}, which triggers a contraction of the myocardium in a coordinated twitch.
3. The volume of blood pumped by the heart during the contraction is the stroke volume. Cardiac output is the product of the stroke volume and the heart rate.
4. Intrinsic regulation is accomplished by preload (the Frank-Starling effect), afterload, and contractility.
5. Extrinsic regulation relies on activity of sympathetic and parasympathetic nerves.

Vascular System 8

CONTENTS

The cardiovascular system transports nutrients to tissues and removes metabolic waste, including heat. The exchange of nutrients and wastes between the blood and the tissues occurs in the small blood vessels, primarily by diffusion. Metabolic wastes are eliminated from the body by the kidneys, lungs, skin, and gastrointestinal tract. Blood flow helps maintain a relatively constant internal environment throughout the body.

Peripheral blood vessel structure varies throughout the circulation. Vascular smooth muscle is arranged helically or circularly around vessels, so that contraction reduces vessel diameter. Vascular smooth muscle contracts by actin-myosin cross-bridging, and intracellular Ca^{++} regulates the strength of contraction. Calcium dynamics is complex because Ca^{++} can enter through voltage-gated channels, can enter through receptor-operated channels, or can be released from the sarcoplasmic reticulum. Most vascular smooth muscle is innervated by sympathetic nerves, and basal sympathetic nerve activity causes a resting level of contraction (vasomotor tone).

Tissue blood flow is controlled by local metabolic needs—acutely, by adjusting vascular resistance, and chronically, by angiogenesis to change capillary density. Tissues with high metabolic rates have high blood flow and high capillary density. Tissues with low metabolic rates have low blood flow and low capillary density. An increase in metabolic rate leads to an increase in tissue blood flow, such as in skeletal muscle during exercise. This mechanism depends on arterial pressure being sufficiently high.

Neural and hormonal regulatory systems help maintain arterial pressure. At rest, the peripheral nervous system (PNS) controls heart rate and the sympathetic nervous system (SNS) controls vascular smooth muscle tone and myocardial contractility. Circulating hormones, such as catecholamines and angiotensin II, provide additional vasoconstriction. Cardiac output is increased by increases in heart rate or cardiac contractility. In addition to maintaining homeostasis, cardiovascular control systems must also adapt to stress, such as exercise.

●●● BLOOD VESSEL HISTOLOGY

Blood vessels have structural characteristics that allow them to be classified as arteries, arterioles, capillaries, venules, and veins. The structure of a blood vessel contributes to its functional characteristics. The anatomic identification of blood vessels is based on the presence of up to three histologic layers: tunica intima, tunica media, and tunica adventitia (Fig. 8-1).

The *tunica intima* (innermost layer) is a layer of endothelial cells that is in contact with the blood. Permeability of this endothelial layer is determined by the endothelial cells, the tight junctions connecting the endothelial cells together, and the presence of pores that extend through the endothelial cell. The tightness of the junctions between endothelial cells varies among tissues. For example, the very tight junctions of cerebral capillaries restrict movement of some drugs to brain cells (the *blood-brain barrier*). In contrast, the endothelial cell pores and relatively loose junctions in the liver and spleen allow easy transit between the blood and tissue spaces in those organs. The endothelium has surface proteins, or adhesion molecules, that allow white blood cells to attach and cross from the circulation into the tissues. The endothelium generates substances such as nitric oxide (endothelial-derived relaxing factor, EDRF), allowing ingested nitroglycerin, friction, and stress to cause vasodilation. Damage to the endothelium may allow blood to enter the middle layer of a blood vessel, creating an aneurysm.

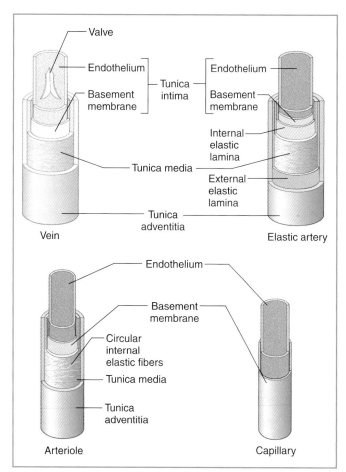

Figure 8-1. The interior of all blood vessels is a continuous endothelial cell layer. For capillaries, this is the only cellular layer. The arteries, arterioles, and veins have in addition a smooth muscle layer that spirals around the blood vessels. The aorta and other large arteries also have elastic tissue.

IMMUNOLOGY

White Blood Cell Adhesion

The capillary endothelial cells express cell adhesion molecules (CAMs) that can serve as points of attachment for the corresponding CAMs on circulating white blood cells. White blood cell adhesion is increased by cytokines released by tissue damage. CAMs are essential for extravasation of white blood cells.

The *tunica media* (middle layer) consists of elastic connective tissue and smooth muscle cells. In the aorta and large arteries, the elastic tissue contributes to the shape of the arterial pressure pulse. Smooth muscle contraction controls the diameter of the vessel and causes a change in blood flow and blood pressure. Smooth muscle is normally partially contracted because of sympathetic nerve activity. Smooth muscle contraction also can be regulated by circulating hormones and (in the smaller vessels) by tissue metabolic factors.

The *tunica adventitia* (outermost layer) consists of a relatively thin layer of connective tissue that provides shape for the blood vessels. This layer also houses the vasa vasorum, the small arteries, and veins that provide nutrients to the cells of the blood vessel.

●●● VASCULAR SEGMENTS

As blood exits the left ventricle, it passes progressively through the aorta, arteries, arterioles, capillaries, venules, veins, and vena cava before returning to the right atrium. These vascular segments have significant functional differences.

Arteries and Arterioles

An extensive network of arteries and arterioles branch off of the aorta and distribute the cardiac output throughout the body. Arteries, particularly the aorta, have an extensive elastic tissue layer. This elastic tissue stretches during ventricular ejection. When the aortic valve closes and ventricular ejection stops, recoil of the elastic tissue slows the fall of arterial pressure during the interval until the next period of ventricular ejection. Blood vessels become stiffer with age and with atherosclerosis, contributing to the rise in systolic arterial blood pressure usually seen in older adults.

Arterioles contain a high proportion of vascular smooth muscle. Arteriolar diameter is a major component of total peripheral resistance, and the contraction of vascular smooth muscle decreases vascular diameter and increases vascular resistance. The degree of contraction of vascular smooth muscle is determined by background activity of the autonomic nervous system, primarily the sympathetic nerves. In addition, circulating hormones such as epinephrine, norepinephrine, and angiotensin can also contract smooth muscle.

Microcirculation Vasculature

The microcirculation consists of the small arterioles, the capillary beds, and the small venules (Fig. 8-2). The smooth muscle of the small arterioles is contracted by sympathetic nerves. The precapillary sphincters (the last band of smooth muscle before the capillaries) respond primarily to local factors. Blood passes from arterioles into capillaries (5 to 10 μm in diameter). The capillary diameter approaches that of the red blood cell (7 μm). Capillaries are the major site of exchange of nutrients and wastes between the blood and the tissues. Capillaries have only a tunica intima (see Fig. 8-1), and the narrow wall facilitates exchange by diffusion.

In tissues such as the skin, blood can also pass from arterioles to venules through metarterioles. Metarterioles are not exchange vessels but serve a separate role. Blood flowing through metarterioles can bypass the true capillaries. This allows a high volume of blood to flow through the skin. Increased blood flow through cutaneous metarterioles helps the body eliminate excess heat, and decreased flow enhances heat conservation.

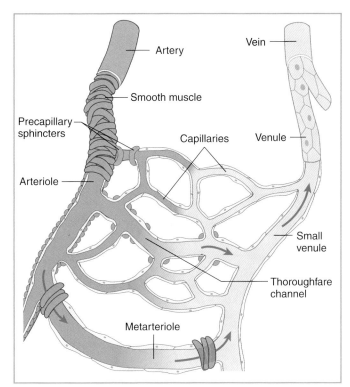

Figure 8-2. The microcirculation is a network of small blood vessels, the smallest of which are the capillaries. Blood flows from the arteries into the arterioles and can pass into the venules through one of three routes: the true capillaries, thoroughfare channels, or metarteriole (arteriovenous bypass) channels. The precapillary sphincter, a circular band of smooth muscle, regulates the flow of blood into the true capillaries.

Venules and Veins

Venules (10 to 100 μm in diameter) collect blood from the capillaries in a convergent flow pattern. Venule smooth muscle is innervated by sympathetic nerves. Along with the veins, venules serve as capacitance (volume storage) vessels, containing two thirds of the circulating blood volume. Permeability of the postcapillary venules is controlled by hormones such as histamine and bradykinin. Postcapillary venules are also the site for the initiation of angiogenesis.

Veins are the capacitance vessels of the circulation. Sympathetic nerve activity constricts the smooth muscle of the veins. This constriction does not impart a physiologically significant resistance to flow, but it does reduce the capacitance of the veins. The consequence of venoconstriction is that the blood storage capacity is diminished and blood flows more easily toward the right atrium. Because of the low venous pressure, venous blood flow is subject to gravitational influences. Valves in the larger veins ensure that blood flow is always toward the heart. Damage to venous valves can cause swellings, such as varicose veins, and lack of leg muscle movement can lead to venous stasis and clotting. During exercise, venous blood flow is assisted by the drop in intra-

thoracic pressure during deep inspiration and by extravascular compression of veins in the exercising skeletal muscle.

Lymphatics

Lymphatics are a network of endothelial tubes that merge to form two large systems that enter the veins. Lymph from the right side of the head, right trunk, and right arm drains into the right lymphatic duct. Lymph from the remainder of the body drains into the thoracic duct, which empties into the thoracic vena cava.

Terminal lymphatics (Fig. 8-3) lack tight junctions, allowing large proteins (and metastasizing cancer cells) to enter the circulatory system through the lymphatic system. Lymph composition closely resembles interstitial fluid composition. In the GI tract, lymphatics allow digested fats to enter the circulation. Lymph is propelled by (1) massaging from adjacent muscle, (2) tissue pressure, and (3) contraction of the lymph vessels. Valves ensure that the flow of lymph is toward the vena cava. Over 24 hours, the volume of lymph flow in the body is equal to approximately 5 L, the same as the total blood volume. Lymph is filtered in lymph nodes before progressing back to the circulation.

●●● HEMODYNAMICS

Hemodynamics describes the physical behavior of blood as a fluid. Hemodynamics examines the interrelationships between flow, pressure gradients, resistance, vessel cross-sectional area, and velocity. These relationships determine arterial pressure, cardiac output, and tissue blood flow, as well as explaining the appearance of murmurs and bruits.

Terms

Q = flow = volume movement with respect to time
P = pressure = force exerted over a surface divided by its area
R = resistance = impediment to flow, expressed in resistance units
V = velocity = distance traveled with respect to time
A = area = cross-sectional area

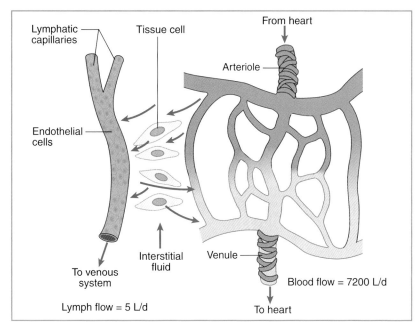

Figure 8-3. Lymphatic vessels originate in the tissues and collect the small volume of fluid that is filtered but not reabsorbed by capillaries. Lymph entering the lymphatic vessels is filtered at a lymph node before being transported into the veins.

Relationship Between above Terms

$$Q = (P_1 - P_2)/R \qquad (1)$$

or, flow = pressure gradient/resistance, or for the peripheral circulation, cardiac output = (mean arterial pressure – right atrial pressure)/total peripheral resistance.

This interaction is complex, since a change in any one component can impact the other two. For example, the regulation of arterial pressure depends on the ability to control both cardiac output and total peripheral resistance:

$$V = Q/A \qquad (2)$$

or, velocity of blood flow = blood flow/cross-sectional area.

Regions with a local narrowing of the blood vessel, such as caused by atherosclerotic plaques, have a high velocity of flow. High-velocity blood flow can generate turbulence, which increases the chance of clot formation. High velocity can also create shear on the vessel wall, and damage to the endothelium contributes to the development of aortic aneurysms.

Lateral pressure, which provides the pressure for vessels that branch from the aorta at right angles, drops when velocity increases. For example, perfusion pressure decreases when an artery branches near the site of a stenosis. In addition, perfusion pressure is decreased in vessels arising from the root of the aorta because of the high velocity of blood flow in this area during ventricular ejection.

Blood vessel radius is a primary determinant of vascular resistance and blood flow. Poiseuille's law identifies four factors that control the flow of fluids through cylindrical tubes: the difference in pressure between the ends of the tube, the fourth power of radius, viscosity, and the length of the tube. Although in the vascular system some underlying assumptions are not met, the equation provides a useful description of the regulation of blood flow. For example, a small change in radius has a marked effect on blood flow, reflecting the fact that flow is proportionate to (radius)[4] (Fig. 8-4).

Resistance to flow is based on the anatomic arrangement of vessels. The renal and splanchnic circulations have the resistances arranged in series. For these vessels, $R_{total} = \Sigma R_{individual}$. Blood flowing through vessels in series has to pass through each vessel in the series, so increasing resistance to blood flow in any one vessel in the series will increase the total resistance to blood flow.

The aorta and most other vascular beds have the resistances arranged in parallel. For these vessels, $1/R_{total} = \Sigma 1/R_{individual}$. In this arrangement, blood has a number of routes to exit the aorta. Opening a new exit route will make it easier for blood to exit the aorta, so adding a new resistance actually decreases the total resistance of the system.

Flow in the vascular system can be organized in laminar or turbulent patterns. Laminar (streamline) flow moves in concentric circles, fastest at the center of tube. Turbulent flow is disorganized and requires more energy to travel the same distance as laminar flow. The chance of turbulent flow increases with increased velocity; e.g., atherosclerotic plaques narrow the blood vessels and can cause turbulence. Decreased blood density, such as caused by anemia, can also cause turbulence. Turbulent flow is audible as a murmur in the heart or bruit in the peripheral circulation.

Viscosity is a measure of the tendency of a fluid to resist displacement. It is due primarily to red blood cells, so blood viscosity is proportional to hematocrit. Viscous drag increases as velocity increases, so high velocity of blood flow in the aorta can tear the endothelial surface and cause a dissecting aneurysm. In capillaries, the apparent viscosity is lower than otherwise predicted owing to the red blood cells

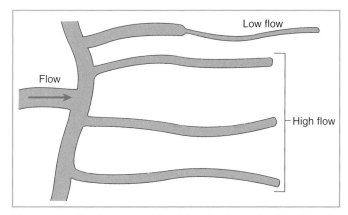

Figure 8-4. Resistance to blood flow is determined by blood vessel diameter and organization. A reduction in diameter reduces flow only through that vessel. The large arteries that exit the aorta are organized as a parallel resistance. Constriction of one of these vessels will reduce flow only to the tissues perfused by that vessel, and shunt flow toward the tissues perfused by the nonconstricted vessels.

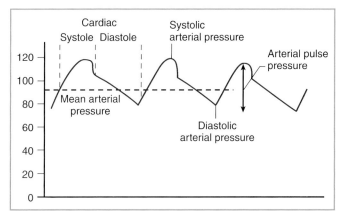

Figure 8-5. The systolic component of the arterial pressure waveform is caused by the ejection of blood from the ventricle and by the stretching of the elastic tissue of the aorta and large arteries. The diastolic component of the arterial pressure waveform is determined by the rate of blood flow from the aorta and by the elastic recoil of the aorta and large arteries.

PATHOLOGY

Cardiac Murmurs

Damage to cardiac valves leads to turbulent blood flow, which can be heard through a stethoscope. The normal heart sounds are used to identify the position (open or closed) of the cardiac valve. Each valve has a location on the chest where it is best heard through the stethoscope. Murmurs that occur when the valve is normally open are attributed to a stenotic or narrowed valve. Murmurs that occur when the valve is normally closed are attributed to regurgitation or to retrograde flow of blood through the valve.

flowing close to the center of the vessel and to plasma flowing adjacent to the endothelial cells.

Pressure-volume curves reflect the compliance, or distensibility, of vessels. Arteries have low compliance. Consequently, small volume changes cause marked pressure changes. Veins have high compliance. Consequently, even large volume changes cause only small changes in pressure. In cardiovascular control, contraction of arterial smooth muscle will affect primarily pressure, whereas contracting venous smooth muscle will affect primarily volume. Vascular compliance characteristics decrease with age owing to "hardening of the arteries," or atherosclerosis.

Laplace's law calculates the force pushing outward against the wall of a vessel. The simplified version of this relationship is

$$T = Pr$$

or, transmural tension equals pressure times radius.

Capillaries have a very small radius and do not rupture when containing blood at 20 mm Hg pressure because of the low transmural tension directed against their walls. In contrast, the increase in diameter in dilated hearts results in an even greater transmural tension on the ventricular wall than would be predicted from the ventricular pressure alone.

Arterial Blood Pressure

Blood in the arteries exhibits a cyclic change in pressure (Fig. 8-5). Arterial pressure is a function of the volume of blood entering the arteries (both stroke volume and heart rate), the volume exiting the arteries (determined by peripheral resistance), and the compliance of the arterial vessels. Arterial pressure is reported as systolic pressure, diastolic pressure, mean arterial pressure, and arterial pulse pressure (Table 8-1).

Systolic arterial pressure is the highest pressure recorded in the arteries during the cardiac cycle. It occurs during ventricular systole and is determined in part by ventricular stroke volume. Diastolic pressure is the lowest pressure recorded in the arteries during a cardiac cycle. It occurs just before the opening of the aortic valve and is determined in part by heart rate and by the rate of blood flow out of the arteries, a function of peripheral resistance.

Mean arterial pressure is the time-average pressure in the arteries. Mean arterial pressure can be approximated as

$$\text{MAP} = P_{\text{diastolic}} + \tfrac{1}{3} \text{ pulse pressure}$$

Pulse pressure is the difference between the peak systolic and the diastolic pressure. The arterial pulse pressure is altered by stroke volume, which preferentially affects systolic pressure; by heart rate and peripheral resistance, which preferentially affect diastolic pressure; and by a decrease in compliance, which increases systolic and decreases diastolic pressures.

Arterial blood pressure can be measured directly or estimated indirectly. Direct measurement is invasive and

TABLE 8-1. Blood Pressure and O_2 Content in the Cardiovascular System

	Systolic (mm Hg)	Diastolic (mm Hg)	Mean (mm Hg)	O_2 Content (mL O_2/100 mL blood)
Right atrium	—	—	0–5	15%
Right ventricle	25–30	0–5	—	15%
Pulmonary artery	25–30	10–15	15–25	15%
Pulmonary capillaries	—	—	10–15	15%–19%
Pulmonary vein	—	—	5–10	19%
Left atrium	—	—	5–10	19%
Left ventricle	100–140	5–10	—	19%
Systemic arteries	100–140	70–90	100	19%
Systemic capillaries	30–40	15–20	17	19%–15%
Extrathoracic veins	—	—	10–20	15%
Intrathoracic veins	—	—	0–10	15%

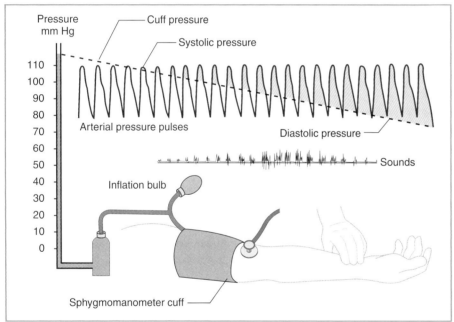

Figure 8-6. Indirect estimation of blood pressure makes use of a sphygmomanometer and a stethoscope. A characteristic sequence of sounds is heard from a stethoscope placed downstream from the sphygmomanometer. The pressure in the blood sphygmomanometer cuff when the first sound is heard is recorded as the systolic arterial pressure. The cuff pressure when the last sound is heard is recorded as the diastolic arterial pressure.

costly. A fluid-filled catheter is introduced into the blood vessel and connected to a pressure transducer and recording device. Alternatively, a small pressure transducer can be inserted directly into the blood vessel, eliminating the need for a catheter. This approach requires careful calibration of the transducer and is subject to possible error due to catheter orientation.

Indirect estimation makes use of a sphygmomanometer (blood pressure cuff) and a stethoscope to identify the Korotkoff sounds (Fig. 8-6). The Korotkoff sounds are an example of a "water-hammer pulse," generated by a moving column of fluid impacting a stationary column of fluid. As the cuff is inflated to a pressure higher than the systolic arterial pressure, the brachial artery is occluded. When cuff pressure falls below systolic arterial pressure, the brachial artery is

occluded for only a portion of the arterial pressure pulse. Turbulence is generated when blood from the heart side of the cuff impacts the stationary blood downstream of the cuff. This results in an audible event and the reappearance of a pulse in the wrist. The cuff pressure at this time is the estimation of systolic arterial pressure. As the cuff pressure is slowly lowered, the brachial artery is occluded for only a portion of the time. The Korotkoff sounds crescendo and become muffled. When the cuff pressure is lower than the diastolic pressure, the brachial artery remains open for the entire arterial pressure pulse, and no sound in generated. The cuff pressure at the time of the last sound is an estimation of diastolic arterial pressure. Normal arterial blood pressure measurement reports both systolic pressure and diastolic pressure.

•••• MICROCIRCULATION

Transcapillary Exchange

Delivery of nutrients to the tissues and removal of waste products from the tissues require both blood flow and exchange between the tissue and the blood. Blood flow in the microcirculation is largely determined by local control but also is influenced by neural and humoral components. Transcapillary exchange of nutrients and wastes is a function of the substance's chemical structure and is governed by the processes of diffusion, filtration, and pinocytosis.

Diffusion is quantitatively the most important process and is described by Fick's law:

$$J = -DA \frac{\Delta c}{\Delta x}$$

where J = net flux of a compound, or diffusional movement; – = movement down the concentration gradient; D = diffusion coefficient, a function of the compound and the barrier; A = surface area available for exchange; Δc = concentration gradient; and Δx = distance.

This equation illustrates that diffusion movement is directly proportionate to surface area and the concentration gradient and that diffusion movement is inversely proportionate to distance. Diffusion is influenced by permeability across the barrier, and for transcapillary exchange, movement is influenced by solubility in lipid cell membrane or water (Fig. 8-7).

Filtration and reabsorption at the capillary occur in accordance with the balance of hydrostatic and osmotic pressures, as described in the Starling hypothesis:

$$\text{Filtration force} = k[(P_c + \pi_i) - (P_i + \pi_c)]$$

where k = permeability coefficient; P_c = hydrostatic (blood) pressure in the capillary; π_i = oncotic pressure in the interstitial fluid; P_i = hydrostatic pressure in the interstitial fluid; and π_c = oncotic pressure in the capillary from plasma proteins.

Filtration occurs at the arteriolar end of the capillaries, and reabsorption at the venular end of the capillaries. The balance of hydrostatic and colloid osmotic pressures favors filtration at the arteriolar end of the capillaries. The drop in pressure along the length of the capillary reverses this balance, and absorption occurs at the venous end of the capillaries (Fig. 8-8). Any change in hydrostatic pressure or colloid osmotic pressure can change the fluid balance between the capillaries in the tissues.

Pinocytosis through cells represents a pathway for the exit for high-molecular-weight proteins, such as albumin. Pinocytosis does not significantly contribute to the reabsorption of proteins owing to the relatively small protein concentration in the interstitial fluid.

Interstitial Fluid Pressure and Volume

Fluid pressure in the interstitial spaces is usually negative (as low as −6 mm Hg). Interstitial fluid is moved back to the

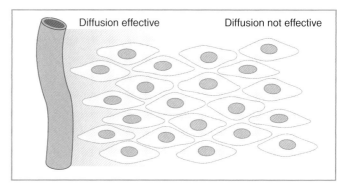

Figure 8-7. Diffusion limits delivery of compounds with poor permeability. The effectiveness of diffusion decreases as the distance from the blood vessel increases.

plasma by reabsorption in the capillaries and by transport within lymph vessels. Lymph flow increases as the accumulation of fluid in the interstitial spaces increases interstitial fluid pressure. Maximum lymph flow can be limited because the interstitial fluid pressure acts to compresses the lymphatic vessels. At this point, any further increase in interstitial fluid pressure also results in compression of the lymph vessels.

Lymph flow is increased by a number of factors: increase in capillary pressure, increase in capillary surface area, increase in capillary permeability, decrease in plasma colloid osmotic pressure, and increase in interstitial fluid protein concentration. As predicted by the Starling hypothesis, all these changes also increase net capillary filtration and increase fluid transfer into the interstitial space. Lymph flow assists in the removal of this excess fluid and prevents excess fluid accumulation.

Edema is an excessive accumulation of fluid in the tissue spaces resulting from an imbalance in microcirculatory fluid exchange. Multiple possible mechanisms can result in edema. Heart failure (congestive heart failure) elevates capillary pressure. Obstruction of the veins increases capillary pressure. Protein wasting syndrome decreases plasma oncotic pressure. Inflammation increases capillary permeability, affecting both the permeability coefficient and the plasma colloid osmotic pressures. Malnutrition and toxic substances decrease albumin synthesis, thereby lowering plasma oncotic pressure. All these events can lead to formation of edema (Box 8-1).

Edema usually does not occur because interstitial fluid pressure is very low. Lymph flow increases as interstitial pressure increases, which drains the interstitial spaces. Increased lymph flow also causes a washout of protein in the interstitial space, decreasing interstitial fluid colloid osmotic pressure. In contrast, chronic lymphatic obstruction traps albumin in the interstitial spaces and increases interstitial fluid oncotic pressure and interstitial fluid volume, leading to edema.

Local Control of Blood Flow

In most tissues, blood flow is tightly coupled to metabolic need. Accumulation of metabolites relaxes vascular smooth muscle, with the subsequent increase in blood flow assisting

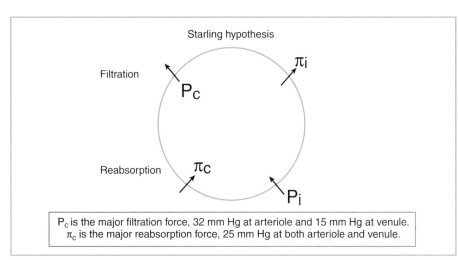

Starling hypothesis

Filtration

P_c

π_i

Reabsorption

π_c

P_i

P_c is the major filtration force, 32 mm Hg at arteriole and 15 mm Hg at venule.
π_c is the major reabsorption force, 25 mm Hg at both arteriole and venule.

A

Figure 8-8. A, Filtration of fluid at the capillary is increased by increases in capillary hydrostatic pressure or interstitial fluid oncotic pressure. Reabsorption is increased by increases in capillary oncotic pressure or by increases in interstitial fluid pressure. **B**, The balance between hydrostatic and colloid osmotic pressures favors filtration at the arteriolar end of the capillaries. The drop in pressure along the length of the capillary reverses this balance, and absorption occurs at the venous end of the capillaries. Any change in hydrostatic pressure or colloid osmotic pressure can change the fluid balance between the capillaries in the tissues.

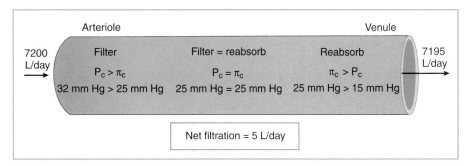

Arteriole

Venule

7200 L/day

Filter
$P_c > \pi_c$
32 mm Hg > 25 mm Hg

Filter = reabsorb
$P_c = \pi_c$
25 mm Hg = 25 mm Hg

Reabsorb
$\pi_c > P_c$
25 mm Hg > 15 mm Hg

7195 L/day

Net filtration = 5 L/day

B

Angiogenesis Inhibitors

Angiogenesis inhibitors have been used experimentally to limit the growth of solid tumors. Cancer cells have a high metabolic rate, and as the tumor grows, new blood vessels must be formed to allow nutrient flow to the tumor. Disruption of blood vessel growth prevents the cancer cells from receiving sufficient blood flow.

in the removal of the excess metabolites. Notable agents that couple metabolism and vasodilation are adenosine, especially for the heart, and H^+, especially for the brain. Depletion of nutrients such as O_2 also relaxes vascular smooth muscle. The vasodilation is limited to the area producing the excess metabolites. As the elevated blood flow washes out vasodilators, vascular resistance returns to normal.

The metabolic regulation of blood flow accounts for observations of active hyperemia, reactive hyperemia, and in part, autoregulation. Active hyperemia is the increase in blood flow in metabolically active tissue. Reactive hyperemia (Fig. 8-9) is the increase in blood flow observed following release of an occlusion. Interruption of blood flow to tissue results in depletion of nutrients and buildup of metabolites. These events cause dilation of the vasculature. After blood flow is restored, there is a period of enhanced blood flow (reactive hyperemia), which helps wash out the accumulated metabolites.

In both active and reactive hyperemia, blood flow is inadequate to match tissue metabolic needs, and the accumulating metabolites cause local vasodilation. Once the metabolites have been washed out, the vasodilatory stimulus is no longer present, and the vascular resistance returns to control levels.

Angiogenesis provides a long-term matching of blood flow with metabolic needs. Capillary density is proportionate to tissue metabolic activity. Tissue hypertrophy and hyperplasia are accompanied by new vessel growth. Angiogenesis inhibitors are used to restrict blood vessel growth in highly metabolic tumors.

Autoregulation is prominent in the cerebral, coronary, and renal circulations. For these tissues, blood flow remains constant over a wide range of blood pressure (Fig. 8-10). Three hypotheses are advanced to account for autoregulation. The metabolic supposition ties blood flow to metabolic needs, so that excess blood flow removes the vasodilator metabolites. The tissue pressure hypothesis proposes that high blood flow increases filtration into interstitial space, causing extravascular compression of the vessels to increase vascular resistance. The myogenic premise states that vascular smooth muscle contracts as a result of high wall tension, as described by Laplace's law. Evidence for the above hypotheses is present in at least one type of tissue.

Box 8-1. MECHANISMS OF EDEMA

Excessive filtration

Capillary permeability
  Histamine
Elevated capillary hydrostatic pressure
  Arteriolar dilation
    Exercise
    Septic shock
  Venous congestion
    Venous blockage
    Cardiac failure
    Varicose veins
Elevated interstitial fluid oncotic pressure
  Protein exudation following histamine release
  Protein leaking following physical damage to capillaries

Impaired reabsorption

Decreased plasma oncotic pressure
  Protein malnutrition
  Liver disease
  Kidney disease
  Hypothyroid myxedema
  Crystalloid resuscitation from hemorrhage

Impaired lymphatic drainage

Physical damage to lymphatics
  Surgery
Blockage of lymph nodes
  Lymphatic filariasis (elephantiasis)

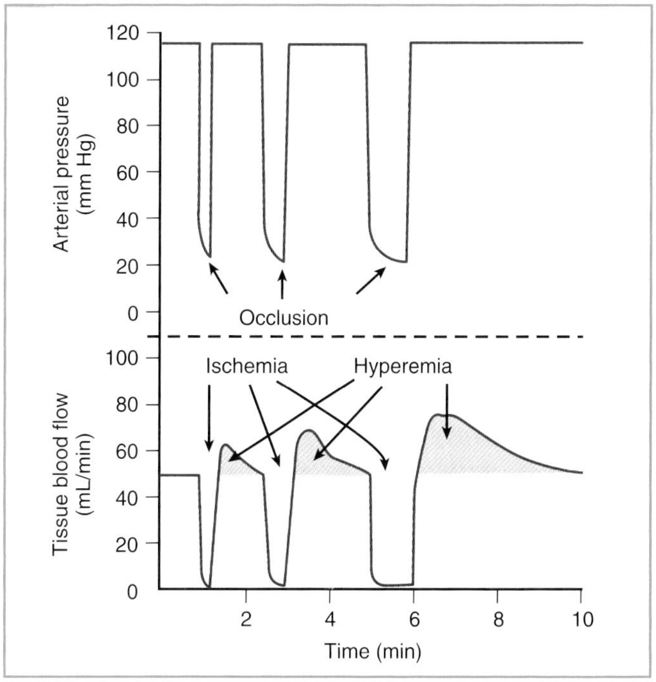

Figure 8-9. Occlusion of blood vessels causes a reduction in arterial pressure and a consequent decrease in tissue perfusion. When the occlusion is released, there is a rebound increase in blood flow that exceeds the starting level. This reactive hyperemic response helps wash out metabolites accumulated during the period of ischemia and is proportionate to the period of time that the tissue blood flow was diminished.

●●● NEURAL AND HORMONAL REGULATION OF VASCULATURE

To be effective, local metabolic control of blood flow requires sufficiently high arterial pressure. Arterial blood pressure is regulated by numerous redundant neural and humoral control systems.

The arterial baroreceptor reflex is a negative-feedback mechanism that helps maintain arterial blood pressure (Fig. 8-11). The arterial baroreceptors are stretch-sensitive nerve endings in the aortic arch and carotid sinus. As stretch receptors, a decrease in blood pressure reduces the rate of firing and an increase in blood pressure increases the rate of firing.

Afferent nerves carry this information to the cardio-vascular control centers of the medulla, where it is integrated.

The SNS and PNS constitute the efferent component of the reflex. The SNS regulates arteriolar resistance, impacting the arterial pressure. The SNS also regulates cardiac contractility, while the PNS regulates heart rate. Finally, the SNS regulates venous capacitance by venoconstriction. A drop in arterial blood pressure leads to an increase in SNS activity and a decrease in PNS activity, both of which should act to help restore blood pressure to normal.

In addition to arterial blood pressure, the circulating blood volume is regulated. Cardiopulmonary "volume" receptors

PHARMACOLOGY

Adrenergic Receptors

Adrenergic receptors are characterized as alpha (α) or beta (β) based on their pharmacologic characteristics. α-Adrenergic receptors are further subdivided into α_1 and α_2 receptors. α_1-Receptors are found on vascular smooth muscle, heart, and prostate, and α_2 receptors are found on presynaptic nerve terminals, platelets, fat cells, and some vascular smooth muscle. β-Adrenergic receptors are subdivided into β_1-receptors on myocardium; β_2-receptors on respiratory, uterine, and vascular smooth muscle, skeletal muscle, and liver; and β_3-receptors on adipose tissue.

are located in the cardiac atria, low-pressure veins, and pulmonary circulation. These volume receptors help regulate urinary volume excretion through both neural and hormonal systems.

Vascular Smooth Muscle Tone

Vascular smooth muscle contraction is determined by the balance of intrinsic, humoral, and nervous system inputs. Basal vascular smooth muscle tone results from a constant

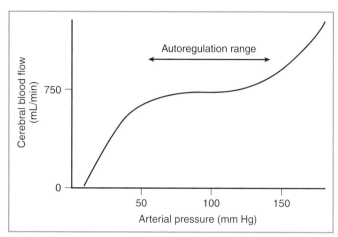

Figure 8-10. Normally, blood flow is proportionate to blood pressure. The brain and some other tissues exhibit autoregulation, whereby blood flow remains fairly constant over a wide range of arterial pressures. Autoregulation is mediated by metabolic control of blood flow and is well developed in the coronary and cerebral circulations.

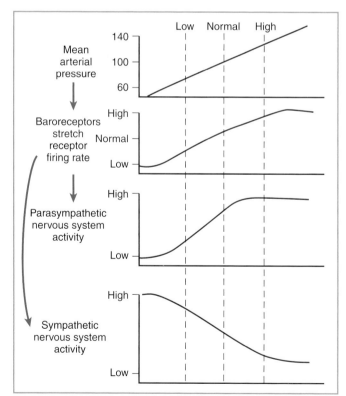

Figure 8-11. The arterial baroreceptors are stretch-sensitive nerve endings in the aortic arch and carotid sinus. A decrease in blood pressure reduces their rate of firing, and an increase in blood pressure increases their rate of firing. The SNS and PNS are the efferent arms of the baroreceptor reflex. A drop in arterial blood pressure leads to a decrease in PNS activity and an increase in SNS activity, both of which should act to help restore blood pressure to normal.

background of autonomic nerve activity, and the degree of contraction is modulated by other factors.

Vascular smooth muscle tone is partially self-determined by the stress-relaxation response. Most vascular smooth muscle tone is due to external factors such as the SNS and PNS (as described above) and humoral agents.

Epinephrine exerts a biphasic cardiovascular effect. Epinephrine stimulates β_2-adrenergic receptors, causing vasodilation. Epinephrine also stimulates α_1-adrenergic receptors, causing vasoconstriction. β_2-Adrenergic receptors are more sensitive than α_1-adrenergic receptors, so vasodilation is seen at low epinephrine doses. α_1-Adrenergic receptors are more numerous than β_2-adrenergic receptors, so vasoconstriction is seen at high epinephrine doses.

Angiotensin II is a powerful vasoconstrictor. Angiotensin II is formed by the sequential actions of renin and angiotensin-converting enzyme. Renin release is the rate-limiting step in angiotensin II formation. Renin is released from the kidney by numerous factors, including hypotension, renal sympathetic activity, and low plasma Na^+.

Humoral vasodilators include histamine, bradykinin, and serotonin. These agents generally act locally. However, in anaphylactic shock, a massive release of histamine from mast cells can cause severe hypotension.

The SNS constricts the vascular smooth muscle of the arteries and the veins by activating α_1-adrenergic receptors. Arteriolar vasoconstriction increases arterial pressure. The vasoconstriction decreases blood flow through vessel and consequently increases the volume of blood remaining in arteries. Venoconstriction decreases venous capacitance. This increases venous return and therefore cardiac output.

The SNS is tonically active; this is called sympathetic vasomotor tone. A decrease in basal SNS activity decreases vasomotor tone and dilates the blood vessels. Sympathetic cholinergic nerves innervate sweat glands and can act indirectly to vasodilate by inducing bradykinin release from sweat glands.

The PNS has a limited role in control of peripheral vasculature. Parasympathetic nerves innervate a limited number of vessels in viscera, the face, and pelvic organs but play an important role in sexual arousal. Acetylcholine causes release of EDRF (nitric oxide) from the vascular endothelial cells and therefore can vasodilate indirectly.

PATHOLOGY

Edema

Edema is the accumulation of free fluid in the interstitial space or within body cavities. Edema can result from excessive filtration of fluid from the capillaries, impaired absorption of fluid back into the capillaries, or impaired drainage of interstitial fluid through the lymphatic vessels.

Central Nervous System Integration

SNS and PNS outflow is coordinated in the cardiovascular centers of the medulla. The dorsolateral medulla initiates responses that raise blood pressure, and the ventromedial medulla initiates responses that lower blood pressure. Medullary cardiovascular centers receive descending input from cerebral cortex, thalamus, hypothalamus, and diencephalon (Fig. 8-12).

A variety of afferent inputs impact cardiovascular control. Arterial baroreceptors regulate both sympathetic and parasympathetic activity. Cardiopulmonary volume receptors selectively control renal sympathetic nerves and also antidiuretic hormone release. Peripheral chemoreceptors of the aortic body and carotid body mediate effects of blood gas changes on the SNS. Central chemoreceptors respond to high CO_2 with general sympathetic activation, as seen in the central nervous system (CNS) ischemic response and in Cushing's reflex. The hypothalamus has some direct effects,

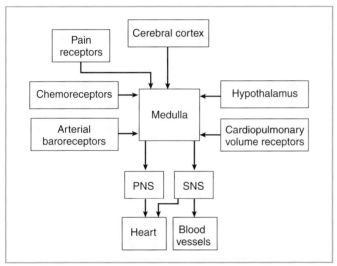

Figure 8-12. The cardiovascular centers of the medulla integrate multiple cardiovascular inputs to regulate SNS and PNS outflow. The arterial baroreceptor and cardiopulmonary volume receptor inputs help maintain a normal blood pressure. Other CNS inputs allow blood pressure to adjust to meet new demands, such as exercise.

notably body temperature–sensitive control of cutaneous circulation. Output from the cerebrum normally is pressor but occasionally is depressor, e.g., blushing and fainting. Pain fibers can elicit diverse cardiovascular responses: skin pain often is pressor and visceral pain often is depressor.

●●● CIRCULATION IN SPECIFIC VASCULAR BEDS

Blood flow serves multiple functions. Matching of blood flow to metabolic needs is complex in organs that have variable metabolic rates, such as skeletal muscle. Local regulation of blood flow is well developed in tissues that have a low tolerance for ischemia, such as the brain and the heart. Some regional circulations serve functions other than tissue nutrition. For example, the cutaneous circulation assists in the regulation of body temperature, the renal circulation transports waste products to the kidneys for elimination, the splanchnic circulation transports absorbed intestinal nutrients, and the pulmonary circulation assists gas exchange. The unique cardiovascular characteristics of tissues are tied tightly to tissue function.

There is extensive sympathetic control of cutaneous vascular smooth muscle and therefore cutaneous blood flow. A decrease in body core temperature leads to vasoconstriction, which decreases the radiant loss of heat. Conversely, an increased body core temperature dilates the arteriovenous anastomoses, increasing cutaneous blood flow, and thereby increasing the radiant loss of heat (Fig. 8-13).

Sympathetic cholinergic nerves innervate cutaneous sweat glands. Activation of these nerves facilitates heat loss through evaporation and indirectly dilates cutaneous vessels via bradykinin release from the sweat glands. CNS output regulates cutaneous vascular smooth muscle in vessels of the head, neck, and shoulders and can cause blushing. A countercurrent heat exchange mechanism in the arms and legs assists thermoregulation. Cool (venous) blood from extremities is warmed as it returns to the body core, and warm (arterial) blood from the body core is cooled as it flows to the extremities. In this way, blood flow to cold extremities, such as feet, hands, and ears, can be maintained to provide adequate delivery of nutrition without compromising temperature regulation.

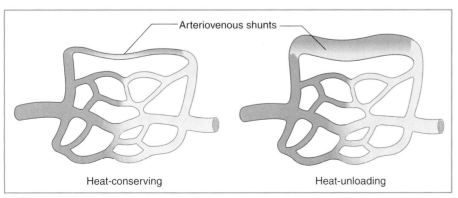

Heat-conserving   Heat-unloading

Figure 8-13. The cutaneous microcirculation consists of capillaries to nurture the skin cells and arteriovenous shunts to assist in thermoregulation. Sympathetic nerves supplying the arteriovenous shunts are controlled by the temperature-sensitive regions of the hypothalamus. Vasodilation of the shunts increases cutaneous blood flow and helps transfer heat away from the body.

Skeletal muscle blood flow is proportionate to metabolic activity. Only 20% of skeletal muscle capillaries are perfused at rest (Fig. 8-14). Skeletal muscle blood flow can increase tenfold during exercise. In resting skeletal muscle, sympathetic adrenergic nerves constrict the vasculature and reduce blood flow. Local metabolic control normally is the most powerful, and local vasodilation can override neural regulation during exercise.

Cerebral circulation provides a constant blood supply to the CNS. Multiple inflows from paired internal carotid arteries, vertebral arteries, and spinal arteries join to form the circle of Willis. The CNS is enclosed in a rigid cranium, so inflow must equal outflow or pressure may increase and damage the CNS tissue. CNS tissue is sensitive to blood flow interruption. After 5 seconds of interruption, a person becomes unconscious, and after 5 minutes, irreversible tissue damage occurs.

Cerebral blood flow regulation is primarily local, so blood flow in discrete brain areas is proportionate to metabolism. CNS autoregulation of blood flow is well developed. The CNS ischemic response is the most powerful activator of sympathetic nerves, occurring when blood pressure falls below 60 mm Hg or increased intracranial pressure prevents blood entry into cranium, called the Cushing reflex.

Splanchnic blood vessels are arranged partly in series, since the GI, spleen, and pancreas capillary beds empty into the hepatic portal vein. Intestinal blood flow is regulated by the SNS. This allows shunting of blood during the fight or flight response. A small amount of local control is seen. Intestinal blood flow also is directly influenced by GI hormones, such as vasoactive intestinal polypeptide (VIP).

Unique blood flow pathways transport intestinal blood to the liver sinusoids before the blood enters the general circulation (Fig. 8-15). Normally 25% of the cardiac output goes to the liver in two vessels. The hepatic portal vein carries three quarters of the blood entering the liver, and the hepatic artery carries the remaining one quarter. The hepatic artery provides most of the O_2 consumed by the liver. Both the hepatic artery and portal vein empty into a hepatic acinus. Blood flows outward from the acinus to sinusoids to hepatic veins.

The hepatic circulation has a low blood pressure. Ascites results from increased liver sinus capillary pressure, usually secondary to increased central venous pressure. The liver is an important capacitance organ and has 15% of total blood volume, half of which can be expelled under stress.

The spleen also has sinuses rather than true capillaries. The spleen stores red blood cells, and it filters and destroys fragile red blood cells. As red blood cells age, they become more rigid. Passage through the spleen deforms the red blood cells and ruptures those that are rigid.

The coronary blood flow is tightly coupled to the workload of the cardiac muscle. Cardiac muscle is almost exclusively aerobic. O_2 extraction by cardiac tissue is high, so increased O_2 delivery is accomplished only by increasing blood flow. Consequently, the myocardium is susceptible to damage if blood flow is interrupted. Autoregulation of coronary blood flow is well developed, with adenosine playing a major role as a local vasodilator metabolite.

Tension developed by the contracting muscle impedes coronary blood flow, particularly to the left ventricular endocardium, during systole. Consequently, left ventricular blood flow is highest during diastole. The right ventricle develops lower pressures and is perfused during ventricular systole (Fig. 8-16). Blood flow to the left ventricle can be compromised by the decreased diastolic duration characteristic of rapid heart rates.

Cardiac vascular smooth muscle is innervated by sympathetic nerves. The major consequence of increased sympathetic activity to the heart, however, is an increase in myocardial blood flow. Increased sympathetic nerve activity increases cardiac work, increases heart rate, and increases contractility. The increased workload on the myocardium

PATHOLOGY

Cushing's Reflex

An increase in intracranial pressure, such as caused by an intracranial hemorrhage, can compress the blood vessels leading to the brain. The increased intracranial pressure reduces cerebral perfusion, and the resultant cerebral ischemia causes massive sympathetic activation. The SNS activity increases systemic blood pressure in an effort to restore cerebral perfusion.

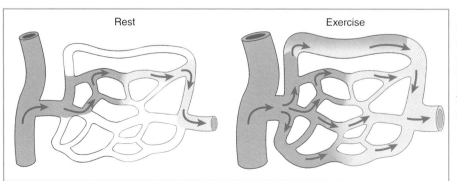

Rest   Exercise

Figure 8-14. At rest, only one fifth of skeletal muscle capillaries are perfused. During exercise, all the capillaries are perfused, and the blood flow through each capillary doubles as a result of local production of metabolites. Together, these changes increase blood flow and delivery of nutrients to exercising skeletal muscle by tenfold.

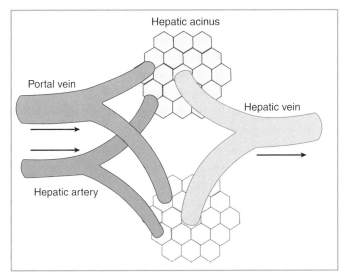

Figure 8-15. The hepatic acinus receives blood flow from both the hepatic artery and the hepatic portal vein. The portal vein carries three quarters of the blood flow to the hepatic acinus, transporting compounds absorbed from the intestines. The hepatic artery carries the remaining quarter to the hepatic acinus, bearing O_2 to support hepatic metabolism. After passing through the acinus, blood flows into the hepatic veins and into the vena cava.

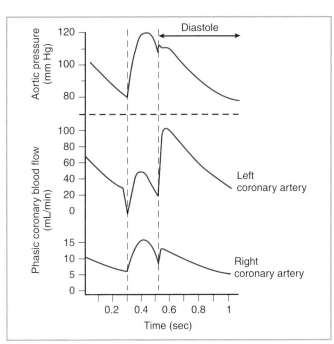

Figure 8-16. Left ventricular blood flow is highest during ventricular diastole. Pressure generated in the wall of the left ventricle during ventricular systole compresses the coronary blood vessels and limits blood flow to the muscle of the left ventricle. During diastole, the coronary blood vessels are no longer compressed and blood flow is restored. This effect is most prominent in the blood vessels supplying the left ventricular endocardial tissue. During rapid heart rates, the diastolic time is shortened, and left ventricular endocardial blood flow may be impaired.

PATHOLOGY

Myocardial Infarction

Oxygen extraction by the myocardium is high in relation to other tissues. The only way to increase the delivery of oxygen to the myocardium is to increase myocardial blood flow. If myocardial blood flow is insufficient to support myocardial metabolic need, an area of ischemia can develop and lead to myocardial infarction. Myocardial infarction can lead to disruption of normal cardiac electrical activity and cause ventricular fibrillation.

causes an adenosine-mediated vasodilation that overwhelms the slight tendency of sympathetics to constrict the myocardial vasculature.

Pulmonary circulation is characterized by low resistance to blood flow, and so pressures are much lower than in the systemic circulation. Pulmonary capillaries are arranged between alveoli so that blood flows in sheets. Pulmonary circulation functions include gas exchange, filtration of clots and other particulate matter, and enzyme activity, notably angiotensin I converting enzyme.

Blood entering the pulmonary circulation is O_2 depleted and resembles systemic venous blood. In contrast, the tracheobronchial tree is nourished by bronchial vessels of the systemic circulation, carrying oxygenated blood. Hypoxia constricts arterioles in the lung, in contrast to the hypoxic vasodilation response in peripheral arterioles. This plays a significant role in matching pulmonary ventilation and perfusion (see Chapter 10).

TOP 5 TAKE-HOME POINTS

1. The arteries are the high-pressure vessels, and the veins are the high-volume (capacitance) vessels.
2. Fluid exchange at the microcirculation depends on the balance of hydrostatic and oncotic pressures in the capillaries and interstitial spaces.
3. Tissue blood flow is regulated to match metabolic need.
4. Arterial blood pressure is controlled by a baroreceptor reflex coupling blood pressure to the activity of the SNS and PNS.
5. Extrinsic regulation is due to the sympathetic nerves and hormones such as angiotensin II and vasopressin.

Integrated Cardiovascular Function

9

The cardiovascular system is a closed circuit. As such, changes at any place in the circuit will have both upstream consequences and downstream consequences. For example, a decrease in cardiac pumping ability will cause a drop in arterial pressure but an increase in venous pressure. Consequently, it is important to understand cardiovascular changes in the context of the entire cardiovascular system.

Figure 9-1 shows the relationships among the parameters describing the cardiovascular system. Beginning from the left, individual tissue blood flow is determined by arterial blood pressure and tissue vascular resistance according to the relationship $Q = \Delta P/R$. Arterial blood pressure is determined by the cardiac output and total peripheral resistance by the same relationship, now rearranged for the whole body as $CO = AP/TPR$. Total peripheral resistance is determined by the balance of neural arteriolar vascular constriction and local arteriolar vasodilation.

Cardiac output is the volume of blood pumped by the heart per minute, the product of heart rate and stroke volume: $CO = HR \times SV$. Heart rate is a function of the pacemaker frequency, determined by both the depolarization threshold and the rate of diastolic depolarization. Chapter 7 described the role of the SNS in accelerating heart rate and of the PNS in slowing heart rate.

Stroke volume is the amount of blood pumped by the heart per contraction (end-diastolic volume – end-systolic volume). The end-systolic volume is a function of ventricular ejection, determined in part by *contractility* and impeded by the *afterload*. The end-diastolic volume (*preload*) is a measure of the filling of the ventricle, determined by ventricular distensibility and the ventricular filling pressure. Ventricular filling pressure is a function of venous capacity and the circulating blood volume.

●●● CONCEPTUAL MODEL OF CARDIOVASCULAR INTEGRATION

The interrelationships of the cardiovascular components can be shown by a conceptual model (Fig. 9-2). In this model, the heart is represented by a pump. Blood is pumped by the heart from the venous reservoir into the arteriolar reservoir. The arteriolar reservoir is narrow and high, reflecting the low compliance of the arteries. The height of the blood in the arterial reservoir reflects the arterial pressure. Blood exiting the arterial reservoir passes through a constriction, representing the total peripheral resistance produced by the arterioles. The volume of blood in the arteries and consequently arterial pressure is a function of the volume of blood entering the arteries (the cardiac output) and the volume of blood exiting the arteries (determined by total peripheral resistance).

Blood flowing past the peripheral resistance enters a venous reservoir. The venous reservoir is wide and low, reflecting the compliance of the veins. The height of the blood in the venous reservoir reflects central venous pressure. Venous pressure represents the balance of the volume entering the veins from the arteries, and the volume flowing from the veins into the right atrium.

The major determinants of arterial pressure are cardiac output and total peripheral resistance. An increase in cardiac output will cause an increase in arterial blood pressure. An increase in total peripheral resistance (arteriolar constriction) will cause a decrease in the volume of blood exiting the arteries and consequently increase arterial blood pressure.

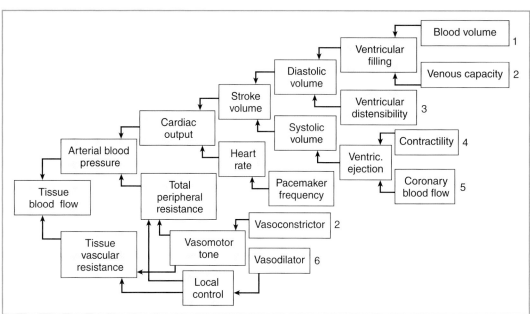

Figure 9-1. Map of the cardiovascular system. This diagram illustrates the causal relationships of various cardiovascular parameters. Blue shaded boxes indicate targets of the sympathetic nervous system. Numbers indicate initial disturbances that can lead to shock.
1, Blood or plasma loss;
2, vasodilation (neurogenic);
3, pericardial tamponade;
4, heart failure;
5, myocardial infarction;
6, peritonitis, anaphylaxis.

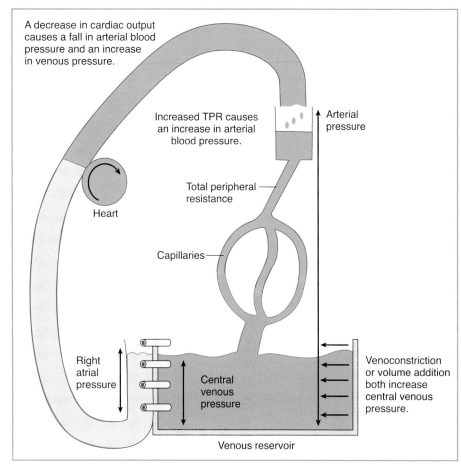

Figure 9-2. Conceptual model of the vascular system. In this diagram, blood flows from the high-pressure arteries through a point of resistance into the capillaries and then into the low-pressure venous reservoir. The heart is represented by a pump that transfers volume from the veins back to the arteries. Arterial blood pressure represents the balance between the inflow volume from cardiac output and the outflow volume past the total peripheral resistance. Venous blood pressure represents the balance of the inflow volume from the capillaries and the outflow volume pumped by the heart and also any changes caused by infusion of new blood or by constriction of the veins.

The increase in arterial pressure is often self-limited. As arterial pressure increases, it is more difficult for the heart to maintain cardiac output (because of the high afterload). This reduces the volume of blood flowing into the arteries. In addition, as arterial pressure increases, the flow past the peripheral resistance increases because of the higher pressure gradient. This increases the volume of blood that flows out of the arteries. Both events act to limit the additional volume of blood contained by the arteries and consequently attenuate the rise in arterial pressure.

The major determinants of venous blood volume, and therefore venous pressure, are total peripheral resistance and cardiac output. An increase in total peripheral resistance (arteriolar constriction) will cause a decrease in the volume of blood exiting the arteries and consequently decrease the volume of blood flowing into the veins. An increase in cardiac output will increase the volume of blood flowing from the veins into the heart and therefore decrease venous blood volume. Venous volume (pressure) can be increased by veno-constriction, which decreases the capacitance of the venous reservoir, or by addition of new volume (transfusion) into the vascular system.

The decrease in venous blood pressure is also self-limited. As venous blood pressure decreases, it is more difficult for the heart to maintain cardiac output (because of the reduced preload). The decrease in venous blood pressure does have a small effect on improving the pressure gradient for blood flow into the veins, but this effect is not physiologically significant.

The major determinants of cardiac output are preload, afterload, and contractility. Two of these determinants are vascular in nature. *Preload* is set by diastolic filling, a function of venous pressure. *Afterload* is tied most closely to arterial blood pressure. *Contractility* is not tied to the vascular system and is a characteristic of the heart alone.

●●● REGULATION

The cardiovascular system acts to deliver nutrients and to remove metabolic wastes from the tissues. The system is organized so that if there is adequate arterial pressure, tissue local control of resistance can match blood flow to tissue metabolic need (see Chapter 8).

Arterial blood pressure is the primary regulated component of the cardiovascular system. The arterial baroreceptor reflex (see Chapter 8) provides acute neural control of arterial pressure. The renal regulation of body fluid volume provides long-term control of arterial pressure (see Chapter 11). Both vascular and renal regulatory systems are augmented by endocrine control, particularly the renin-angiotensin system and antidiuretic hormone (ADH).

Blood volume is regulated to a lesser degree by an equivalent reflex, the cardiopulmonary volume receptor reflex. Control of blood volume is augmented by renal sympathetic nerves and endocrine agents such as atrial natriuretic hormone, urodilatin, and ADH. All these agents alter the renal handling of water and Na$^+$ and are described in more detail in Chapter 11.

●●● ARTERIAL HYPOTENSION AND SHOCK

Figure 9-1 also provides mechanistic insights into the multiple causes of hypotension and shock. Hypotension is caused by a cardiac output that is inadequate to maintain arterial pressure. By definition, the normal baroreceptor and other cardiovascular regulatory mechanisms could not provide compensation for the initial disturbance, or hypotension

would not occur. In using the figure, begin on the far right, and follow the sequence of events by moving to the left. Boxes not directly involved in the sequence represent possible points of compensatory changes.

Hemorrhage or plasma loss both lead to a reduction in circulating blood volume. Reduced blood volume causes a drop in ventricular filling pressure, a decrease in end-diastolic pressure, and a consequent fall in stroke volume, cardiac output, arterial pressure, and tissue perfusion. Patients in hemorrhagic shock have low blood pressure and low cerebral perfusion, causing anxiety and confusion. Compensations include activation of the SNS, leading to an increase in contractility, heart rate, and peripheral resistance. Patients in shock consequently also have an elevated heart rate and SNS-mediated cold, pale, damp (diaphoretic) skin. Vascular recovery is augmented by SNS-mediated reduction in venous capacitance and reabsorption of interstitial fluid into the vascular space, both of which help attenuate the drop in venous pressure.

Pericardial tamponade results from fluid accumulation in the pericardium acting to limit the expansion of the ventricle during the diastolic filling phase of the cardiac cycle. As shown in Figure 9-1, the reduction in diastolic volume causes a decrease in stroke volume, a decrease in cardiac output, a decrease in arterial pressure, and a decrease in tissue perfusion. The clinical presentation of patients with pericardial tamponade is similar to that of patients in hemorrhagic shock. Patients have low blood pressure and low cerebral perfusion (anxiety, confusion). Compensations include activation of the SNS, leading to an increase in contractility, heart rate, and peripheral resistance. Patients in shock consequently also have an elevated heart rate, and SNS-mediated diaphoretic skin. One difference between hemorrhage and pericardial tamponade is the ventricular filling pressure. In hemorrhage, it is low. In tamponade, it is high, and patients exhibit signs of venous congestion (elevated jugular venous pressure, hepatic enlargement).

Myocardial infarction is one of a number of clinical events that can impair myocardial contractility. Reduced contractility causes a reduced ventricular ejection, an increase in end systolic volume and reduced stroke volume, cardiac output, arterial blood pressure, and tissue perfusion. Again, the clinical presentation of patients with impaired contractility is similar to that of patients in hemorrhagic shock. Patients have low blood pressure and low cerebral perfusion, causing

Myocardial Infarction

Myocardial infarction results from inadequate perfusion of a region of the heart muscle, usually because of blockage in the coronary arteries. The damaged region of the heart shows a loss of contractility and also abnormal electrical behavior. Consequently, myocardial infarction can lead to ventricular failure, or the site of injury can serve as an abnormal electrical focus, causing ventricular fibrillation.

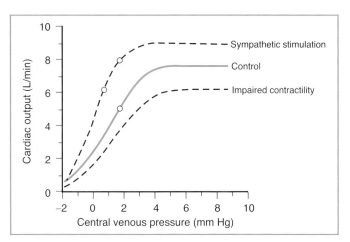

Figure 9-3. Cardiac function curves. The Frank-Starling relationship describes the increase in cardiac output due to an increase in preload on the ventricles. This cardiac function curve is shifted upward by agents that increase contractility, and downward by events that impair contractility.

anxiety and confusion. Compensations include activation of the SNS, leading to an increase in heart rate and peripheral resistance. Patients experiencing a myocardial infarction consequently have an elevated heart rate and diaphoretic skin. As is the case for pericardial tamponade, the ventricular filling pressure is high, and patients exhibit signs of venous congestion. The reduced contractility is usually limited to one ventricle. If the left ventricle is impaired, pressures in the pulmonary venous vasculature increase, and congestive heart failure develops. If contractility in the right ventricle is impaired, pressures in the systemic veins increase, causing an elevated jugular venous pressure and hepatic enlargement and possibly the formation of ascites.

Anaphylactic shock results in marked vasodilation secondary to the mast cell release of histamine. This dilates both arteriolar and venous smooth muscle. The arteriolar smooth muscle dilation causes a drop in total peripheral resistance and consequently a drop in arterial blood pressure. This is an unusual case of a high cardiac output associated with a low arterial pressure owing to the massive drop in peripheral resistance.

Disruption of sympathetic nervous system output alters numerous cardiovascular target organs and causes a pronounced hypotension from multiple causes. Clinical cases involving sympathetic nervous system dysfunction include neurogenic shock and vasovagal syncope. Decreased cardiac sympathetic activity slows heart rate and reduces ventricular contractility, both of which reduce cardiac output. Reduced sympathetic nerve activity to the vasculature causes both venodilation and arteriolar dilation. The venodilation decreases ventricular filling pressure and exacerbates the reduction in cardiac output. The arteriolar dilation reduces peripheral resistance and causes a drop in blood pressure.

●●● CARDIAC AND VASCULAR FUNCTION CURVES

As illustrated above, the relationships between cardiac output and venous pressure are particularly complex. On the one hand, an increase in venous pressure causes an increase in preload and therefore cardiac output (i.e., cardiac output and venous pressure are directly related: as one goes up, the other goes up). On the other hand, a decrease in cardiac output will cause an increase in venous pressure (i.e., venous pressure

and cardiac output are inversely related: as one goes up, the other goes down). The need to separately track cause and effect is eliminated by simultaneously plotting cardiac and vascular function curves on the same graph.

Cardiac Function Curve

Cardiac output is directly proportional to right atrial (vena cava) pressure (Fig. 9-3). The Frank-Starling relationship describes how increased preload increases cardiac pumping ability, represented by the cardiac function curve. The volume of blood actually pumped also depends on contractility and afterload, since the aortic valve must open before the heart can eject blood. The consequences of changing contractility or changing afterload are represented by shifting the curve. An increase in performance (positive inotropic effect) is graphed as an upward shift of the cardiac function curve. A decrease in performance (negative inotropic effect) is seen as a downward shift in the cardiac function curve. The actual cardiac performance is dependent on venous pressure (preload), and contractility and afterload. Venous return ultimately limits cardiac output, because the heart cannot pump any volume that does not enter the right atrium.

Vascular Function Curve

Venous pressure is inversely proportional to cardiac output. Decreased cardiac output increases venous blood volume, graphed in the vascular function curve. The graphing of this curve does not follow standard approaches in that the cause (independent variable) is placed on the y-axis and the effect (dependent variable) on the x-axis. This is done so that right atrial pressure remains on the x-axis and cardiac output on the y-axis, as was done for the cardiac function curve (see Fig. 9-3).

The vascular function curve is affected by volume within the system and by systemic vascular resistance (Fig. 9-4). The implications of the vascular function curve are illustrated by events that change cardiac output, such as ventricular fibrillation and subsequent cardiopulmonary resuscitation (CPR). Ventricular fibrillation decreases cardiac output to zero. During this time, arterial pressure falls, since no new blood is being pumped into the arteries, and central venous pressure rises, as blood accumulates in the veins. Arterial pressure continues to fall, and venous pressure continues to rise, until both pressures reach about 7 mm Hg, called the mean circulatory filling pressure.

The external chest compression of CPR forces blood from the ventricles into the arteries. Arterial pressure begins to rise as arterial blood volume increases. Venous pressure begins to fall as CPR transfers blood from the veins to the arteries and consequently venous volume decreases.

The vascular function curves are shifted by changes in the volume of blood in the veins, the venous smooth muscle tone,

and by the total peripheral resistance. An increase in venous volume causes a parallel rightward shift in the vascular function curve. For any level of cardiac output, venous pressure will be higher. Changes in venous tone have identical effects to those of changing venous volume. As shown in Figure 9-2, constriction of the venous chamber causes an increase in venous pressure for any level of cardiac output. Changes in total peripheral resistance cause a different kind of shift in the vascular function curve. When TPR decreases, arterial pressure falls and venous pressure rises. This is true as long as cardiac output is higher than zero. When cardiac output is zero, TPR does not alter venous pressure, although it will change the time that it takes for blood to drain from the arteries into the veins.

When the cardiac and the vascular function curves are plotted on the same graph, they intersect (Fig. 9-5). This intersection establishes a value of cardiac output and venous pressure that will be maintained. Lasting changes in cardiac output or venous pressure can only be accomplished by shifting either the cardiac function curve or the vascular function curve. This principle is illustrated by considering the integrated cardiovascular effects of myocardial infarction, hemorrhage, and exercise.

Myocardial infarction causes a drop in cardiac output and an elevation in venous pressure. The reduction in the pumping ability of the ventricle is due to myocardial ischemia damaging or killing a portion of the ventricular myocytes. As ventricular pumping ability is impaired (curves B and C in Fig. 9-5), cardiac output falls and venous pressure increases. Damage to the left ventricle leads to an elevation in pulmonary venous pressure and, if severe, an increase in pressure in the pulmonary capillaries. Damage to the right ventricle leads to an elevation in central venous pressure and an increased pressure in the hepatic sinusoids. The elevation in venous pressure results in an increase in ventricular

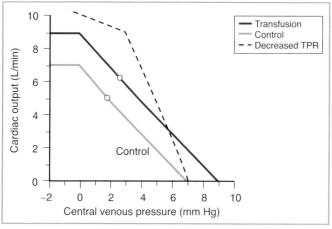

Figure 9-4. Vascular function curves. The vascular function curve describes the decrease in central venous pressure caused by an increase in cardiac output. A change in volume in the system causes a parallel shift in the vascular function curve. The change in total peripheral resistance does not influence the mean circulatory filling pressure (when cardiac output is zero), but it does causes a change in the curve at any other level of cardiac output.

PATHOLOGY

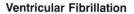

Ventricular Fibrillation

Ventricular fibrillation is uncoordinated contraction of individual regions of the myocardium. As a consequence, cardiac output falls to zero. Cardiopulmonary resuscitation (CPR) relies on external chest compression to generate a pressure within the ventricular chamber. When performed by a trained provider, CPR can produce a cardiac output of 1.5 L/min, about 30% of normal. This low level of cardiac output may be sufficient to provide blood flow to the brain and heart, enabling those organs to survive until the ventricle can be defibrillated.

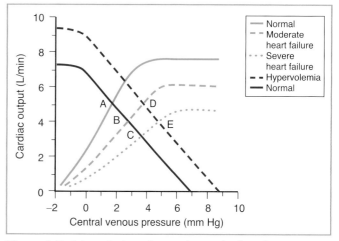

Figure 9-5. Integrated cardiac and vascular function curves. Simultaneously plotting the cardiac and the vascular function curves on the same axis illustrates the complex relationship between cardiac output and central venous pressure. In this graphic, cause and effect are not illustrated. To maintain a change in cardiac output or in central venous pressure, either the cardiac or the vascular function curve has to be shifted.

diastolic filling pressure, which should help recover some of the cardiac output. Over time, renal retention of volume may help increase venous pressure (points D and E in Fig. 9-5), and cardiac output may recover further.

Exercise causes an increase in cardiac output with little change in venous pressure. During exercise, the SNS causes a positive inotropic effect on the ventricles, which increases cardiac output. During whole body exercise, the local vasodilation overcomes any SNS vasoconstriction, and total peripheral resistance actually decreases. The decrease in total peripheral resistance further augments the increase in cardiac output by preventing an increase in arterial pressure during the period of high cardiac output.

●●● EFFECTS OF RESPIRATION ON CARDIOVASCULAR FUNCTION

Intrathoracic pressure influences venous return and consequently cardiac output and arterial pressure. Inspiration drops intrathoracic pressure, dilates the thoracic vena cava, and acutely decreases atrial filling. Cardiac output falls, and consequently arterial pressure falls. The drop in arterial pressure reduces stretch on the arterial baroreceptors, causing a reflex increase in heart rate. Exhalation reverses the above steps. These cyclic changes in heart rate appear as a "normal sinus arrhythmia" on the ECG.

The Valsalva maneuver is an exaggerated exhalation, usually a sustained, forced exhalation against a closed glottis. During a maintained increase in intrathoracic pressure, venous return is interrupted, and cardiac output falls. The subsequent fall in arterial pressure reduces cerebral blood flow. If the elevated thoracic pressure is maintained, blood pressure will be insufficient to support CNS metabolism, producing syncope, which interrupts the voluntary abdominal compression and allows normal (baroreceptor) control of arterial pressure to be reestablished.

●●● EFFECTS OF ACCELERATION AND GRAVITY ON CARDIOVASCULAR FUNCTION

Body position accentuates the effect of gravity on venous return. Orthostatic hypotension can occur when a person arises suddenly from a prone position or as blood pools in the legs of soldiers at parade attention for long periods. The reduced venous return leads to the drop in blood pressure. The response is augmented on hot days, when enhanced blood flow to the skin contributes to the drop in arterial pressure. The hypotension is also augmented by drugs that block the action of the sympathetic nerves. As with the Valsalva maneuver, syncope causes the body to assume a prone position, which eliminates the gravity-induced circulatory problem.

Prolonged bed rest causes a redistribution of circulating blood volume away from gravity-dependent regions, such as the legs, and toward the trunk. This increase in central venous volume causes a diuresis due to increased venous (atrial) pressure and stretch of the cardiopulmonary receptors. Patients confined to bed rest remain in negative fluid balance for up to 3 days, with a net loss of body fluid volume. Patients who stand up after prolonged bed rest experience orthostatic hypotension.

Acceleration can also induce venous pooling and syncope. This is prevented by augmenting the flow of blood from the legs toward the heart. For astronauts, this involves positioning the legs at chest level relative to the acceleration force during lift-off. For military fighter pilots, "gravity" suits provide pneumatic external compression of the lower body to minimize pooling of blood in the extremities during acceleration.

●●● INTEGRATION AND REDUNDANCY OF CARDIOVASCULAR CONTROL

Arterial blood pressure is regulated by neural and endocrine mechanisms and augmented by exchange between the vascular and other body fluid spaces. Neural control is mostly by the SNS, with a minor role played by the PNS in controlling heart rate and some local vascular beds. Endocrine agents that control vascular smooth muscle tone include the vasoconstrictors catecholamines, angiotensin II, and ADH and the vasodilator nitric oxide. Physical mechanisms include exchange of fluid between the plasma and the interstitial fluid at the capillaries of the microcirculation, and the loss of plasma from filtration at the renal glomerulus. The renal regulation of blood pressure is augmented by the same agents that constrict vascular smooth muscle—the catecholamines, angiotensin II, and ADH—as well as the steroid hormone aldosterone. It is useful to understand the vascular control systems on the basis of both the pressure range over which they operate and the time frame in which they operate.

Cardiovascular control systems can be grouped by the pressure range over which they act. Baroreceptor control operates in the normal arterial pressure range and is important in compensating for both increases and decreases in blood pressure. Some vascular control systems become important only during a drop in arterial pressure. During hypotension, angiotensin II and fluid translocation are important compensatory mechanisms. Severe hypotension activates the CNS ischemic response, a massive activation of the SNS. Renal regulation of fluid volume is effective over the entire range of arterial pressures (Fig. 9-6).

Cardiovascular control systems can also be grouped by the time delay before they become effective (Fig. 9-7). Nervous system reflexes are the most rapid, causing a physiologic response within seconds. Peptide and catecholamine hormones become effective within minutes. Fluid translocation effects are noticeable after 10 minutes. Steroid hormones take hours to exert effects. Renal fluid retention requires days to alter arterial pressure. Consequently, acute cardiovascular responses center on the autonomic nervous system, and chronic cardiovascular disorders are tied more closely to body fluid regulation.

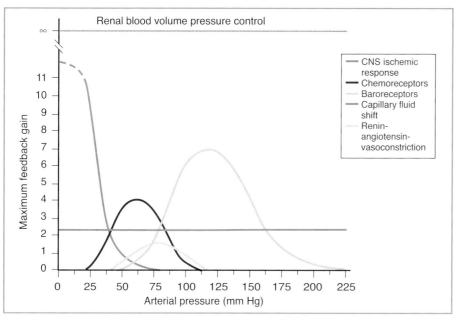

Figure 9-6. Cardiovascular control mechanisms can be organized according to blood pressure. At a normal arterial blood pressure level of 100 mm Hg, blood pressure is controlled acutely by the arterial baroreceptors and chronically by the renal regulation of blood volume. As blood pressure falls, the renin-angiotensin system, then chemoreceptors, and finally the central nervous system ischemic response become important regulators. The renal regulation of body fluid volume and capillary fluid shift is effective at all levels of arterial blood pressure.

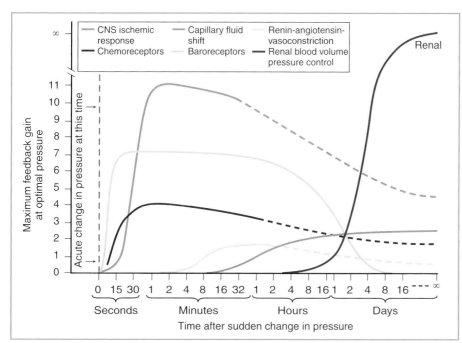

Figure 9-7. Cardiovascular control mechanisms can be organized according to time to onset. The nervous system is activated within 1 minute following an acute change in blood pressure. Endocrine control systems become effective in minutes to hours, and the renal regulation of body fluid volume requires days.

●●● CARDIOVASCULAR ADJUSTMENT TO EXERCISE

Aerobic exercise causes an increase in metabolism that has to be matched by an increase in cardiac output. At the tissue level, an increase in metabolites causes a vasodilation that increases tissue blood flow and also decreases total peripheral resistance. Arterial pressure changes only slightly during exercise because the increase in cardiac output is matched by a drop in peripheral resistance.

Exercise induces a marked and maintained increase in cardiac output. During exercise, overflow from the CNS motor cortex activates the medullary pressor center. The consequent increase in SNS and decrease in PNS activity enhances myocardial contractility and increases heart rate. Exercise enhances venous return through both local dilatation of exercising muscle beds and SNS-mediated venoconstriction of capacitance vessels. The rhythmic compression of skeletal muscle helps propel blood through the veins.

During exercise, cardiac output is preferentially directed to the exercising muscle and heart. There is a locally mediated dilatation of coronary and exercising skeletal muscle and an SNS-mediated constriction of the splanchnic and the nonexercising muscle vascular beds. During prolonged exercise, the temperature regulatory centers of the hypothalamus dilate the cutaneous vessels, which assists in removal of excess heat.

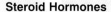

Steroid Hormones

Steroid hormones alter DNA transcription as their major mechanism to produce biological effects. The processes of transcription and translation require time. Consequently, the time frame for steroid hormone biological activity is normally expressed in terms of hours. There is recent experimental evidence of steroid hormones interacting with membrane-bound proteins, which can produce measurable effects within minutes.

After strenuous exercise ends, local control keeps skeletal muscle vasodilated, but stopping activity causes the removal of the motor cortex drive on the medullary pressor center. Consequently, venous return falls and blood pressure falls. This initiates a baroreceptor reflex increase in heart rate until arterial pressure can be maintained. If the high rate of heat loss continues, hypothermia can result.

●●● TOP 5 TAKE-HOME POINTS

1. The balance between cardiac output and central venous pressure depends on (1) myocardial contractility, (2) arterial vascular resistance, (3) venous capacitance, and (4) the volume of blood in the circulation.
2. The arterial baroreceptor reflex and the autonomic nervous system are the major players in the acute regulation of blood pressure.
3. The renal regulation of body fluid volume is the dominant long-term regulator of blood pressure.
4. If blood pressure is maintained, local control of vascular resistance allows tissues to match perfusion and metabolic need.
5. Multiple endocrine and neural cardiovascular regulatory systems interact to maintain a constant arterial blood pressure.

Pulmonary System

10

CONTENTS

Lungs facilitate exchange of O_2 and CO_2 between tissues and the atmosphere. O_2 uptake is necessary to support aerobic (oxidative) metabolism, and CO_2 is eliminated as a metabolic waste product. Inspiration brings atmospheric air into the alveoli for exchange. Diffusion drives O_2 from the alveoli into the blood and CO_2 from the blood into the alveoli. After exchange, the arteries transport oxygenated blood from the heart to the tissues. Oxygen diffuses from tissue capillaries through interstitial fluid, cell membranes, cytoplasm, and finally reaches the mitochondria. Carbon dioxide follows the reverse path, entering blood at the tissue capillaries. The veins bring CO_2-rich blood back to the heart and lungs for elimination in the expired air.

The lungs fill the thoracic cavity, and although they are not physically attached, the lungs and chest wall move together during respiration. The interpleural space is a thin region between the pleura lining the lungs and the pleura lining the interior of the chest wall. This pleural fluid effectively couples the movement of the lungs to the movement of the chest wall.

Within the thorax, the elastic recoil of the lungs pulls the lungs away from the chest wall. Conversely, the recoil of the thorax pulls the chest wall away from the lungs. These opposing forces cause the interpleural pressure to be negative, about −4 mm Hg at rest, and even more negative during inspiration.

Alveoli must remain open to participate in gas exchange. The alveoli are interconnected with elastic tissue, so inflation of one alveolus helps expand the adjacent alveoli (interdependence). Surfactant reduces surface tension generated by the air-water interface. The surfactant-mediated decreases in surface tension are greater in uninflated alveoli, again preventing collapse and closure.

Ventilation and perfusion are matched to facilitate gas exchange. Alveolar hypoxia causes pulmonary vascular smooth muscle to vasoconstrict and to direct pulmonary blood flow away from areas of poor ventilation. Low CO_2 in the airways causes constriction of the bronchiole smooth muscle, directing ventilation to alveoli that are better perfused.

Control of respiration involves a basic rhythm generated by the brainstem that is modified by multiple neural inputs. Respiration is controlled by both central CO_2 sensors and peripheral CO_2 and O_2 sensors. Pulmonary stretch receptors reflexly inhibit inspiration and prevent overinflation of the lungs. There is no hormonal control of respiration. Hormones do, however, control constriction of bronchiole smooth muscle. Histamine and acetylcholine constrict the bronchioles, important in anaphylactic shock. Epinephrine and norepinephrine dilate the bronchioles. Descending input from higher central nervous system (CNS) structures provides additional respiratory control, particularly during exercise.

The lungs are not a classical endocrine organ, but participate in two important endocrine actions. Angiotensin converting enzyme is localized on the pulmonary capillary endothelium, and catalyzes the formation of the vasoconstrictor peptide, angiotensin II. Histamine is released from mast cells in the lung during anaphylactic shock.

●●● PULMONARY SYSTEM PHYSIOLOGY MAP

The physiologic map of the pulmonary system is complex, reflecting the various factors involved in exchanging gas between the outside air and the tissues (Fig. 10-1). The central point of pulmonary function is the exchange across the barrier that separates the alveolar air and the pulmonary capillary blood. This process is driven by diffusion and consequently determined by the components of Fick's law of diffusion: the diffusion coefficient reflecting solubility, the surface area available for exchange, the concentration gradient, and the distance over which the compound must move.

In Figure 10-1A, the focus is on alveolar partial pressure (1) and the movement of air between the alveoli and the atmosphere. This movement is determined by the partial pressure (composition) of the gas entering the alveoli (2), and the alveolar minute ventilation (3), the rate at which air enters the alveoli. Air movement within the respiratory system is complicated because air flow is achieved by a "push-pull exchange" process rather than by a "flow-through" process. In this exchange process, the inspired air mixes with air already within the body (4), and the volume of new air

flowing into the mouth is greater than the volume of new air that flows into the alveoli. Pulmonary ventilation has to account for dead space ventilation of airways that do not participate in gas exchange. These events contribute to the drop in oxygen partial pressure (P_{O_2}) as air flows toward the alveoli.

The maximal inspired volume is determined by the physical size of the lungs and the compliance of the lungs. Normal ventilation is less than the maximum and is determined by airway resistance and by the pressure gradient between the atmosphere and the alveoli.

The map in Figure 10-1B begins at alveolar partial pressure, but the focus shifts to the transport of O_2 and CO_2 in the blood and the exchange at the tissue level. Oxygen transport in the blood is accomplished primarily through the red blood cell (RBC) protein hemoglobin, with a very small amount of O_2 being carried dissolved in the plasma. Blood CO_2 transport is primarily in the form of bicarbonate, with smaller amounts being carried on the hemoglobin protein and dissolved in the plasma.

Gas exchange between the mitochondria in the tissues and the blood in the systemic capillaries is again accomplished by diffusion and described by the components of Fick's law of diffusion: the diffusion coefficient reflecting solubility, the

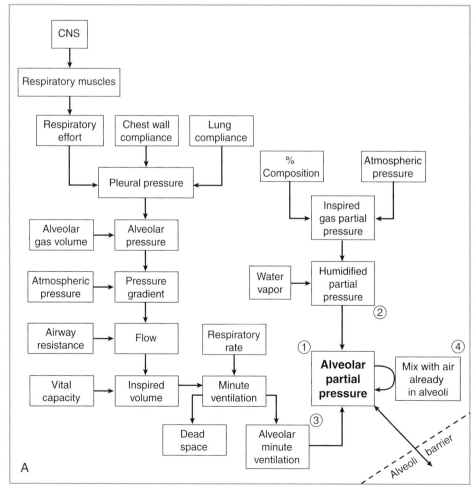

Figure 10-1. Map of the respiratory system. Gas exchange across the alveolar/pulmonary capillary barrier is the focal point for pulmonary function. **A,** Gas composition and the volume of air exchange determine the alveolar gas composition.

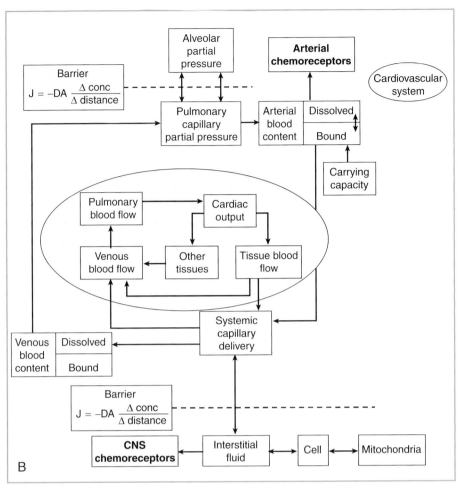

Figure 10-1. *Continued.* **B,** The focus shifts to blood flow (pink shaded area) and blood-carrying capacity. The two points of homeostatic regulation, the arterial chemoreceptors and the CNS chemoreceptors, are shown in shaded boxes.

surface area available for exchange, the concentration gradient, and the distance over which the compound must move.

There are three regulated variables controlled by a negative feedback system in the pulmonary system: arterial blood partial pressure of O_2 (Pa_{O_2}), arterial blood partial pressure of CO_2 (Pa_{CO_2}), and CNS tissue pH. The gas composition of arterial blood is monitored by chemoreceptors located at the carotid bodies and the aortic bodies. Afferent nerves from these chemoreceptors synapse in the respiratory centers of the pons and the medulla. The CNS chemoreceptors monitor brain pH as a measure of CO_2 levels. Any increase in CO_2 in the CNS or arterial plasma will cause an increase in ventilation. A pronounced drop in arterial O_2 partial pressure also can cause an increase in ventilation. The increase in ventilation should facilitate pulmonary uptake of O_2 and elimination of CO_2, returning the body gas levels to their normal values.

●●● STRUCTURE AND FUNCTION OF THE RESPIRATORY SYSTEM

The lungs lie within the thoracic cavity on either side of the heart. They are cone shaped, with the apex rising above the first rib and the base resting on the diaphragm. The right lung is divided into three lobes, and the left lung into two lobes.

The mediastinum separates the two lobes from each other and from the heart, thoracic blood vessels, esophagus, and part of the trachea and bronchi (Fig. 10-2).

Air travels progressively through the nose and pharynx, then the trachea, bronchi, and bronchioles before entering the alveoli. The airways branch into progressively smaller airways, and each dividing point is called a "generation." Alveoli are reached after 20 to 25 generations. Larger airways are kept open by cartilage, and small airways and alveoli are kept open by transpulmonary pressures and by connections to adjacent alveoli. Goblet cells line the airways and secrete mucus. Mucus helps keep the airways moist and traps inspired particulate matter. Ciliated epithelia propel mucus toward the pharynx. Mucus and trapped particles are either expelled by coughing or swallowed.

The trachea and bronchi contain smooth muscle. Airway smooth muscle normally is relaxed. Hormones released from pulmonary mast cells can cause a strong contraction, particularly histamine and the slow reactive substance of anaphylaxis. This release is characteristic of allergic reactions. The presence of irritants also causes release of constrictor hormones.

Vagal parasympathetic stimulation (acetylcholine) contracts airway smooth muscle. Sympathetic nerves and the circulating catecholamine hormones epinephrine and norepinephrine relax airway smooth muscle. This airway dilation

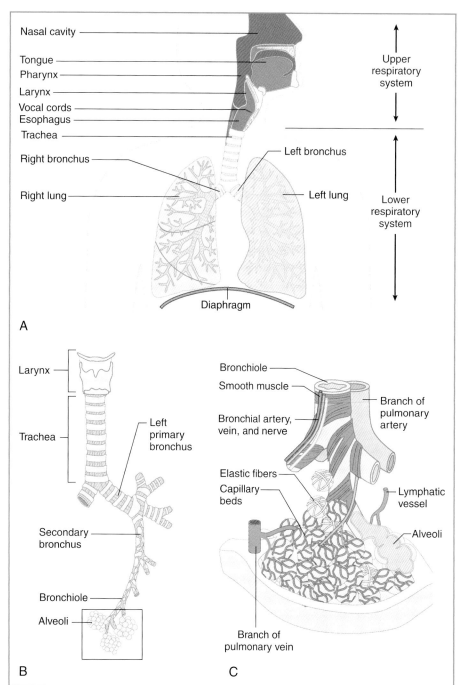

Figure 10-2. Functional anatomy of the pulmonary system. **A**, Air entering the lungs passes first through the upper airways and then through the trachea and the lower airways before reaching the alveoli. **B**, Progressive branching of the tracheobronchial tree ends in the alveoli. **C**, Pulmonary vascular supply includes the bronchial circulation, which originates from the aorta, and the pulmonary circulation, which originates from the pulmonary artery.

assists the increase in ventilation that accompanies a sympathetic "fight or flight" response.

Upper Airways and Larynx

The upper airways include nasal cavities, the pharynx, and the larynx. The mouth can be considered part of the upper airway because it is a secondary route for air to pass to the trachea.

Inspired air is warmed and humidified while passing through the nose. Particulate matter is filtered while passing through the nose. Turbulent air flow causes precipitation of particles as they contact the mucous layer. In addition, nose hairs help filter larger particles. Inspired particles smaller than 5 μm can pass through the nose. These particles can precipitate in bronchioles or alveoli or remain suspended and be expired (e.g., 60% of cigarette smoke is expired). The sneeze reflex is initiated by irritation of the nasal passages and helps clear the nasal passages of foreign matter. The mouth is less effective in warming, filtering, and humidifying air during high-volume breathing. Consequently, a larger percentage of particulate matter enters the lower airways and becomes trapped in the mucous layer during mouth breathing.

The pharynx is a cone-shaped passageway extending from the nose to the larynx. It is a common pathway for both the respiratory and the digestive systems. The epiglottis forms the barrier between the pharynx and the larynx. When food or liquids are swallowed, the epiglottis seals the larynx and prevents aspiration of food and liquid into the lower airways.

Speech is a combination of phonation, pitch, articulation, and resonance. Phonation is accomplished by vibration of the vocal cords of the larynx. Pitch of sound is altered by stretching or relaxing the vocal cords. Pitch of sound is also altered by changing the shape and mass of the vocal cord edges. Articulation of sound is accomplished by the lips, tongue, and soft palate of the mouth. Resonance of sound is controlled by the mouth, nose, nasal sinuses, pharynx, and thoracic cavity.

Lower Airways

The lower airways, or tracheobronchial tree, connect the larynx and the alveoli. Gas exchange between the inspired air in the pulmonary capillaries occurs in the respiratory bronchioles, the alveolar ducts, and the alveolar sacs.

The trachea is a flexible, muscular air passage held open by cartilaginous rings. Although the trachea is primarily a passageway, air entering the body is further humidified and warmed during its passage through the trachea. The trachea ends at the branching point leading to the left to the left primary bronchus and to the right to mainstem bronchi.

The mainstem bronchi undergo series of branchings into progressively smaller airways. The small bronchioles do not possess cartilage and can collapse and trap air in the smaller airways when intrapleural pressure is high. The terminal bronchioles are the last airways of the conducting system. The remaining airways are the respiratory zone, which participates in gas exchange.

Alveoli are the functional components of the lung. The total surface of the alveolus is approximately 800 square feet, or about the size of a tennis court. Alveoli are specialized for gas exchange. The epithelia of the alveoli consist of type I and type II pneumocytes. The inner wall of the alveoli is lined with surfactant secreted by type II pneumocytes. Oxygen passing from alveolar air into the pulmonary capillary passes sequentially through a fluid and surfactant layer lining the alveoli, alveolar epithelia, epithelial basement membrane, interstitial space, capillary basement membrane, and finally capillary endothelium.

Pleura

Pleurae are serous membranes that separate the lungs and the wall of the thoracic cavity. The visceral pleura covers the surface of the lungs, and the parietal pleura covers the inside of the thorax, mediastinum, and diaphragm. A thin film of serous fluid fills the space between the two pleurae. This pleural fluid couples the movement of the lungs and chest wall, so that changes in chest wall shape cause a corresponding change in lung shape. Normally the pressure in the interpleural space is negative and keeps the lungs inflated so that they fill the thoracic space.

Entry of air into the interpleural space (pneumothorax) allows the lung to collapse and the chest wall to expand. Lungs can be "reinflated" by removing pleural air. The mediastinum usually limits lung collapse to one side.

Muscular Structure

Ventilation results from the action of skeletal muscles to alter the thoracic space. Normal breathing uses the diaphragm for inspiration, and expiration is accomplished passively by recoil of elastic tissue of the lung. The diaphragm is a dome-shaped muscle that makes up the base of the thoracic cage. The dome of the diaphragm extends upward into the thoracic space. During inspiration, the diaphragm contracts and flattens, expanding the volume of the thoracic space. The subsequent drop in interpleural pressure causes the lungs to expand, pulling the lungs downward toward the abdominal space.

Forced breathing is facilitated by a variety of accessory muscles (Table 10-1). Forced inspiration causes a further increase in the volume of the thoracic space by pulling the ribs upward and outward. Forced expiration reverses the direction and decreases the thoracic space by pulling the ribs downward and inward.

PATHOLOGY

Infant Respiratory Distress Syndrome
Fetal production of surfactant occurs early in the third trimester. Babies born before 28 weeks of gestation do not have sufficient surfactant to allow the airway to remain open, and infant respiratory distress syndrome develops. The lack of surfactant greatly increases the work of breathing and increases the probability that the alveoli will collapse from increased surface tension.

PATHOLOGY

Pneumothorax
An opening in the thoracic cage, combined with the negative intrapleural pressure, allows air to enter the pleural space. The lungs will collapse because of their elastic recoil, and the chest wall will expand outward. Contraction of the diaphragm then causes air to enter the intrapleural space rather than to inflate the lungs. A puncture of the trachea or tearing of the bronchi allows air to enter the intrapleural space during inspiration, but the air cannot be expelled during expiration, creating a *tension pneumothorax*.

TABLE 10-1. Accessory Muscles of Respiration

Forced Inspiration	Forced Expiration
External intercostals	Internal intercostals
Sternocleidomastoids	Abdominals
Scalenes	
Anterior serrati	

ANATOMY

Intercostal Muscles

The internal intercostal muscles and the external intercostal muscles are arranged at right angles to each other. Contraction of the internal intercostals elevates the ribs away from the thoracic cavity. Contraction of the external intercostal muscles pulls the ribs into the thoracic cavity.

VENTILATION

Air movement during both inspiration and expiration requires the creation of a pressure gradient. The initial event in inspiration is contraction of the diaphragm, which causes an increase in the volume of the thoracic space and a decrease in the interpleural pressure (B_1 to B_2 in Fig. 10-3). The expansion of the lungs causes alveolar pressure to drop below atmospheric pressure (A_2), creating a pressure gradient that is diminished (A_3) as air flows into the alveoli (C_1 to C_2). Inspiration (air flow) ends when intra-alveolar pressure equals atmospheric pressure. By the end of inspiration, interpleural pressure is at its most negative, but alveolar pressure has returned to atmospheric pressure because of the increase in lung volume.

The sequence is reversed during expiration as air moves from the alveoli to the atmosphere. Relaxation of the diaphragm causes a decrease in the volume of the thoracic cage, and interpleural pressure becomes less negative. Compression of the lungs causes alveolar pressure to become positive (1 cm H_2O) relative to the atmosphere. Again, air moves down the pressure gradient, now exiting the lungs. Expiration ends when intra-alveolar pressure equals atmospheric pressure.

Lung Volumes and Compliance

Pulmonary ventilation is divided into four volumes and four capacities, as illustrated in Figure 10-4. The volumes are (1) inspiratory reserve volume—the difference between a normal and a maximal inspiration, (2) tidal volume—the amount of air moved during a normal, quiet respiration, (3) expiratory reserve volume—the difference between a normal and a

maximal expiration, and (4) residual volume—the amount of air remaining in the lungs after a maximal expiration. The first three volumes can be measured by spirometry. Residual volume cannot be determined by spirometry but can be measured by helium dilution or determined by plethysmography.

Capacities are the sum of two or more respiratory volumes. The normal resting point of the lung is at the end of a normal, quiet expiration. Functional residual capacity is the volume of air remaining in the lungs after this normal, quiet expiration and is equal to (expiratory reserve volume + residual volume). Inspiratory capacity is the volume of air that can be inspired following a normal, quiet expiration and is equal to tidal volume + inspiratory reserve volume. Vital capacity is the volume of air under voluntary control, equal to (inspiratory reserve volume + tidal volume + expiratory reserve volume). Vital capacity measurement requires maximal effort on the part of the patient and is often called forced vital capacity. Total lung capacity is the amount of air contained within a maximally inflated lung (all four volumes combined).

Spirometry measures all volumes and derived capacities except residual volume and the two capacities that include residual volume—total lung capacity and functional residual capacity (see Fig. 10-4). Normal values are a function of height, sex, age, and, to a lesser degree, ethnic group. Changes in volumes and capacities are indicative of pulmonary dysfunction.

Timed vital capacity, obtained during a forced expiration following a maximal inspiration, is also an important clinical test. FEV_1 (forced expiratory volume in 1 second) usually is 80% of vital capacity. FEV_3 (forced expiratory volume in 3 seconds) usually is 95% of vital capacity. Equivalent diagnostic information is obtained from measurement of peak expiratory flow rates (Fig. 10-5).

Clinical assessment of pulmonary function commonly uses flow-volume loops to illustrate simultaneously the patient data obtained by spirometry and FEV. Flow-volume loops plot the spirometry data on the x-axis, with the residual volume at the far right and the total lung capacity at the far left. The velocity of air flow is plotted on the y-axis, with zero air flow plotted in the middle of the y-axis, inspiratory flow being downward from zero and expiratory flow being upward from zero.

The expiratory portion of the loop provides the peak expiratory flow, and the slope of the right side of the expiratory flow loop provides an effort-independent flow rate. This portion of the loop is effort independent because the increase in intrathoracic pressure during forced expiration will collapse bronchi that lack cartilaginous support.

Pulmonary function tests help distinguish between two major classes of pulmonary disease: restrictive and obstructive. The flow-volume tracings for these two types of disease are shown in Figure 10-6.

Restrictive diseases limit expansion of the lungs, because of either damage to the lungs (fibrosis) or limitation in thoracic expansion (musculoskeletal). Patients with restrictive disease have low total lung capacities and low vital capacities. The peak velocity of flow and the FEV are low, but the FEV_1

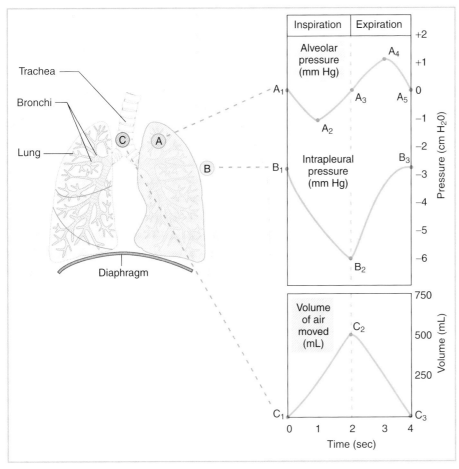

Figure 10-3. Interpleural and alveolar pressure changes during the respiratory cycle. During inspiration, interpleural pressure decreases due to expansion of the thoracic cage. Lung expansion causes alveolar pressure to become negative relative to the atmosphere, and air enters the lungs. Inspiration stops when the entering air causes alveolar pressure to rise to atmospheric pressure. During expiration, the cycle is reversed, with the decrease in lung size causing an increase in alveolar pressure. As air flows out of the lungs, alveolar pressure returns to atmospheric pressure.

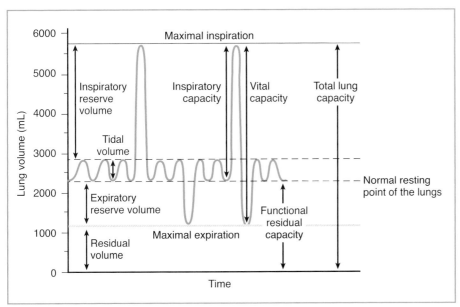

Figure 10-4. Spirometry allows measurement of lung volumes. Spirometry allows determination of three lung volumes and their associated capacities. Spirometry cannot determine residual volume or any capacity-containing residual volume.

is normal. Patients with restrictive disease can move only a small volume of air but can move that small volume fairly well. These patients often breathe with lower tidal volumes but higher frequencies in order to maintain adequate minute alveolar ventilation.

Obstructive diseases limit airflow, either because of narrowing of the airways themselves (asthma) or because of obstruction by a tumor or foreign body. Patients with obstructive disease have high total lung capacity but low vital capacity. Inspiration may be normal, but expiration is

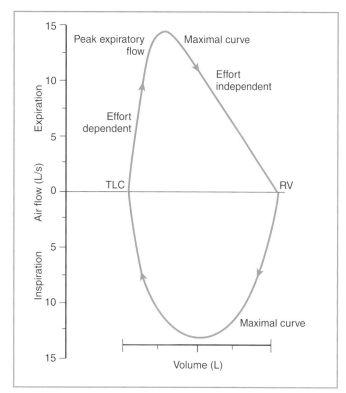

Figure 10-5. The flow-volume curve plots the spirometry values against the velocity of air flow. Peak expiratory air flow occurs early during the expiratory cycle, with the later portions of the curve being independent of effort. The effort-independent portion of the curve reflects elastic recoil of the lung and the critical closing pressures.

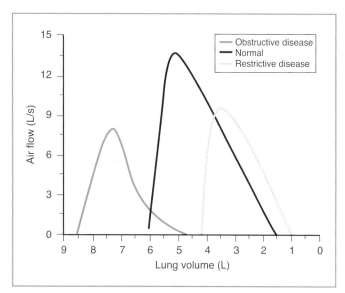

Figure 10-6. Obstructive pulmonary disease and restrictive pulmonary disease cause characteristic shifts in the flow-volume relationship. Obstructive diseases are characterized by elevated lung volume due primarily to the elevated residual volume. Restrictive diseases are characterized by reduced lung volume due primarily to reduced vital capacity. Both diseases show a decrease in the peak velocity of air flow.

impaired. This causes air to become "trapped" in the lungs and increases the residual volume. Peak velocity is low because of the airway obstruction, and impairment of exhalation causes a "scooped" slope of the second half of the expiratory flow-volume loop. Attempts to increase exhalation only cause a further increase in intrathoracic pressure, collapsing the small bronchioles. Patients with obstructive disease often breathe with higher tidal volumes and lower frequencies in order to maintain adequate alveolar minute ventilation.

●●●● SURFACTANT AND PULMONARY COMPLIANCE

Compliance is the change in volume divided by the change in pressure. For the lungs, measured compliance is due to both compliance of the lungs and compliance of the thorax. Hysteresis, or wandering, is a change in measured compliance during inspiration and expiration. Hysteresis is due to the viscous properties of the lungs and surface tension within the alveoli.

Surfactants act like a detergent to reduce the surface tension of the fluid lining the alveoli. Surfactants are secreted by type II granular pneumocytes. Surfactant contains a variety of phospholipids, particularly dipalmitoyl lecithin and sphingomyelin. Reduced surface tension is essential to allowing a functional air-water interface on the surface of the alveoli (Fig. 10-7).

Diseases can alter compliance. Compliance is reduced in disease states such as fibrosis and surfactant deficiency. For these individuals, a much larger inspiratory effort is required to inflate the lungs. At the other extreme, compliance is increased is disease states such as emphysema. For these individuals, inflation of the lungs is relatively easy, but elastic recoil is less effective in assisting expiration.

Alveoli

Minute ventilation is the tidal volume times the respiratory rate, usually, 500 mL × 12 breaths/min = 6000 mL/min. Increasing respiratory rate or tidal volume will increase minute ventilation. Dead space refers to airway volumes not participating in gas exchange. Anatomic dead space includes air in the mouth, trachea, and all but the smallest bronchioles, usually about 150 mL. Physiologic dead space also includes alveoli that are ventilated but do not exchange gas because of low blood flow (usually, 0 mL in normal humans). Tidal volume must exceed dead space or functional alveoli will not be ventilated with fresh air.

Only air delivered to the terminal bronchioles and alveoli is available for gas exchange. Alveolar minute ventilation is less than minute ventilation and is calculated as ([tidal volume − dead space] × respiratory rate) or ([500 mL − 150 mL] × 12 breaths/min) = 4200 mL/min. Increasing tidal volume increases alveolar ventilation more effectively than does increasing respiratory rate (see the earlier discussion of restrictive and obstructive disease).

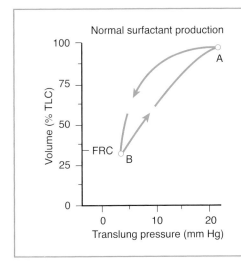

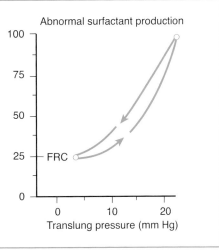

Figure 10-7. Surfactant causes hysteresis during the respiratory cycle. Surfactant reduces surface tension in the inflated alveoli, delaying closure during the expiratory portion of the respiratory cycle. In the absence of surfactant (e.g., respiratory distress syndrome), a greater increase in pressure is needed to move a normal volume of air, the functional residual capacity is decreased, and hysteresis is not as evident.

●●● WORK OF RESPIRATION

The movement of air requires work, defined for the respiratory system as pressure times volume (Fig. 10-8). Respiratory work has three components: resistance to air flow, expansion of the elastic tissue of the lung, and expansion of the chest wall. Work due to resistance to air flow is increased by bronchiole constriction, increased by turbulent flow when flow velocity is high, and decreased by reducing air viscosity (e.g., helium use in SCUBA diving). Work due to expansion of the elastic tissue of the lungs is increased in fibrosis. Work due to expansion of the chest wall is also increased in fibrosis.

Expiration normally is passive and requires no additional work. Active expiration requires additional work and involves the accessory muscles of breathing. Active expiration also increases the possibility of the increase in intrathoracic pressure collapsing the small bronchi, so the additional muscular effort yields only a small improvement in ventilation.

The metabolic costs of respiration are considerable. Normal breathing can account for up to 5% of total body O_2 consumption. During exercise, the proportion can increase to up to 30%. Importantly, in disease states, the metabolic costs of respiration can become unsustainable. In these cases, patients may be placed on a respirator to reduce the total body metabolic load while the underlying cause of the increased respiratory work is corrected.

●●● GAS EXCHANGE

Gas exchange is driven by diffusion. Consequently, movement of gas is always down a concentration (partial pressure) gradient. Oxygen is less soluble than CO_2, and consequently oxygen diffusion requires a higher pressure gradient in both the lungs and the tissues. The effectiveness of diffusion diminishes as the distance to be traveled increases. Normally, the distance between alveolar air and blood is small, and O_2 and CO_2 diffuse with little trouble. However, diseases such as

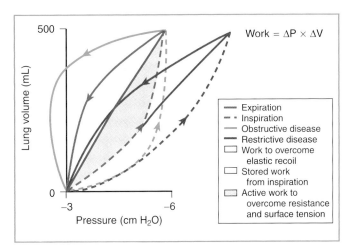

Figure 10-8. Respiratory work has multiple components. The work of breathing includes work against the elastic recoil of the lung, work to overcome airway resistance, and work to overcome surface tension. The work of breathing is increased in restrictive disease because of the necessity to overcome elastic recoil. The work of breathing is increased in obstructive disease because of the necessity to overcome airway resistance. In severe obstructive disease, additional work may be needed for expiration.

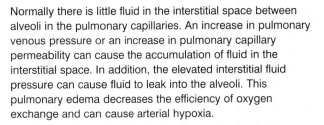

PATHOLOGY

Pulmonary Edema

Normally there is little fluid in the interstitial space between alveoli in the pulmonary capillaries. An increase in pulmonary venous pressure or an increase in pulmonary capillary permeability can cause the accumulation of fluid in the interstitial space. In addition, the elevated interstitial fluid pressure can cause fluid to leak into the alveoli. This pulmonary edema decreases the efficiency of oxygen exchange and can cause arterial hypoxia.

pulmonary edema increase the distance between alveolar air and blood and can impede gas movement.

Air–Alveolar Gas Mixing

Inspired air has a total pressure of 760 mm Hg at sea level (1 atmosphere). Nitrogen accounts for 79% of the air, or about 597 mm Hg partial pressure. Oxygen accounts for 21% of the air, or a partial pressure of 159 mm Hg. Water vapor accounts for 0.5% of the air, or a partial pressure of 4 mm Hg. Carbon dioxide accounts for 0.04% of the air, or a partial pressure of 0.3 mm Hg (Fig. 10-9).

Air entering the trachea is humidified, increasing the water vapor partial pressure but not changing the total atmospheric pressure. Consequently, the partial pressure of the other gases is decreased. In humidified air in the larger airways, water vapor partial pressure increases to 47 mm Hg, and O_2 partial pressure decreases to 150 mm Hg. When entering the alveoli, inspired humidified air mixes with CO_2-rich humidified air already present in the alveolus, so the partial pressure of the other gases is further diluted. Oxygen partial pressure decreases to 104 mm Hg, and CO_2 partial pressure (PCO_2) is 40 mm Hg. Water vapor partial pressure remains at 47 mm Hg.

Expired air is a mixture of dead space air and alveolar air (Fig. 10-10). Dead space air exits first, so gas pressures represent those listed above for the trachea. End tidal air samples more closely represent the values of alveolar air. Consequently, end tidal air sampling is used to estimate mixed venous blood CO_2 levels.

Alveolar–Blood Gas Exchange

The alveolus–capillary exchange surface area is large, facilitating diffusion. Gas exchange occurs in the terminal portions of the pulmonary air spaces, the respiratory bronchiole, alveolar ducts, and alveoli. Alveolar gases must diffuse through a series of barriers (Fig. 10-11):

1. Fluid lining the alveoli, including surfactant
2. Alveolar epithelial cells
3. Epithelial basement membrane

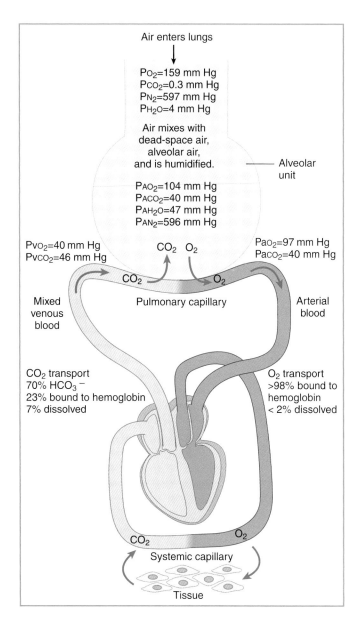

Figure 10-9. Inspired air is humidified and mixed with dead-space air before reaching the alveolus. Arterial blood gas values are slightly less than those in the alveolar air because of the small amount of shunt blood flow. Mixed venous blood gas values reflect the gas partial pressure in the tissues. a, arterial; A, alveolar; v, venous.

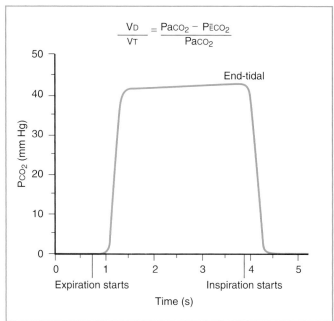

Figure 10-10. During expiration, the first gas leaving the body is dead space that has not participated in gas exchange and consequently contains no CO_2. The remainder of the gas leaving the body reflects air that originated in the alveoli. End-tidal CO_2 partial pressure is normally a good measure of alveolar CO_2 and therefore of arterial PCO_2. VD, dead space volume; VT, tidal volume; $P\bar{E}CO_2$, average expired gas CO_2 pressure.

4. Interstitial space, which normally contains a small volume of fluid
5. Capillary basement membrane
6. Capillary endothelial cells

Abnormalities in alveolar–blood gas exchange are tied to the components of the diffusion equation. Increased diffusion distance decreases gas exchange. This increased distance can be due to edema in interstitial spaces. Decreased available surface area decreases gas exchange, such as in emphysema or following surgical removal of one lobe of the lung. Decreased solubility decreases gas exchange. Solubility for a given gas is constant, and solubility is grouped with gas molecular weight as the diffusion constant. Solubility is an important consideration for O_2 exchange, since O_2 is much less soluble than CO_2. Finally, CO is highly soluble and is not normally present in the blood, allowing clinical use of CO to estimate lung-diffusing capacity.

A decreased pressure gradient will decrease gas exchange. Oxygen has a much higher pressure gradient, which partially offsets the higher solubility for CO_2. Oxygen exchange is usually the limiting factor for survival in chronic pulmonary disease. When O_2 exchange is facilitated by enhancing inspired O_2 content, CO_2 can become the limiting factor for survival in chronic pulmonary disease.

●●● PULMONARY CIRCULATION

The lungs receive the entire output of the right ventricle. Consequently, pulmonary blood flow is equal to cardiac output, about 5 L/min.

The normal transit time for blood through the pulmonary capillaries is about 0.75 seconds. Gas equilibration between the alveolar air and the pulmonary capillary takes about 0.25 seconds for O_2 and about 0.05 seconds for CO_2. This means that there is a large "safety factor" ensuring that gas equilibrates with pulmonary blood. Even during exercise, pulmonary capillary transit times remain sufficient to ensure adequate exchange. The longer time for O_2 equilibration, however, means that in disease states, O_2 exchange becomes limited more quickly than does CO_2 exchange.

Pulmonary vascular resistance is much lower than systemic vascular resistance, and blood pressures in the pulmonary system are much lower than the corresponding systemic vascular segments. Pulmonary arterial pressure is about 25/15 mm Hg, pulmonary capillary pressure about 12 mm Hg, and pulmonary venous pressure about 8 mm Hg. These pressures are recorded during the passage of a Swan-Ganz catheter from the systemic veins into the pulmonary artery (Fig. 10-12).

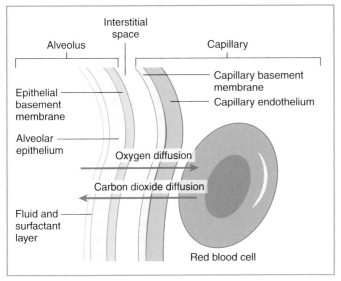

Figure 10-11. Oxygen entering the pulmonary capillaries crosses a surfactant-containing layer of fluid, alveolar epithelium, alveolar basement membrane, interstitial space, capillary basement membrane, and capillary epithelium before reaching the plasma. Carbon dioxide travels in the opposite direction.

Figure 10-12. A Swan-Ganz catheter is introduced into a large vein and advanced in the direction of blood flow. Vena cava and right atrial pressures are about 0–5 mm Hg. Right ventricular pressure is 25/0 mm Hg, pulmonary artery pressure is 25/15 mm Hg. Inflation of the balloon on the catheter allows recording of the pulmonary artery wedge pressure, about 8 mm Hg, which is a good estimate of pulmonary venous blood pressure.

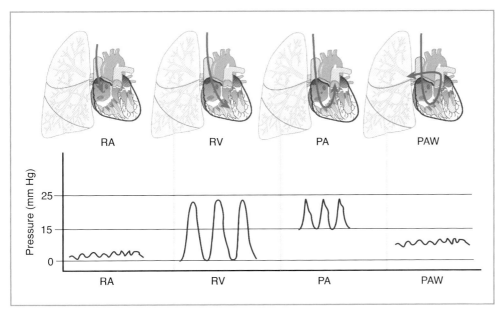

A small amount of systemic arterial blood flow, the bronchial circulation, supplies nutrient flow to the trachea, bronchi, and large thoracic blood vessels. Most of the bronchial circulation empties into the pulmonary veins, representing a source of O_2-depleted blood that mixes with blood that absorbed O_2 while passing through the pulmonary capillaries. This flow is part of normal right-to-left shunt flow and accounts for the pulmonary venous blood having a slightly lower O_2 saturation than would otherwise be expected.

In contrast to the systemic circulation, extravascular compression from the alveoli represents a significant component to pulmonary vascular resistance. This extravascular compression can come from interpleural pressures in the case of vessels outside the lungs, or from alveoli for pulmonary capillaries. At lung volumes approaching residual volume, the higher (less negative) interpleural pressure provides compression on the vessels outside the lung and increases pulmonary vascular resistance. At lung volumes approaching total lung capacity, expansion of alveoli provides compression of the pulmonary capillaries and increases pulmonary vascular resistance. The lowest total vascular resistance is at lung volumes approaching the functional residual capacity.

The relatively low pressures in the pulmonary vasculature render pulmonary blood flow susceptible to changes due to gravity (Fig. 10-13). Pulmonary blood flow is highest in the base of the lungs (zone 3). If pulmonary venous pressure falls below alveolar pressure, the alveoli can limit blood flow (zone 2). If alveolar pressure exceeds pulmonary artery pressure, the alveoli can completely obstruct pulmonary blood flow (zone 1). Zone 1 represents a nonfunctional

portion of the lung and does not occur physiologically. In disease states characterized by low pulmonary vascular pressure (e.g., hemorrhagic shock) or high alveolar pressure (i.e., positive pressure ventilation), zone 1 can develop and impair gas exchange.

Pulmonary vascular smooth muscle can play an important role in shunting blood away from unventilated portions of the lungs. In the lungs, hypoxia causes vasoconstriction (in contrast to the vasodilation in systemic vasculature). This allows pulmonary blood flow to be shunted to regions of the lung that are better ventilated. Hypoxic pulmonary vasoconstriction is the principal mechanism balancing pulmonary perfusion and alveolar ventilation.

●●● VENTILATION-PERFUSION BALANCE

Effective gas exchange requires a balance of alveolar ventilation and pulmonary blood flow. Regional differences in both alveolar ventilation and perfusion exist in the lung, with the base of the lung receiving the highest proportion of both ventilation and perfusion.

The ratio of ventilation to perfusion (V/Q ratio) indicates the efficiency of gas exchange for that portion of the lung. Minute alveolar ventilation is about 5 L/min, and cardiac output is also about 5 L/min, so the body V/Q ratio is close to the optimal value of 1. Different regions of the lung can show different V/Q ratios. The apex of the lung has a high V/Q ratio, and the base of the lung has a low V/Q ratio.

Normal and abnormal ventilation-perfusion ratios are illustrated in Figure 10-14. If ventilation is zero, the ratio is zero, no gas exchange occurs, and alveolar gas content reflects pulmonary venous gas content only. Low V/Q ratios are described as a physiologic shunt. If perfusion is zero, the ratio is infinity, again no gas exchange occurs, and alveolar gas content reflects inspired air gas only. High V/Q ratios are described as physiologic dead space.

●●● BLOOD TRANSPORT OF OXYGEN AND CARBON DIOXIDE

Oxygen is transported in blood either bound to hemoglobin or dissolved in the plasma. Blood O_2 content, normally 20 mL O_2/100 mL blood, includes both the dissolved and hemoglobin-bound O_2 stores. The dynamics of dissolved O_2 transport are simple, since the amount dissolved is determined by the O_2 partial pressure. The dynamics of O_2 transport by hemoglobin are more complex, related to the nonlinear relationship of P_{O_2} and hemoglobin content.

Oxygen transport is illustrated graphically in Figure 10-15. The y-axis is P_{O_2}, in mm Hg. The x-axis shows the three compartments: alveolar O_2, dissolved O_2, and hemoglobin-bound O_2. The hemoglobin-carrying capacity is shown by the volume of the colored area.

Ninety-eight percent of O_2 transported in the blood is bound to hemoglobin (see Fig. 10-15). Hemoglobin O_2-carrying ability is 99% saturated at P_{O_2} of 100 mm Hg. Mixed

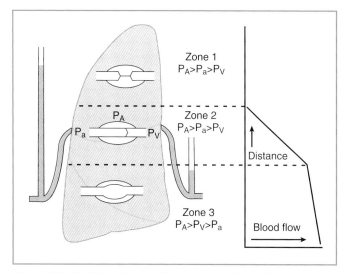

Figure 10-13. Blood flow in the lungs is affected by gravity and alveolar pressure. The base of the lungs receives the greatest amount of blood flow. Blood flow to the higher portions of the lungs is diminished because of lower pulmonary arterial pressure due to the effects of gravity. Alveolar pressure can limit perfusion if it exceeds pressure in the vascular system. This is unusual, but it can occur when alveolar pressure is very high or pulmonary vascular pressure is very low.

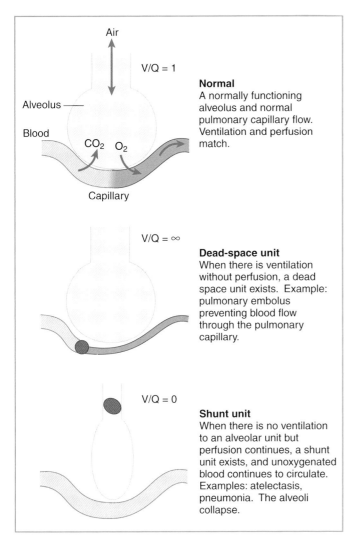

Figure 10-14. Abnormalities in ventilation and perfusion can diminish gas exchange. Normal respiratory function requires both ventilation and perfusion, and has a V/Q ratio of 1. Obstruction of the blood vessel creates a dead-space unit that is ventilated but not perfused and has a V/Q ratio of ∞. Obstruction of the airway creates a shunt unit that is perfused but not ventilated and has a V/Q ratio of 0.

BIOCHEMISTRY

Hemoglobin

Hemoglobin consists of four of polypeptide chains, each of which has a heme group that can bind oxygen. The binding of oxygen changes the quaternary structure of the hemoglobin molecule and accounts for the sigmoid shape of the oxyhemoglobin dissociation curve.

venous blood has a P_{O_2} of 40 mm Hg. Even though the P_{O_2} has fallen by more than 50%, the amount of O_2 bound to hemoglobin is still 75% of the amount in arterial blood. Decreases in blood hemoglobin concentration cause a decrease in blood O_2-carrying capacity. The remaining 2% of

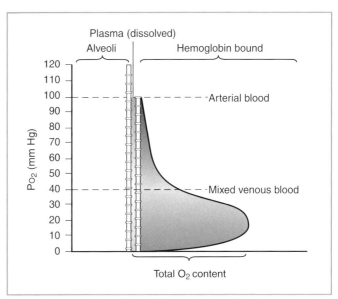

Figure 10-15. Blood O_2-carrying capacity includes dissolved O_2 and O_2 bound to hemoglobin. When alveolar partial pressure of O_2 is 100 mm Hg, 98% of the blood O_2 content is bound to hemoglobin and only 2% is dissolved in the plasma. At this point, the hemoglobin is 100% saturated, and any further increase in alveolar partial pressure of O_2 can only increase the amount of O_2 carried dissolved the plasma. In the systemic capillaries, P_{O_2} falls to 40 mm Hg, reducing the total amount of O_2 bound to hemoglobin to 75%. A decrease in the amount of hemoglobin, or in O_2-binding capacity, can decrease the arterial O_2 content.

O_2 transported in the arterial blood is dissolved in plasma. The amount dissolved in plasma can be increased by increasing alveolar P_{O_2} levels. Clinically, this is achieved by supplementing the inspired O_2 levels up to 100% O_2, or by placing the patient in a hyperbaric chamber and increasing the total atmospheric pressure.

Agents that decrease the affinity of hemoglobin for O_2 help unload O_2 in systemic capillaries (called a shift to the right of the dissociation curve, or an increased P50) (Fig. 10-16). These agents include decreased pH, increased temperature, and increased DPG, a product of red blood cell metabolism.

Carbon dioxide is transported in blood in three forms. Seventy percent of the blood CO_2 is HCO_3^-. The combination of CO_2 and water to form H^+ and HCO_3^- is a reversible reaction catalyzed by RBC carbonic anhydrase. Carbon dioxide diffuses rapidly, so plasma and RBC CO_2 pools are in equilibrium. Twenty-three percent of blood CO_2 is bound to hemoglobin, and 7% of blood CO_2 is dissolved in the plasma.

Oxygen and CO_2 each decrease hemoglobin affinity for the other gas, but not by competing for the same binding site. The Bohr shift describes the decrease in O_2 affinity caused by the binding of CO_2 to hemoglobin. As a consequence of this effect, hemoglobin O_2 affinity is increased in pulmonary capillaries as CO_2 is lost to the lungs, and hemoglobin O_2 affinity is decreased in the tissue capillaries as CO_2 is gained from the tissues. This effect facilitates the loading of O_2 onto

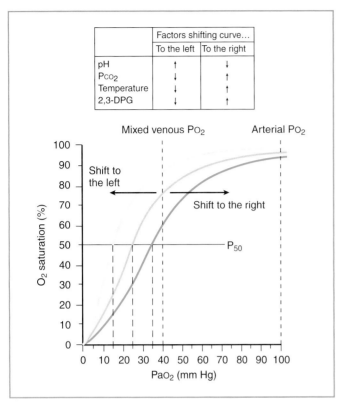

	Factors shifting curve...	
	To the left	To the right
pH	↑	↓
Pco2	↓	↑
Temperature	↓	↑
2,3-DPG	↓	↑

Figure 10-16. Hemoglobin affinity for O_2 can be altered. The hemoglobin affinity for O_2 is decreased by factors that occur during exercise: a decrease in pH, an increase in Pco_2, or an increase in temperature. Prolonged hypoxia generates 2,3-DPG, which also decreases hemoglobin affinity for O_2. Each of these changes allows a greater proportion of the bound O_2 to dissociate from hemoglobin and be delivered to the tissues. The decrease hemoglobin affinity for O_2 is called a shift to the right of the oxyhemoglobin dissociation curve, or an increase in P50, the Po_2 at which 50% of the hemoglobin is saturated with O_2.

hemoglobin in the pulmonary capillaries and the unloading of O_2 at the systemic capillaries.

The Haldone effect describes the decrease in CO_2 affinity caused by the binding of O_2 to hemoglobin. Hemoglobin CO_2 affinity is increased in systemic capillaries as O_2 is lost to the tissues, and hemoglobin CO_2 affinity is decreased in pulmonary capillaries as O_2 is gained from the alveoli. This effect facilitates the loading of CO_2 onto hemoglobin in the systemic capillaries and the unloading of CO_2 from hemoglobin at the pulmonary capillaries.

●●● REGULATION OF PULMONARY FUNCTION

Neural respiratory control centers are located in the pons and the medulla. The dorsal respiratory neurons in the nucleus of the tractus solitarius of the medulla generate the basic pattern of inspiratory activity. Ventral respiratory neurons, located in the nucleus ambiguus and nucleus retroambiguus, control ventilation during active breathing. Stimulation increases inspiratory rate above that set by the dorsal respiratory

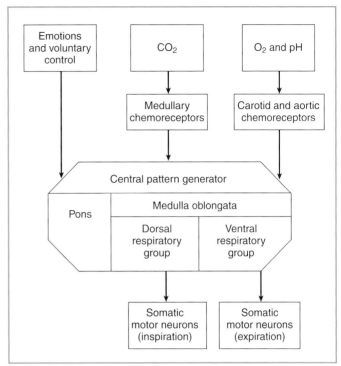

Figure 10-17. The pons and medulla of the brainstem generate a basic respiratory rhythm. This rhythm is modified by a negative feedback control tied to the peripheral chemoreceptors (CO_2 and O_2) and central chemoreceptors (CO_2 only). The control of ventilation is further regulated by descending inputs from higher CNS centers, particularly the motor cortex, limbic system, and autonomic nervous system.

neurons. Stimulation also causes an active expiration, which increases respiratory efficiency (Fig. 10-17).

The pneumotaxic center of the pons controls both rate and pattern of respiration. Descending inputs act to inhibit the dorsal respiratory centers. These function to end the inspiratory cycle. Shortening the period of inspiration acts to increase respiratory rate. The apneustic center of the lower pons also causes inspiration but appears to be of limited physiologic significance.

Neural receptors in the lungs can modify the basic respiratory rhythm. Stretching of receptors in the bronchi and bronchioles initiates the Hering-Breuer reflex, which ends inspiration and acts to prevent overfilling of the lungs. The pulmonary vasculature is surrounded by J receptors, whose activation by pulmonary congestion causes an increase in breathing rate.

Respiration is controlled by negative feedback reflexes (Fig. 10-18). Plasma Po_2 and Pco_2 are sensed in arterial blood by aortic body and carotid body chemoreceptors. Afferent impulses from the chemoreceptors travel by the vagus and glossopharyngeal nerves. Pco_2 (pH) in the CNS is sensed by the medullary chemosensitive area. This region has connections to other brainstem respiratory centers. There are no O_2 sensors in the CNS.

Respiration is also controlled by inputs from motor cortex and cardiovascular centers. Respiration is integrated with

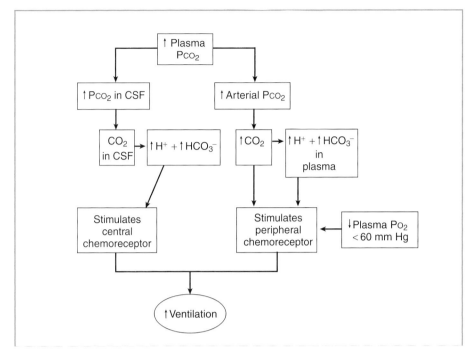

Figure 10-18. Carbon dioxide normally regulates ventilation at both CNS and peripheral chemoreceptors. An increase in arterial P_{CO_2} will stimulate peripheral chemoreceptors and increase ventilation. An increase in CNS P_{CO_2} will cause acidosis, which will increase ventilation. In both cases, an increase in ventilation will enhance respiratory loss of CO_2 and restore blood and tissue P_{CO_2} to normal.

speaking. Respiration increases during exercise appear to be a learned, anticipatory response (feed-forward reflex) mediated through connections with the motor cortex.

Regulation of Blood Oxygen

Peripheral chemoreceptors are the only mechanism for O_2 to influence respiration. Decreased arterial P_{O_2} reflexly stimulates respiratory activity. This stimulus is particularly strong when arterial P_{O_2} drops below 60 mm Hg. Above Pa_{O_2} of 80 mm Hg, O_2 has little effect on respiratory drive. Normal Pa_{O_2} is 95 mm Hg, so O_2 control of respiration is normally of minor importance.

Ascent to altitude decreases ambient atmospheric pressure and P_{O_2}, so O_2 can act as a respiratory stimulus at high altitudes. In addition, in chronic disease, the pH change due high CO_2 is compensated and low O_2 can become the dominant respiratory stimulus.

Regulation of Blood Carbon Dioxide

Carbon dioxide is the dominant regulator of respiration. Carbon dioxide levels are sensed at both peripheral chemoreceptors and central chemoreceptors. Central chemoreceptors are the more sensitive acute controller of respiration but do not respond directly to plasma P_{CO_2}. Normally, peripheral chemoreceptors in the aortic body and carotid body play a minor role in regulating respiration.

Carbon dioxide must first diffuse through the blood-brain barrier before stimulating the CNS chemoreceptors (Fig. 10-19). Cerebrospinal fluid CO_2 then dissociates into H^+ and HCO_3^-. Cerebrospinal H^+ is adequate stimulus for the chemoreceptors. Plasma H^+ cannot cross the blood-brain

barrier and does not directly affect the CNS chemoreceptors. Prolonged pH change alters the HCO_3^- actively pumped out of the cerebrospinal fluid, so the pH stimulus diminishes after a few days.

There is a significant synergistic interaction between respiratory stimulation due to increased CO_2 and decreased O_2 (Fig. 10-20). An increase in CO_2 will potentiate the ventilatory stimulus normally caused by hypoxia. A decrease in O_2 will potentiate the ventilatory stimulus caused by an increase in CO_2. The physiologic consequence of this interaction is that combined hypoxia and hypercapnia provide an exceptionally potent stimulus for ventilation.

Integrated Control of Respiration

The pons and medulla generate a normal cyclic pattern of respiration. This pattern is altered by both homeostatic and adaptive reflexes. Homeostatic reflexes involve the central and peripheral chemoreceptors, where the O_2 and CO_2 stimulation of respiration is synergistic. Hypercapnia stimulates respiration, and hypoxia stimulates respiration. Combined moderate hypoxia and moderate hypercapnia synergistically stimulate respiration. Adaptive reflexes involve higher CNS centers, activated during exercise, or during activation of the sympathetic nervous system. In addition, hypotension stimulates respiration, as does increased body temperature.

Pulmonary Mechanisms in Acid-Base Regulation

Elimination of the acid CO_2 is directly proportionate to ventilation. Consequently, a mismatch between ventilation

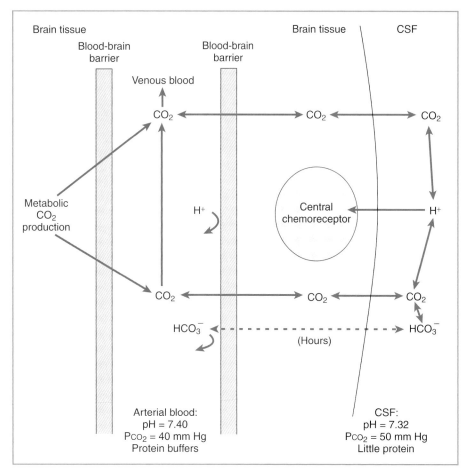

Figure 10-19. Central chemoreceptors respond to blood and CSF acidosis. Carbon dioxide easily crosses the blood-brain barrier, where it can dissociate into H^+ and stimulate ventilation. CSF has a very poor pH buffering capacity, and CNS CO_2 and acidosis both can stimulate ventilation.

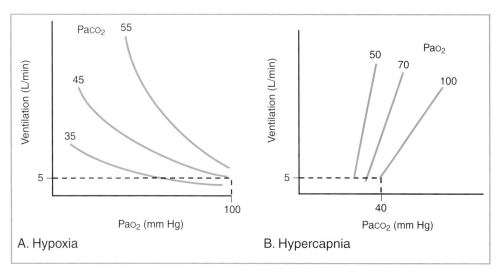

Figure 10-20. Hypoxia and hypercapnia synergistically stimulate ventilation. Hypoxia (**A**) alone will stimulate ventilation. This effect is enhanced when accompanied by an elevation in P_{CO_2}. Similarly hypercapnia (**B**) alone will stimulate ventilation. This effect is enhanced when accompanied by a decrease in P_{O_2}.

and metabolic CO_2 production produces an acid-base disturbance. Hyperventilation produces a respiratory alkalosis. Underventilation produces a respiratory acidosis. Acid-base disturbances due to nonrespiratory causes will alter respiration, since pH is tied closely to the chemoreceptors, particularly in the CNS. Excess metabolic acid production may be compensated by increased ventilation. Conversely, metabolic alkalosis may be offset by decreased ventilation. Acid-base regulation is discussed in more detail in Chapter 17.

●●● TOP 5 TAKE-HOME POINTS

1. The pulmonary system is specialized for O_2 absorption and transport to the tissues and for CO_2 transport from the tissues back to the lungs for elimination from the body.

2. Exchange of air between the atmosphere and the alveoli is complicated by the organization of air delivery as a "push-pull" system, in which inspired air mixes with air already present in the lungs.

3. Movement of gas between the tissues and the alveoli is accomplished by diffusion down concentration gradients. This is facilitated by matching of ventilation and perfusion in the lung, red blood cell transport specializations, and matching perfusion and metabolic consumption at the tissues.

4. Homeostatic respiratory control is centered primarily on CO_2, with hypoxia becoming important only when arterial P_{O_2} falls below 60 mm Hg.

5. Higher CNS centers can alter basic respiratory control during exercise.

Renal System and Urinary Tract

11

CONTENTS

⬤⬤⬤ RENAL SYSTEM STRUCTURES

The renal system consists of the kidneys, ureters, bladder, and urethra. The kidney contains the nephron, the functional unit of the renal system. The nephron consists of the glomerular and peritubular capillaries and the associated tubular segments. The glomerular tuft (glomerulus) contains capillaries and the beginning of the tubule system, Bowman's capsule.

Tubule fluid, an ultrafiltrate of plasma, is formed at the renal glomerulus and passes through the tubules. The composition of the filtrate is modified by secretion and reabsorption as it passes through the tubules of the renal cortex and medulla, ending with the collecting ducts. A second capillary bed, the peritubular capillaries, carries the reabsorbed water and solute back toward the vena cava. Filtrate from the tubules collects at the renal calyx and is transported by the peristaltic action of the ureter to the bladder. The bladder stores urine until elimination from the body through the urethra.

Kidneys

Renal Cortex and Medulla

Each kidney can be visually and functionally divided into an outer cortex and an inner medulla. The renal cortex contains all the glomeruli, a large portion of the peritubular capillaries, as well as the proximal tubule, distal tubule, and cortical portion of the collecting duct. The renal medulla contains the vasa recta, the loop of Henle, and the medullary portion of the collecting duct. The renal medulla has a pyramidal structure, with the collecting ducts emptying into the renal calyces (Fig. 11-1).

Blood Vessels and Renal Tubules

The kidneys have an extensive vascular supply and receive about 20% of the cardiac output. The renal vascular pattern is unusual in that blood flows through two capillary beds, one with high pressure (glomerular) and the second with low pressure (peritubular), connected in series. Blood enters the kidney via the renal artery and, after a series of divisions, arrives at the glomerulus. Blood entering the glomerular capillaries must first pass through an afferent arteriole. Blood exiting the glomerular capillaries passes through a second arteriole, the efferent arteriole. Blood then flows through the peritubular capillaries, which include the vasa recta that extend into the renal medulla. Blood leaves the peritubular capillaries, collects in progressively larger venules and veins, and then exits the kidney via the renal vein.

Filtrate formed in Bowman's capsule remains separated from the body fluid spaces by a layer of epithelial cells that extends through the remainder of the urinary system.

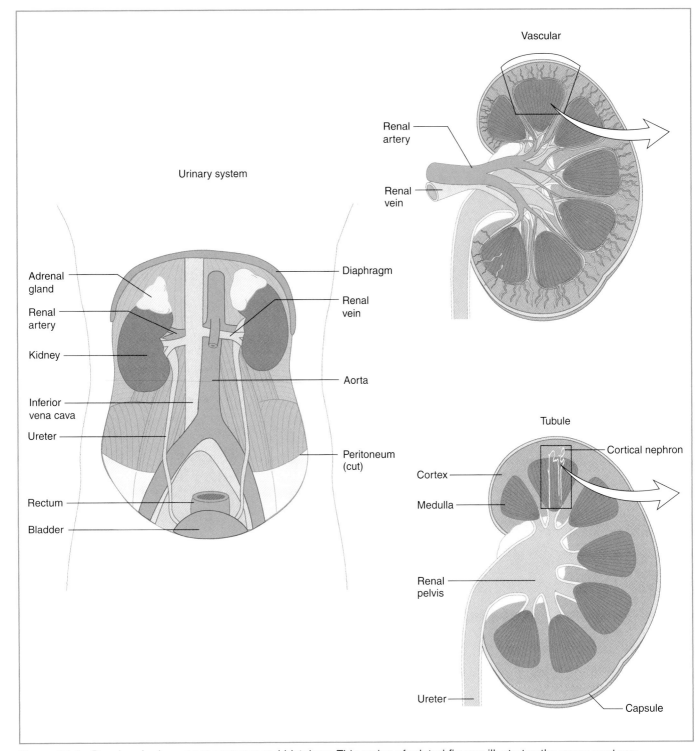

Figure 11-1. Renal and urinary tract anatomy and histology. This series of related figures illustrates the gross anatomy extending down to the fine anatomy of the glomerular capillaries and the renal tubule system.

Consequently, renal filtrate and urine are functionally outside the body, similarly to the fluids of the GI tract. Renal tubules consist of a single layer of epithelial cells that selectively secrete or reabsorb compounds. Tubular transport represents a mechanism to reabsorb water and solutes filtered at the glomerulus before they are excreted from the body in the urine. The ureter, bladder, and urethra also have an epithelial lining, but the epithelial cells do not allow transport of water or solutes. Consequently, filtrate that exits the renal collecting duct and collects in the renal pelvis is identical to the final urine.

The tubular segments originate at the glomerulus. The glomerular filtrate travels progressively through Bowman's capsule, the proximal tubule, loop of Henle, distal tubule,

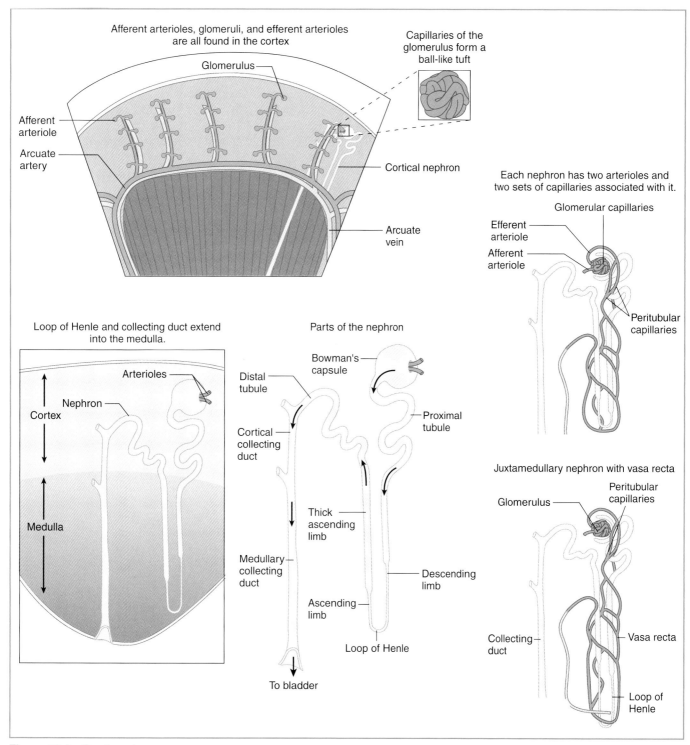

Figure 11-1. *Continued.*

connecting segment, and collecting duct. Upon exiting the tubules, the tubular fluid passes into the renal papilla and exits the kidney via the ureter.

Tubule segments are anatomically adjacent to the vascular supply for that nephron. The junction of glomerulus and the macula densa of the distal tubule that originated from that glomerulus forms the juxtaglomerular apparatus. This arrangement allows negative feedback control of glomerular filtrate formation at the individual nephron level.

Ureters, Bladder, and Urethra

The ureters originate at the renal hilus and conduct urine from the kidney to the bladder. Anatomically, the ureters consist of an epithelium-lined lumen surrounded by smooth muscle, nerves, blood vessels, and connective tissue. Peristalsis, originating in the renal calyx, propels urine toward the bladder.

The bladder is a highly distensible organ lying behind the symphysis pubis. The wall of the bladder consists of an epithelial layer, a mesh-like arrangement of smooth muscle (detrusor) layer, and a thin connective layer containing nerves and blood vessels. This anatomic arrangement allows the wall of the bladder to distend to a large volume without generating much tension. Inflow to the bladder comes from the ureters, which connect with the bladder at the ureterovesical junction. Urine passing from the bladder into the urethra must pass through the smooth muscular internal bladder sphincter.

The urethra extends from the bladder to the surface of the body. It consists of an epithelium-lined lumen and a smooth muscle layer. Urine exiting the urethra must pass through the muscular external sphincter.

●●● FUNCTION OF THE ELIMINATION SYSTEM

The kidneys balance the excretion of substances as urine against the accumulation from either ingestion or production. The kidneys clear the blood of unwanted substances, such as nitrogenous waste products.

Filtration at the renal glomerulus is the first step in urine formation (Fig. 11-2). The kidneys filter a volume equal to plasma volume every 24 minutes. A volume equal to that of total body water is filtered every 6 hours. Glomerular filtrate is similar to plasma but is called an ultrafiltrate because it lacks cells and high-molecular-weight proteins. Glomerular filtrate is modified as it passes through the renal tubules (see Fig. 11-2B). Reabsorption of filtrate components is movement from the filtrate into the peritubular capillaries. This process enhances conservation of glucose, peptides, and electrolytes. Secretion of plasma components enhances elimination of organic acids and bases (and some drugs). The modified glomerular filtrate is excreted as urine.

The balance between hydrostatic pressure and oncotic pressure in the glomerular capillaries determines filtration at the renal glomerulus. An ultrafiltrate, lacking high-molecular-weight proteins, passes into Bowman's capsule. This ultrafiltrate is modified by diffusion, osmosis, and carrier-mediated transport across the renal epithelial cells as it passes through the tubular system.

Net movements of compounds occur across the tubules by both reabsorption and secretion (Fig. 11-3). Reabsorption from the filtrate back into the plasma of the peritubular capillaries is both active and passive. Reabsorbed compounds pass either through the tight junctions in a paracellular pathway or may be transported across the cell in the transcellular pathway. In contrast, secretion from the plasma of the peritubular capillaries into the filtrate is usually active, with the notable exception of K^+ secretion in the distal tubule.

Interstitial fluid osmolarity varies across the kidney. Interstitial fluid of the renal cortex is isotonic and surrounds the glomeruli, proximal tubules, distal tubules, and early portions of the collecting ducts. In contrast, medullary interstitial fluid is hypertonic (relative to plasma) and bathes the vasa recta, loops of Henle, and late portions of collecting ducts. There is a continuous gradient of interstitial fluid osmolarity in the renal medulla, from the slightly hypertonic juxtacortical regions to the highly hypertonic tip of the renal papilla. The regulation of medullary interstitial fluid osmolarity is discussed in the section on Urinary Concentration and Dilution.

Nephron structure is tied in part to the location of the glomeruli in the cortex. Superficial (outer cortical) nephrons generally have short loops of Henle and are less effective at salt and water conservation. Juxtamedullary nephrons generally have long loops of Henle that extend to the tip of the renal papilla, and they are more effective at salt and water conservation. Renal prostaglandins preferentially increase blood flow to the deeper cortical layers, allowing prostaglandins to enhance renal salt and water conservation without affecting total renal blood flow.

Renal Blood Flow

Blood entering the kidney passes through two capillary beds in series. The balance of Starling forces determines transcapillary fluid movements. Because of the high glomerular capillary pressure, only plasma filtration occurs at the glomerular capillaries. The lower capillary pressure in the peritubular capillaries results in only reabsorption occurring at the peritubular capillaries. The vasa recta arise from juxtamedullary glomeruli, allowing a small amount (5%) of renal blood flow to perfuse the renal medulla.

Urine formation can be described as the sequential partitioning of renal blood flow (Fig. 11-4). Total renal blood flow averages about 1100 mL/min. Of the renal blood flow, about 57% of it is plasma, so renal plasma flow is approximately 625 mL/min. About 20% of the plasma entering the kidney is filtered at the renal glomerulus, a glomerular filtration rate (GFR) of 125 mL/min. Between 80% and 99% of the glomerular filtration is reabsorbed, so the final urinary flow rate varies between 0.4 mL/min to 20 mL/min, and usually averages about 1 mL/min.

Renal blood flow is about 25% of resting cardiac output. In contrast to most other organs, renal blood flow is not closely tied to renal metabolic needs. Consequently, renal venous Po_2 is higher than mixed venous Po_2. Autoregulation allows

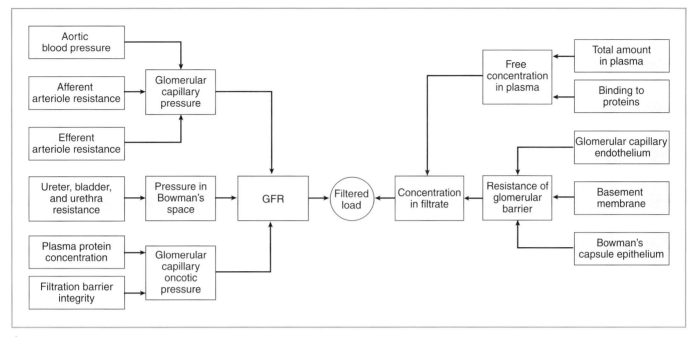

A

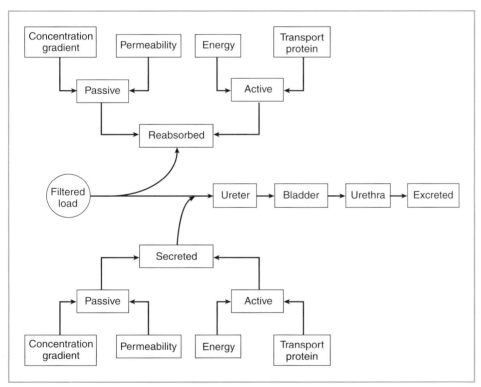

B

Figure 11-2. The renal physiology map illustrates major renal processes. Conceptually, renal processes can be split into those creating the filtered load at the renal glomerulus and those modifying the filtered load as it passes through the renal tubule system.

renal blood flow to remain "constant" over a wide range of arterial pressures. Renal blood flow autoregulation, however, is a consequence of GFR autoregulation and is not tied to renal metabolic rate.

The renal cortex is better perfused than the renal medulla. All renal blood flow goes to a glomerulus. Blood exiting the renal glomerulus goes to the cortical peritubular capillaries, to the medullary peritubular capillaries, or to the medullary vasa recta (a small portion).

Clearance

Renal clearance uses the rate at which a compound is "cleared" from the body, i.e., is excreted in the urine, to determine aspects of renal function. The practical aspect of the clearance

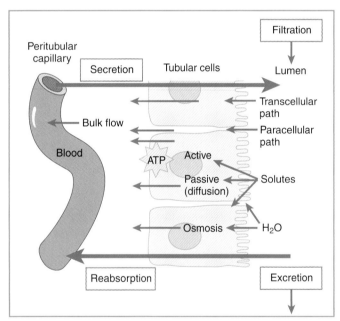

Figure 11-3. Urine formation reflects the processes of filtration, reabsorption, and secretion. Filtration at the renal glomerulus is the first step in urine formation. Reabsorption is the movement of compounds from the filtrate across the tubule epithelium and back into the peritubular capillaries. Secreted compounds move from the peritubular capillaries into the lumen of the tubules. The glomerular filtrate, after it is modified by reabsorption and secretion, is then excreted from the body as urine.

principle is that by applying it to select compounds, one can estimate glomerular filtration rate and renal plasma flow. Below is the equation for calculating clearance (Fig. 11-5).

Clearance
  = urine flow rate × urine concentration/plasma concentration

Glomerular filtration rate can be estimated from the clearance equation if that substance entered the urine only through filtration at the glomerulus. Two common compounds that exhibit this property are inulin and mannitol. Some compounds are reabsorbed by one tubule region and secreted in another tubule region. If the rate of reabsorption is equal to the rate of secretion, there is no net tubule transport in the kidney and this compound can be used to estimate GFR. Urea and creatinine, both endogenous compounds, share this characteristic and sometimes are used to estimate GFR.

Glomerular filtration represents the major excretion process for creatinine. Consequently, a decrease in GFR causes a proportionate increase in plasma creatinine concentration (Fig. 11-6). Reducing GFR by 50% causes plasma creatinine to increase by twofold. Reducing GFR to 25% of normal causes plasma creatinine to increase by fourfold. Changes in plasma creatinine provide a clinical measure of renal function.

Renal plasma flow can be estimated from the clearance equation if that substance is 100% cleared from plasma. There are numerous compounds that can approximate this criterion, such as para-aminohippuric acid (PAH) and Diodrast. In reality, compounds are at best only 90% extracted by the kidney, and a small amount of the compound that entered the kidney is returned to the body by the renal veins. Consequently, the clearance calculation is called effective renal plasma flow, and it is a slight underestimation of true renal plasma flow. The true renal plasma flow can be calculated as the PAH clearance divided by the extraction ratio for PAH.

Free water clearance is based on a comparison of urine osmolarity and plasma osmolarity. This determination provides a measure of the individual's water balance. An individual is in positive free water clearance if the urine is dilute compared with the plasma. Conversely, negative free water clearance occurs when the urine is hypertonic compared with plasma. Free water clearance can be calculated as

$$C_{H_2O} = \text{urine flow rate} - C_{osm}$$

Figure 11-4. Urine formation reflects the sequential partitioning of renal blood flow.

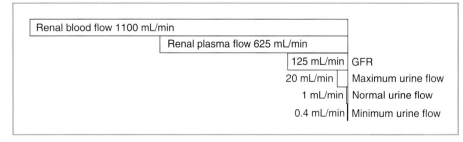

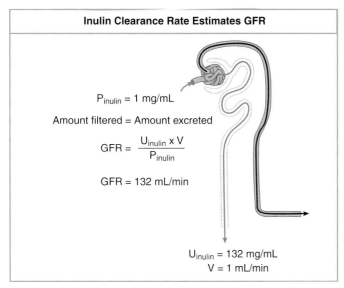

Inulin Clearance Rate Estimates GFR

$P_{inulin} = 1\ mg/mL$

Amount filtered = Amount excreted

$$GFR = \frac{U_{inulin} \times V}{P_{inulin}}$$

$GFR = 132\ mL/min$

$U_{inulin} = 132\ mg/mL$
$V = 1\ mL/min$

A

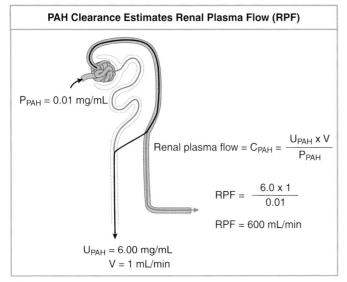

PAH Clearance Estimates Renal Plasma Flow (RPF)

$P_{PAH} = 0.01\ mg/mL$

$$Renal\ plasma\ flow = C_{PAH} = \frac{U_{PAH} \times V}{P_{PAH}}$$

$$RPF = \frac{6.0 \times 1}{0.01}$$

$RPF = 600\ mL/min$

$U_{PAH} = 6.00\ mg/mL$
$V = 1\ mL/min$

B

Figure 11-5. The clearance principle allows estimation of GFR and renal blood flow. Compounds excreted in the urine (U) originate within the body. Clearance (C) calculates the flow of plasma necessary to deliver that amount of the compound to the kidney. **A,** Inulin enters the urine only through the process of glomerular filtration. Consequently, the clearance of inulin can be used to calculate glomerular filtration rate (GFR). **B,** Para-aminohippuric acid (PAH) enters the urine through the processes of glomerular filtration and active secretion. Consequently, the clearance of PAH can be used to estimate renal plasma flow. This calculation is an underestimation of the true renal plasma flow, because PAH is not 100% extracted from the plasma flowing into the kidney. The term "effective renal plasma flow" is sometimes used to describe the PAH clearance estimation.

Plasma osmolarity is much less variable than urine osmolarity. Consequently, free water clearance is empirically estimated as being positive when the urine osmolarity is less than 280 mOsm, and negative when urine osmolarity is greater than 330 mOsm.

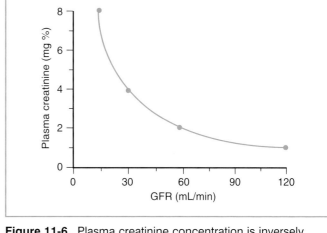

Figure 11-6. Plasma creatinine concentration is inversely proportionate to glomerular filtration rate.

Transcapillary Fluid Exchange

Fluid movement at each capillary bed depends on the balance of fluid pressures and osmotic pressures (Fig. 11-7 and Table 11-1). Glomerular capillary blood pressure reflects resistance to flow at afferent and efferent arterioles. Preglomerular (primarily afferent arteriole) constriction decreases flow of blood into the glomerular capillaries and decreases glomerular capillary blood pressure. Postglomerular (primarily efferent arteriole) constriction decreases the flow of blood out of the glomerulus and increases glomerular capillary pressure.

Glomerular capillary blood pressure reflects the opposing influence of afferent and efferent arteriolar resistance (see Fig. 11-7). Afferent arteriolar constriction increases vascular resistance and decreases glomerular capillary pressure. Activation of renal sympathetic nerves constricts preferentially the afferent arteriole. Efferent arteriolar constriction increases vascular resistance and increases glomerular capillary pressure. The efferent arteriolar smooth muscle is particularly sensitive to the vasoconstrictor action of angiotensin II.

Peritubular capillary blood pressure reflects the influence of preperitubular vessel constriction. Afferent arteriolar constriction decreases renal blood flow and decreases peritubular capillary pressure. Efferent arteriolar constriction decreases renal blood flow and decreases peritubular capillary pressure. Peritubular capillary blood pressure represents the combined influence of afferent and efferent arteriolar constriction (Fig. 11-8).

Plasma oncotic pressure is due to the presence of albumin and other large molecular proteins that cannot freely cross the capillary wall. At the glomerulus, an ultrafiltrate of plasma enters Bowman's capsule, but albumin remains in the glomerular capillaries. Consequently, glomerular filtration causes an increase in the oncotic pressure of blood exiting the glomerular capillaries.

The increase in oncotic pressure in the glomerular capillaries can reduce the net filtration pressure in the glomerulus. For example, in hypotensive shock, there is a reduced rate of renal blood flow. In this case, GFR is reduced because of the combined reduction in glomerular capillary hydrostatic pressure and the low flow–induced increase in glomerular capillary oncotic pressure. Conversely, if glomerular blood flow (per minute) is high, the volume filtered (per milliliter of blood) decreases, attenuating the normal increase in plasma oncotic pressure and increasing GFR. If the glomerular barrier is damaged so that the glomerular capillaries become permeable to albumin, the normal reabsorptive oncotic force is diminished and GFR is increased.

The oncotic pressure in Bowman's capsule usually is 0 because the ultrafiltrate in Bowman's capsule does not contain much albumin. The interstitial fluid oncotic pressure is low around the peritubular capillaries because of the small amount of albumin that is present in the interstitial fluid.

The filtration coefficient reflects restriction on movement of particles into the ultrafiltrate (Fig. 11-9). The negatively charged basement membrane hinders filtration of negatively charged proteins and represents the major impediment to filtration. In addition, capillary endothelial pores and podocyte (Bowman's capsule epithelium) pores and fibers of the basement membrane restrict movement based on molecular weight.

The filtration coefficient is variable, and it changes in some disease states. A decreased pore size is caused by contraction of endothelial cells. Endothelial contraction can be caused by angiotensin II, norepinephrine, prostaglandins, and

bradykinin. Diseases that cause a thickening of the basement membrane also diminish filtration.

A loss of the negative charges on basement membrane, such as by glycosylation of the basement membrane proteins or by antigen-antibody reactions, allows some proteins to

PATHOLOGY

Malignant Hypertension

Malignant hypertension is characterized by a progressive increase in blood pressure over a short time. Plasma angiotensin II levels rise in concert with the increase in blood pressure. Angiotensin is not the cause of the hypertension, but rather the angiotensin II constriction of the efferent arteriole helps preserve glomerular filtration and renal function during this disease process.

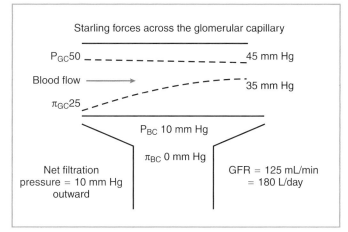

Figure 11-8. Hydrostatic and oncotic pressures determine filtration across the glomerular capillary (GC). Glomerular capillary filtration depends on the balance of the hydrostatic and the oncotic pressures. Hydrostatic pressure at the afferent end of the glomerular capillaries is high and decreases slightly along the length of the glomerular capillary. Plasma oncotic pressure in the glomerular capillary increases along the length of the glomerular capillary as plasma is filtered, but the large proteins remain within the capillary. The net balance of pressures ensures that only filtration occurs in the glomerular capillaries.

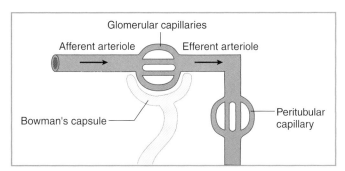

Figure 11-7. Arteriolar resistance determines renal blood flow and glomerular filtration rate. Blood flows sequentially through the afferent arteriole, glomerular capillaries, efferent arteriole, and finally peritubular capillaries. Vascular smooth muscle of the afferent and efferent arterioles regulates renal blood flow, glomerular capillary pressure, and peritubular capillary pressure (see Table 11-1).

TABLE 11-1. Renal Blood Flow and Glomerular Filtration Rate

	Renal Blood Flow	Glomerular Capillary Pressure	Glomerular Filtration Rate	Peritubular Capillary Pressure	Peritubular Reabsorption
Afferent constriction	↓	↓	↓	↓	↑
Efferent constriction	↓	↑	↑	↓	↑
Afferent dilation	↑	↑	↑	↑	↓
Efferent dilation	↑	↓	↓	↑	↓

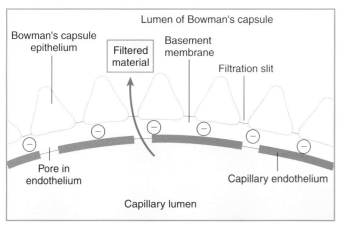

Figure 11-9. The glomerular filtration barrier impedes filtration of large proteins. Plasma in the glomerular capillaries must pass through the capillary endothelium, a basement membrane, and Bowman's capsule epithelium before it becomes glomerular filtrate. The negatively charged basement membrane impedes the movement of proteins into the glomerular filtrate.

PATHOLOGY

Poststreptococcal Glomerulonephrosis

About 7 days after a streptococcal infection, the kidneys exhibit glomerulonephrosis. The increase in urine volume and protein excretion in the urine are caused by destruction of the glomerular basement membranes by antibodies generated in response to the infection.

pass into the urine (proteinuria). Two common causes of proteinuria are diabetes and streptococcal infection.

In summary, fluid movement across the capillary is based on the combination of hydrostatic and oncotic pressures. Filtration occurs at the glomerular capillaries owing to the high capillary pressure and the normal oncotic pressure. Consequently, 20% of the plasma that enters the kidney is filtered. Reabsorption occurs at the peritubular capillaries owing to the lower capillary pressure and the higher plasma oncotic pressure. For this reason, 80% to 99.5% of ultra-filtrate formed in the glomerulus is reabsorbed.

Tubular Secretion and Reabsorption

Transport proteins and tightness of tight junctions determine the transport characteristics of the renal tubules. Transport of solutes can be passive, active, or secondary active. Passive movement is by diffusion, and the direction is down the electrochemical gradient. Transport proteins can facilitate this movement. Active transport occurs against an electrochemical gradient. This movement utilizes energy, obtained from hydrolysis of ATP (primary active transport) or by coupling movement to the simultaneous movement of Na^+ (secondary active transport, Na^+-coupled cotransport). Movement of water is always passive, utilizing osmotic gradients.

Tubular epithelial cells are specialized into an apical (facing the tubular lumen) surface and a basolateral (facing the interstitial fluid and peritubular capillaries) surface. The tight junctions that join epithelial cells together provide a physical boundary between the apical and basolateral surfaces. The permeability of the tight junctions varies along the length of the renal tubules. The proximal tubule and descending limb of the loop of Henle have "leaky" tight junctions that allow passage of water and solute. The ascending limb of the loop of Henle and later tubule segments have "tight" tight junctions that restrict the movement of electrolytes and water. These "tight" tight junctions allow transepithelial concentration gradients, electrical gradients, and osmotic gradients to be created by the selective transport of solutes or water through the cells.

Apical microvilli act to increase surface area and assist diffusion and transport, particularly in the proximal tubule cells. Mitochondrial density varies by tubule segments, correlating with the metabolic activity of the cell.

RENAL TUBULAR SEGMENTS

Renal tubule segments are characterized by their transport capabilities. Secretion and reabsorption across the tubules depends on transport proteins on the apical and basolateral membrane surfaces. Figure 11-10A–D illustrates some of the important epithelial transport processes in regions of the renal tubules. In these drawings, the tubule fluid is on the left side and is bordered by the apical membrane of the cell. The interstitial fluid (and peritubular capillaries, not shown) is on the right side of the figures and is bordered by the basolateral surface of the cells. Na^+/K^+-ATPase is on the basolateral surface of all the cells.

Proximal Convoluted Tubule

The proximal convoluted tubule (see Fig. 11-10A) reabsorbs 65% of the filtered water, Na^+, Cl^-, and K^+. The epithelia of the proximal tubule have "leaky" tight junctions and can maintain only a small transepithelial membrane potential.

Most of the energy consumed by the proximal tubule is tied to Na^+ reabsorption. On the apical surface, Na^+ enters the cell by facilitated diffusion and can be inhibited by amiloride. The Na^+/K^+-ATPase on the basolateral surface prevents intracellular Na^+ accumulation.

Glucose and amino acids are reabsorbed by Na^+-coupled transport in the proximal tubule (see Fig. 11-10A). A family of transport proteins on the apical surface of the epithelial cell uses the diffusion of Na^+ down its electrochemical gradient as the energy source. Transport of glucose across the basolateral surface occurs by facilitated diffusion.

HCO_3^- is reabsorbed as major anion early in the proximal tubule through a variety of mechanisms. The apical Na^+/H^+ antiport secretes H^+ into the lumen, where it combines with filtered HCO_3^- to form CO_2. The CO_2 can freely diffuse from the lumen into the cell, where it dissociates back to H^+ and HCO_3^-. The H^+ is recycled and again secreted into the lumen.

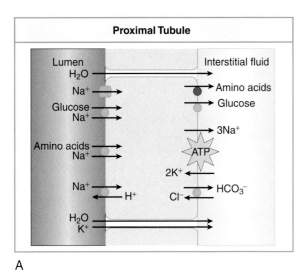

A

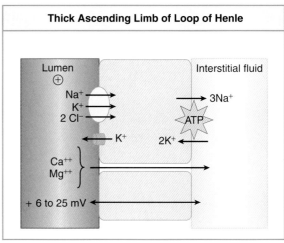

B

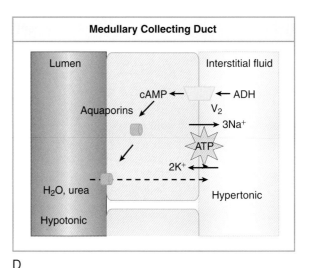

C   D

Figure 11-10. Specific transport proteins on the apical or the basolateral tubular epithelial cell surfaces mediate reabsorption and secretion.

The HCO_3^- is transported out of the cell across the basolateral surface by an HCO_3^-/Cl^- exchange. The H^+ secretion causes the luminal pH to drop to 7.2 in the proximal tubule.

The reabsorption of Na^+ and HCO_3^- causes a slight drop in the filtrate osmolarity. The osmotic gradient between the filtrate and the renal interstitial fluid, combined with the "leaky" tight junctions, allow water to be reabsorbed. This water reabsorption then causes an increase in the concentration of all the other filtrate components. This concentration gradient provides a driving force to allow reabsorption by diffusion.

K^+ reabsorption in the proximal tubule is primarily paracellular, driven by a concentration gradient caused by water reabsorption. A small amount of K^+ is actually secreted in late proximal tubule, but a net 70% of the filtered K^+ load is reabsorbed in the proximal tubule. Cl^- is absorbed passively in later proximal tubule by both a chemical gradient and a transluminal electrical gradient.

The proximal tubule normally reabsorbs 100% of filtered glucose, amino acids, and small peptides. On the apical surface, this movement is due to Na^+-coupled cotransport. Consequently, amino acid and glucose reabsorption show saturation kinetics (see Fig. 11-11). The transport maximum for glucose is only about three times higher than the normal filtered load. If plasma glucose increases enough to increase the filtered load above this level, some of the filtered glucose will not be reabsorbed and will be excreted in the urine.

The cells of the proximal tubule also secrete organic acids and bases (transporter not shown). This secretion is the basis for the use of PAH for the clearance estimation of renal plasma flow. In addition, this secretion can be a major route for the elimination of certain drugs, such as penicillin, from the body.

Loop of Henle

The loop of Henle carries filtrate from the proximal tubule to the renal medulla and back to the renal cortex. There are three functional divisions: the thin descending limb, thin ascending limb, and thick ascending limb.

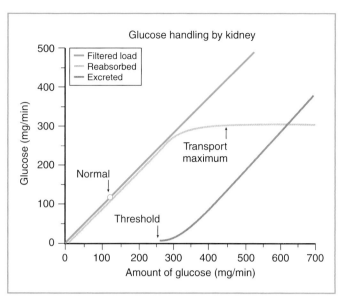

Figure 11-11. Glucose reabsorption depends on transport proteins in the proximal tubule. When the filtered load of glucose is less than 200 mg/min, the amount of glucose filtered and the amount reabsorbed is equal, and no glucose is excreted. The number of transport proteins determines the transport maximum for glucose, usually around 300 mg/min. If plasma glucose concentration rises so that the filtered glucose load exceeds the transport maximum, then some glucose remains behind in the lumen of the proximal tubule. This excess glucose will be excreted in the urine. The splay in the glucose transport curve occurs because of variability in the transport rate of glucose in individual proximal tubule segments.

PATHOLOGY

Diabetes Mellitus

Diabetes mellitus results from either a deficiency in insulin production (type I) or an impaired tissue response to insulin (type II). Both forms of the disease are characterized by persistently high blood glucose levels. When the glomerular filtered load of glucose exceeds the reabsorptive capacity of the renal tubules, glucose remains in the filtrate, where it acts as an osmotic particle causing diuresis.

The thin descending limb of the loop of Henle has leaky "tight" junctions. This allows water to leave by passive diffusion as the tubule segment enters the hypertonic renal medulla. In addition, urea and Na^+ diffuse from medullary interstitial fluid into the lumen of the tubule. The thin ascending limb of the loop of Henle is distinguished from the descending limb in that the tight junctions are now "tight" and water impermeable. As the name suggests, at the transition from descending to ascending, the tubule segment makes a 180-degree turn and the filtrate is now being carried back toward the cortex.

The epithelia of the thick ascending limb of loop of Henle also contain "tight" tight junctions. The most important transport protein in this segment is the apical $Na^+/K^+/2\ Cl^-$

PHARMACOLOGY

Potassium-Sparing Diuretics

The entry of Na^+ through the apical channel on the distal tubule principal cell creates the electrical gradient that causes K^+ secretion. Any diuretic that increases the amount of Na^+ delivered to the distal tubule will cause K^+ loss in the urine. Only diuretics such as spironolactone that interfere with Na^+ reabsorption by the principal calls will not cause K^+ secretion, and such diuretics are said to be potassium sparing.

transporter (see Fig. 11-10B), which can be blocked by furosemide or bumetanide. The back-leak of K^+ across a channel on the apical surface causes a lumen-positive (6 to 25 mV) transluminal potential. This transepithelial potential then drives the paracellular absorption of calcium and magnesium. The solute transport without water movement results in a drop in the filtrate osmolarity to 100 mOsm, so the ascending limb of the loop of Henle is sometimes called the diluting segment. The solute transport into the interstitial space without water movement also is one of two mechanisms causing hypertonicity of renal medullary interstitial fluid.

Distal Convoluted Tubule and Early Cortical Collecting Duct

The tight junctions of the cells lining the distal tubule are "tight," so water and electrolytes cannot diffuse across the tubule and the filtrate remains hypotonic. In the early portion of the distal tubule, an apical Na^+/Cl^- transporter causes further reabsorption of ions. Thiazide diuretics block this reabsorption.

The principal (most common) cells of later distal tubule and cortical collecting duct have a complex mechanism mediating the aldosterone-sensitive secretion of K^+. The apical surface has an Na^+ channel, allowing the absorption of Na^+. The apical and basolateral cell membranes have identical K^+ channels. As Na^+ enters across the apical membrane, the transepithelial potential becomes negative (up to –50 mV). This transepithelial potential is the driving force for K^+ secretion. The magnitude of the transepithelial potential determines whether potassium is secreted back into the lumen across the apical surface or K^+ moves across the basolateral surface. The net effect of these transport processes is that as Na^+ is reabsorbed, K^+ is secreted.

Distal tubule K^+ delivery is low because of the K^+ reabsorption in the thick ascending limb of Henle, so active K^+ secretion in the distal tubule determines urinary K^+ loss. Blockade of electrogenic Na^+ reabsorption decreases transluminal potential, so K^+ secretion is impaired. This is the mechanism of action of K^+-sparing diuretics such as amiloride.

Another type of cell found in the cortical collecting duct is the intercalated cell. These carbonic anhydrase–rich cells secrete H^+ and decrease transluminal potential. The loss of the negative transluminal potential caused by H⁺ secretion accounts for the decreased K⁺ secretion in acidosis (see Fig. 11-11).

Collecting Duct

Antidiuretic hormone (ADH) binds to a vasopressin II receptor on the basolateral surface of the collecting duct cells, causing a cAMP-mediated translocation of aquaporins to the apical surface of the collecting duct cell. These aquaporins increase the permeability of the apical membrane to water, promoting their reabsorption. In the medullary portion of the collecting duct, ADH also increases the permeability to urea, promoting urea reabsorption. The reabsorption of urea is the

second mechanism that contributes to the creation of the hypertonic medullary interstitial fluid.

Summary of Tubule Transport

Figure 11-12 and Table 11-2 summarize renal epithelial transport. The proximal tubule epithelia (see Fig. 11-12A) have extensive apical microvilli, enhancing the surface area available for the reabsorption of electrolytes, water, glucose, and amino acids. The proximal tubule also secretes hydrogen ions, organic acids, and organic bases. The thin descending limb of the loop of Henle (see Fig. 11-12B) has thin epithelial cells, consistent with only passive movement of ions, water, and urea. The epithelia of the thick ascending limb of the loop

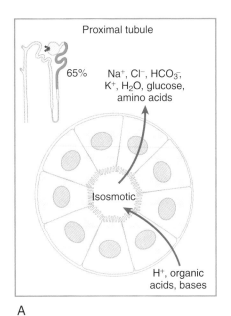
A

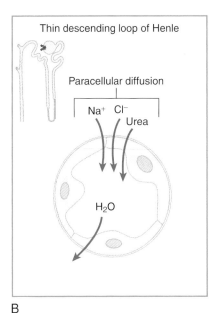
B

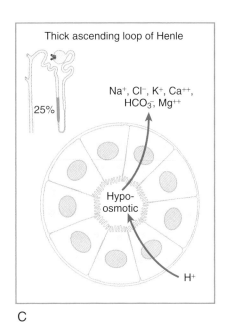
C

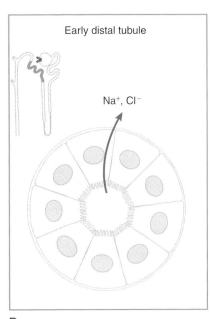
D

E

Figure 11-12. Histologic appearance reflects transport characteristics of the renal tubule segments.

TABLE 11-2. Renal Tubule Segment Transport

	Proximal Tubule	Descending Limb of Loop of Henle	Ascending Limb of Loop of Henle	Distal Tubule	Collecting Duct
Water	Reabsorb	Reabsorb		Reabsorb (ADH)	Reabsorb (ADH)
Na^+	Reabsorb (SNS, angiotensin II)		Reabsorb	Reabsorb (aldosterone)	Reabsorb
K^+	Reabsorb		Reabsorb	Secrete (aldosterone)	Secrete (aldosterone)
Urea	Reabsorb				Reabsorb (ADH)
Bicarbonate	Reabsorb		Reabsorb	Reabsorb/secrete	
Creatinine	—		—	—	—

ADH, antidiuretic hormone; SNS, sympathetic nervous system.
Regulation shown in parentheses.

of Henle (see Fig. 11-12C) have numerous mitochondria and apical microvilli, consistent with the metabolically coupled reabsorption of sodium, chloride, potassium, calcium, bicarbonate, and magnesium. The thick ascending limb of the loop of Henle also secretes hydrogen ion. The early distal tubule epithelia (see Fig. 11-12D) participate in the reabsorption of sodium and chloride. The late distal tubule (see Fig. 11-12E) has principal cells involved in the reabsorption of Na^+ and the secretion of K^+, as well as intercalated cells involved in hydrogen and bicarbonate transport. The collecting duct epithelia exhibit an ADH-regulated transport of water and urea.

RENAL HANDLING OF WATER AND ELECTROLYTES

An alternative perspective of tubule transport is obtained by examining the amount of the filtered load that enters the Bowman's capsule that remains in the filtrate after it is modified in each tubular segment. Figures 11-13 through 11-16 trace the reabsorption and secretion of H_2O, Na^+, K^+, and urea along the renal tubules.

The normal filtered load for water is 125 mL/min, the GFR. Normal water excretion varies from 0.4% to 20% of this total (see Fig. 11-13). About 66% of this load is reabsorbed by a paracellular route (through the tight junctions) in the proximal tubule by osmotic movement, following the osmotic gradient created by the reabsorption of Na^+ and HCO_3^-. An additional 5% to 10% is reabsorbed in the descending limb of the loop of Henle, in response to the osmotic gradient between the filtrate and the hypertonic interstitial fluid of the renal medulla. Beginning at the ascending limb, the tight junctions connecting the tubule cell do not allow the paracellular movement of water. Consequently, there is no further water reabsorption in the ascending limbs and early distal tubule. Water reabsorption in the later distal tubule and collecting duct occurs via an ADH-sensitive transcellular route, mediated by aquaporins in the water channels. In the absence of ADH, the segments remain impermeable, and the rate of water passing through the collecting duct is about the same as the amount that passed through the ascending

limb of the loop of Henle. In the presence of ADH, the distal tubule and collecting duct become water permeable, and the water is reabsorbed osmotically as the tubule fluid comes into equilibrium with the renal interstitial fluid.

The normal Na^+ filtered load is 18 mEq/min, approximately 99% of which is reabsorbed (see Fig. 11-14). Approximately 66% of the Na^+ filtered load is reabsorbed in the proximal tubule, including some that is reabsorbed during the Na^+-coupled absorption of glucose and amino acids. The tubular Na^+ load actually increases in the descending limb of Henle owing to paracellular diffusion into the filtrate from the Na^+-enriched renal medullary interstitial fluid. Na^+ load decreases in the thick ascending limb of the loop of Henle because of the activity of the $Na^+/K^+/2$ Cl^- transporter. Final Na^+ reabsorption occurs in the distal tubule through the NaCl symport and aldosterone-sensitive reabsorption by the principal cells.

The potassium filtered load is approximately 0.5 mEq/min, most of which is reabsorbed by the end of the loop of Henle (see Fig. 11-15). Approximately 66% of the K^+ filtered load is reabsorbed in the proximal tubule, mostly by a paracellular route. There is little K^+ reabsorption in the descending limb of the loop of Henle. The $Na^+/K^+/2$ Cl^- transporter in the thick ascending limb reabsorbs most of the remaining K^+, in part because of the much greater proportion of Na^+ present in the filtrate and because the protein has to reabsorb one K for every Na transported. The potassium that appears in the final urine is due to aldosterone-sensitive K^+ secretion in the late distal tubule. The maximal K^+ reabsorption rate in the proximal tubule and loop of Henle is close to the filtered load. Consequently, any increase in K^+ filtered load, such as from an increase in plasma K^+ concentration, will cause some K^+ to remain in the filtrate that exits the loop of Henle and be excreted. This is analogous to the urinary glucose excretion occurring in diabetics when the glucose filtered load exceeds the proximal tubule glucose transport capacity.

The urea filtered load is 0.6 mmol/min, approximately 50% of which is reabsorbed across the tubules (see Fig. 11-16). About 25% of the filtered load is reabsorbed across the proximal tubule, mostly by a paracellular route. Urea diffuses into the filtrate from the urea-enriched medullary

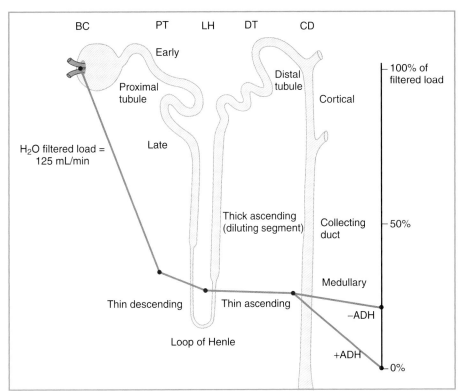

Figure 11-13. Ninety-nine percent of water is reabsorbed as filtrate passes through the renal tubules. Final water excretion rate varies between 0.4 and 20 mL/min and is determined by ADH acting on the collecting duct.

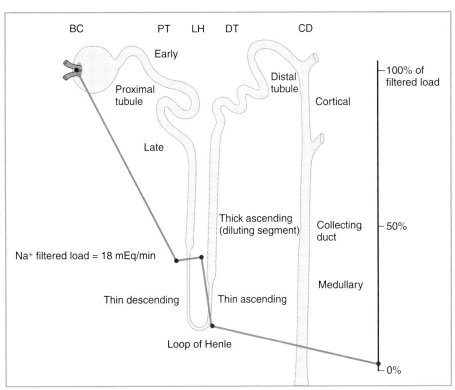

Figure 11-14. Ninety-nine percent of filtered Na^+ is reabsorbed as filtrate passes through the renal tubules. Reabsorption occurs primarily in the proximal tubule (66%) and loop of Henle (20%).

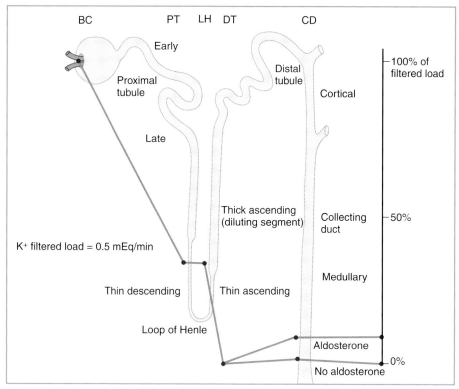

Figure 11-15. Ninety-nine percent of filtered K^+ is reabsorbed as filtrate passes through the renal tubules. Reabsorption occurs primarily in the proximal tubule (66%) and loop of Henle (33%). Filtrate leaving the loop of Henle is potassium depleted. Potassium appearing in the urine can be up to 10% of the filtered load, and is due primarily to distal tubule potassium secretion.

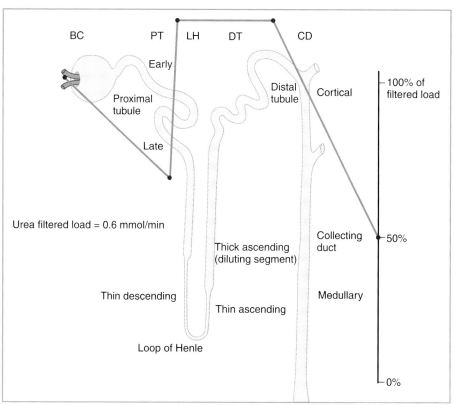

Figure 11-16. Fifty percent of filtered urea is reabsorbed as filtrate passes through the renal tubules.

interstitial fluid in the descending limb, increasing above the original filtered load. The tight junctions of the ascending limb and early distal tubule prevent any further urea movement. The collecting duct has ADH-sensitive urea permeability, particularly the medullary portions of the collecting duct. Urea is reabsorbed in the collecting duct so that the final urea excretion is 50% of the filtered load.

Water reabsorption, as well as solute reabsorption and secretion, results in a change in the composition of the tubule fluid, as shown in Figure 11-17. In this figure, the y-axis is "concentration (times that of filtrate)." The concentration of a compound can change either because the amount of the compound has changed or the amount of water has changed. Inulin and creatinine are not transported across the tubules, so changes in inulin concentration can be used to track water reabsorption. About 66% of the filtered water is reabsorbed in the proximal tubule, causing a threefold increase in the concentration of inulin. In the late distal tubule and collecting duct, inulin concentration increases further owing to ADH-mediated water reabsorption. The reabsorption of 99% of the filtered water load causes inulin concentration to increase 100-fold by the end of the collecting duct.

The reabsorption of Na^+/K^+ and Cl^- in the proximal tubule is proportionate to water reabsorption; therefore, their concentration does not change. In the descending limb of the loop of Henle, there is passive diffusion of Na^+/K^+ and Cl^- into the tubular filtrate. In the thick ascending limb of the loop of Henle, there is active reabsorption of sodium, potassium, and chloride, and consequently a decrease in their concentration. There is some Na^+ and Cl^- reabsorption in the later tubular segments, and aldosterone-sensitive potassium secretion.

PAH is secreted in the proximal tubule; consequently, its concentration increases more rapidly than that of creatinine and inulin. The remaining changes in PAH concentration are due to the passive movement of water.

About 50% of the filtered urea load is reabsorbed in the proximal tubule. The large increase in urea concentration in the descending limb of the loop of Henle is due to diffusion of urea from the medullary interstitial fluid into the tubule. In the collecting duct, urea is reabsorbed along with water; consequently its concentration does not increase as rapidly as does that of inulin.

●●● URINARY CONCENTRATION AND DILUTION

The balance of water and solute reabsorption rates determines urine osmolarity. Water reabsorption is driven by an osmotic gradient, particularly evident as filtrate passes through tubule segments of the hypertonic renal medulla. Reabsorption and secretion characteristics are specific for each solute and can result from both passive (diffusion) and active transport.

Renal cortex interstitial fluid is isotonic with plasma, around 300 mOsm. Renal medullary interstitial fluid is hypertonic to plasma, up to 1600 mOsm (Fig. 11-18). The accumulation of

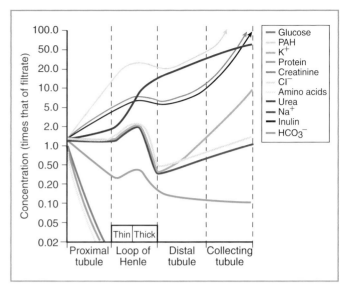

Figure 11-17. Summary of transport across the renal tubules. The lines marked creatinine and inulin illustrate the changes in the concentration of these compounds caused by water reabsorption. For all other compounds, the change in concentration reflects both water and solute movement. See text for explanation.

solute particles in the renal medulla is due to (1) solute reabsorption in the ascending loop of Henle and (2) reabsorption of urea in the inner medullary collecting duct under the influence of ADH. In addition, renal medullary blood flow does not disrupt gradient. This is because the vasa recta allow countercurrent exchange of osmotic particles as blood passes into the medulla and because only 5% of renal blood flow goes to the medulla.

Glomerular ultrafiltrate is isosmotic with plasma (step 1 in Fig. 11-18). The ultrafiltrate, however, lacks large plasma proteins and blood cells. Proximal tubule filtrate also is isosmotic with plasma (step 2 in Fig. 11-18). This is because the "leaky" tight junctions allow osmotic movement of water to match the reabsorption of solute ($NaHCO_3$) in this tubule segment. An increase in the number of osmotic particles in proximal tubular filtrate can decrease water reabsorption. Consequently, blockade of HCO_3^- reabsorption by carbonic anhydrase inhibitors also causes an osmotic diuresis.

The descending limb of the loop of Henle conducts filtrate to the hypertonic renal medulla. The leaky "tight" junctions allow movement of both solute and water. Consequently, filtrate osmolarity is increased as tubular fluid comes into equilibrium with the hypertonic medullary interstitial fluid (step 3 in Fig. 11-18). In addition, urea enters tubular fluid from the medullary interstitial fluid.

In the thick ascending limb of the loop of Henle, the tight "tight" junctions are impermeable to water. The active Na^+, K^+, $2\ Cl^-$ transport (step 4 in Fig. 11-18) decreases osmolarity to below plasma osmolarity by end of thick limb (step 5 in Fig. 11-18). Urea becomes the major remaining osmotic particle.

The "tight" tight junctions of the distal tubule and connecting segment allow tubular fluid osmolarity to differ

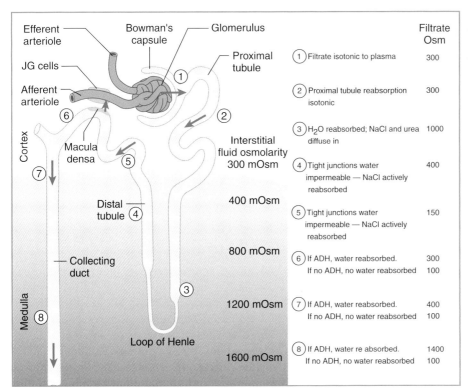

Figure 11-18. Filtrate osmolarity varies along the length of the renal tubules because of both water reabsorption and solute transport.

from interstitial fluid osmolarity. Distal tubular fluid osmolarity (step 6 in Fig. 11-18) can fall as low as 100 mOsm owing to selective Na/Cl reabsorption and the absence of water reabsorption.

In the collecting duct, tight junctions remain tight, preventing the paracellular movement of water and solutes. The collecting duct carries fluid through the renal medulla. Transcellular water permeability of the collecting duct is under the control of ADH and determines the final urine osmolarity. ADH stimulates the insertion of water channels—aquaporins—on the collecting duct apical membrane. Consequently, ADH increases water permeability and therefore enhances water reabsorption. ADH also increases urea permeability and reabsorption in the medullary collecting duct.

Medullary interstitial fluid osmolarity sets the upper limit on urine osmolarity around 1600 mOsm. Additional Na/Cl reabsorption from the hypotonic distal tubule filtrate sets the lower limit on urine osmolarity. In the absence of ADH, there is little water reabsorption, so distal tubular filtrate osmolarity (150 mOsm) is further reduced to 100 mOsm by active Na/Cl transport. Excessive ADH stimulates water reabsorption along the entire length of the collecting duct, so urine osmolarity equilibrates with medullary interstitial fluid osmolarity, around 1600 mOsm.

●●● URINARY ACID-BASE REGULATION

Renal acid/base excretion complements pulmonary CO_2 elimination to regulate body acid-base balance. Normally, there is a net acid production by the body, and urine pH is slightly acidic to keep the body in pH balance. Acids excreted in the urine include H^+, ammonium, phosphate, and sulfate. When the urine pH becomes alkaline, the urinary base is predominantly HCO_3^-. The total urinary acid excretion has to account for all these compounds, and it is calculated as

Total urinary acid excretion
= [(phosphate + sulfate) + ammonium] – bicarbonate

Plasma HCO_3^- levels are normally 24 mEq/L, and plasma H^+ levels are 0.0006 mEq/L. This means that glomerular filtrate contains over 10,000 times as much HCO_3^- as H^+. To produce acidic urine, the first step has to be bicarbonate reabsorption.

The primary pH function of the proximal tubule is HCO_3^- reabsorption, a process facilitated by the presence of the enzyme carbonic anhydrase in both the lumen and the cell. Carbonic anhydrase catalyzes the reaction $H^+ + HCO_3^- \rightleftharpoons CO_2$. An apical Na^+/H^+ antiport secretes H^+ into the tubule lumen, where H^+ combines with HCO_3^- to form CO_2. CO_2 diffuses across the apical membrane into the proximal tubule cell, where it dissociates back to H^+ and HCO_3^-. The H^+ is again pumped across the luminal membrane, and the HCO_3^- pumped on basolateral surface by $Na^+/3HCO_3^-$ symport, and is returned to the body in the renal venous blood. The H^+ secretion decreases the luminal fluid pH to 7.2, acidotic relative to plasma.

The proximal tubule also produces ammonia (NH_4^+). In this inducible reaction, glutamine is metabolized within the cell to form NH_3. NH_3 is uncharged, so it diffuses into tubular lumen. Within the lumen, secreted H^+ binds to NH_3 to form NH_4^+. The charged NH_4^+ does not freely diffuse, and remains in lumen (ammonia trapping). This process is important because the H^+ bound to NH_3 does not alter the pH of the luminal fluid. The activity of the enzymes regulating glutamine metabolism into ammonia is increased in chronic acidosis. Consequently, ammonia excretion is an important mechanism allowing excess acid secretion in chronic acidosis.

HCO_3^- becomes concentrated in the descending limb of the loop of Henle as water is reabsorbed. In the thick ascending limb, NH_4^+ can substitute for K^+ in the $Na^+/K^+/2$ Cl^- transporter.

The distal nephron pH is regulated primarily by the intercalated cells. These cells have the same transporters as seen on proximal tubule cells. There are two populations of intercalated cells, specialized for either HCO_3^- or H^+ secretion, determined by which transport proteins are on the cell apical surface. The pH of the plasma determines which population of cells will be activated.

In acidosis, increased entry of CO_2 from the basolateral side of the cell can cause net Na^+/HCO_3^- reabsorption from the filtrate and an increase in acidity of the urine. Na^+/H^+ exchange is enhanced, and the H^+ secreted into the lumen is trapped in the lumen by ammonia or phosphate buffers. Na^+/HCO_3^- is cotransported on the basolateral surface. Conversely, in alkalosis, decreased entry of CO_2 from the basolateral surface can promote net HCl reabsorption. This response involves primarily a decrease in the luminal Na^+/H^+ exchange and an increase in the luminal HCO_3^-/Cl^- exchange.

●○● ● REGULATION OF RENAL FUNCTION

Intrinsic—Tubuloglomerular Feedback and Glomerulotubular Balance

Intrarenal control of renal function is by tubuloglomerular feedback and by glomerulotubular balance. In tubuloglomerular feedback, Na/Cl delivery to the distal tubule serves as a signal to provide negative feedback control of GFR (Fig. 11-19). In glomerulotubular balance, filtration at the glomerulus alters the oncotic pressure of the plasma that exits the glomerulus and flows into the peritubular capillaries. This consequently alters the balance of transcapillary fluid exchange in the peritubular capillary bed.

Distal tubule NaCl delivery is proportionate to glomerular filtration rate. Tubuloglomerular feedback adjusts GFR to maintain a relatively constant rate of distal tubule NaCl delivery. A drop in the delivery of Na^+ or Cl^- to the distal tubule is sensed at the macula densa. This signal is transmitted to the afferent arteriole. The afferent arteriole dilates, which increases glomerular capillary pressure. The afferent arteriole cells release renin, leading to intrarenal angiotensin II formation. Angiotensin II constricts preferentially the efferent arterioles, as the efferent arterioles are much more sensitive to angiotensin II. Efferent arteriolar constriction increases glomerular capillary pressure. Both vascular changes combine to cause an increase in GFR, which restores distal tubule Na^+ or Cl^- delivery.

Tubuloglomerular feedback results in the regulation of GFR. A drop in arterial blood pressure causes both a decrease

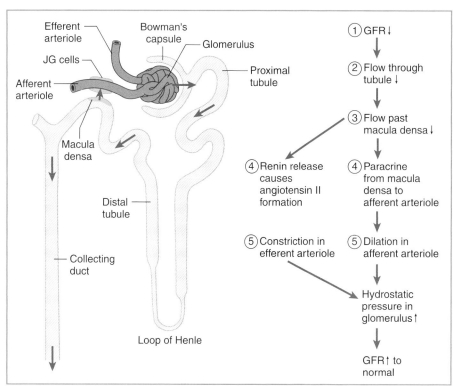

Figure 11-19. Tubuloglomerular feedback regulates glomerular filtration rate. The juxtaglomerular apparatus consists of the afferent arteriole, efferent arteriole, and distal tubule associated with that glomerulus. If the delivery of Na/Cl to the distal tubule fails, the afferent arteriole will dilate and renin will be released, causing formation of angiotensin II and consequent constriction of the efferent arteriole. These vascular changes cause an increase in glomerular filtration rate and increase the filtered Na/Cl load, restoring Na/Cl delivery to the macula densa.

in GFR and a decrease in renal blood flow. The drop in GFR causes a tubuloglomerular feedback–mediated arteriolar dilation, restoring GFR and also increasing renal blood flow. Consequently, the regulation of GFR also results in the autoregulation of renal blood flow.

Glomerulotubular balance ties peritubular capillary filtrate reabsorption to glomerular filtration rate. An increase in filtration at the glomerulus enhances filtrate reabsorption at the peritubular capillaries. Increased GFR increases the oncotic pressure of the blood exiting the glomerulus. When that blood enters the peritubular capillaries, the higher oncotic pressure increases reabsorption of filtrate from the renal tubules. An increase in GFR causes a proportionate increase in fluid reabsorption from the proximal tubules and loop of Henle. This balance is not perfect, so increase in GFR does increase fluid delivery to the late tubule segments

Extrinsic—Neural and Hormonal Control

Extrarenal neural and endocrine control helps integrate renal function. Neural control is predominantly through sympathetic nervous system constriction of the renal afferent arteriole. Renal sympathetic nerves are preferentially activated by reflex inputs from high-pressure arterial baroreceptors and low-pressure cardiopulmonary volume receptors. An increase in renal sympathetic activity constricts the afferent arteriole, decreasing both renal blood flow and GFR. In addition, renal sympathetic nerves are one of the factors controlling renin release. Neural reflexes initiated by decreased blood volume also release ADH from the supraoptic nucleus, reducing short-term fluid loss.

A variety of endocrine agents alter renal excretion. Angiotensin II constricts preferentially the efferent arteriole, maintaining GFR even when arterial blood pressure is low. Blockade of angiotensin II formation in disease states can cause renal failure. Aldosterone promotes K^+ secretion by the principal cells in the later tubular segments, and aldosterone has smaller effects on Na^+ handling by the principal cells. Atrial natriuretic polypeptide (ANP, ANF) promotes tubular Na^+ secretion, but the physiologic significance of this action has yet to be determined. ADH promotes water conservation in the medullary collecting duct.

The neural and endocrine modification of urinary excretion exists only in the presence of normal renal perfusion pressure. Importantly, renal perfusion pressure is the dominant long-term determinant of filtrate formation. An increase in renal perfusion pressure causes pressure diuresis and pressure natriuresis. Conversely, a reduction in renal perfusion pressure promotes both water and sodium retention (Table 11-3).

●●● EXCRETION

Urine production by the kidneys is (relatively) constant. Filtrate passes from the renal collecting ducts into the renal calyces. There is a spontaneous peristalsis every 10 to 150

seconds that originates in the renal pelvis and assists the flow of urine into the ureters. The frequency of these contractions is increased by parasympathetic nerve activity and decreased by sympathetic nerve activity.

Activation of afferent (pain) nerves in the ureters initiates a ureterorenal reflex that decreases urine production. This reflex can be activated by obstruction of the ureters and causes ureter constriction and afferent arteriolar constriction to decrease urine production.

The bladder stores urine until it is eliminated from the body by micturition. The smooth muscle of bladder wall is the detrusor muscle. There are both sensory and motor components to pelvic nerves supplying the bladder. Parasympathetic activity to the detrusor muscle causes contraction. The smooth muscle of the internal sphincter at the neck of the bladder normally is contracted, and the external sphincter consists of skeletal muscle under voluntary control, innervated by the somatic motor neurons of the pudendal nerves (Fig. 11-20).

Once bladder filling increases wall tension above a threshold, a micturition reflex is initiated. The wall tension initiates a spinal reflex, causing activation of the parasympathetic nerves supplying the detrusor muscle. The resulting contraction further increases wall tension, supporting increased activity of the reflex and further contraction. The reflex also causes relaxation of the internal sphincter. If the external sphincter is voluntarily relaxed, micturition occurs. If the external sphincter remains contracted, the process

TABLE 11-3. Acute* Versus Chronic Regulation of Na^+, K^+, and Body Fluid Volume

	Acute*	Chronic
Na^+	Excrete: aldosterone, angiotensin II, SNS, blood pressure Conserve: ANP, urotensin II	Excrete: ADH (dilutional) Conserve: aldosterone
K^+	Excrete: aldosterone, filtered load	Excrete: aldosterone, filtered load
Body fluid volume	ADH	Renal perfusion pressure

ADH, antidiuretic hormone; ANP, atrial natriuretic polypeptide; SNS, sympathic nervous system.
*Minutes, except hours for aldosterone.

PHARMACOLOGY

Diuretics

Blood volume is tightly coupled with blood pressure. A reduction in circulating blood volume occurs when extracellular fluid is depleted by diuretics. Consequently, diuretics can be used to manage hypertension.

Urinary Incontinence

Damage to the spinal cord causes a loss of descending control of micturition. If the afferent and efferent nerves between the spinal cord and the bladder remain intact, it is still possible to generate a spinal reflex to initiate micturition.

repeats until (1) the tension plateaus (for a minute or so), (2) the reflex fatigues, or (3) the bladder relaxes. If emptying did not occur, the process will begin again after a few minutes. Urination is facilitated by abdominal contraction that compresses the bladder and increases wall tension, initiating the reflex.

●●● RENAL ENDOCRINE FUNCTION

The kidneys also function as an endocrine organ, secreting the enzyme renin and the hormone erythropoietin. The kidney additionally produces agents that act within the kidney itself—renin and prostaglandins. Finally, vitamin D_3, which enhances Ca^{++} absorption, is activated to 1,25-dihydroxycholecalciferol (calcitriol) by the renal proximal tubules.

Renin is synthesized and released from cells lining the afferent arteriole. Renin is released in response to diminished stretch (hypotension), sympathetic nerve activity, decreased distal tubule Na^+ delivery to the macula densa, and epinephrine through β-adrenergic receptor stimulation. Renin is an enzyme that catalyzes formation of angiotensin I from the plasma protein angiotensinogen. Angiotensin I is cleaved by angiotensin-converting enzyme to form the vasoconstrictor peptide angiotensin II. Angiotensin-converting

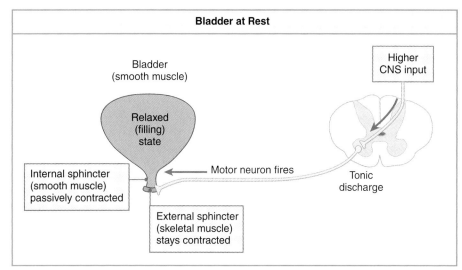

A

Figure 11-20. A spinal reflex mediates micturition. Filling of the bladder increases bladder wall tension. Afferent sensory signals from the bladder cause a sympathetically mediated contraction of the bladder wall. This contraction further increases wall tension, until the tension plateaus, the reflex fatigues, or the bladder sphincters relax and micturition occurs.

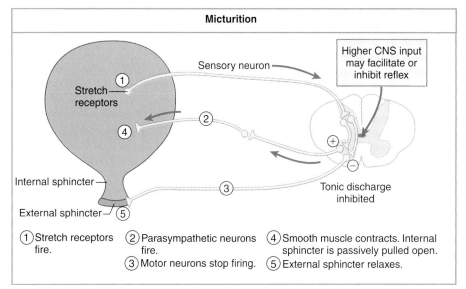

B

enzyme is found in high concentration in pulmonary epithelial cells. Angiotensin II acts within the kidney to constrict the efferent arteriole, outside the kidney to constrict vascular smooth muscle, and on the adrenal cortex to release aldosterone.

The kidney is the primary source of erythropoietin, the hormone that regulates red blood cell synthesis. Renal hypoxia stimulates erythropoietin release.

The kidneys can synthesize prostaglandin E_2, prostacyclin, leukotrienes, and thromboxanes. Prostaglandins dilate renal vascular smooth muscle and consequently increase renal blood flow. The rate of renal prostaglandin production normally is low, but prostaglandin production is increased during periods of renal ischemia. Consequently, blockade of renal prostaglandin production normally has little effect on renal blood flow, but during renal ischemia, blockade of renal prostaglandin production can cause a marked decrease in renal blood flow.

RENAL METABOLIC FUNCTION

Renal blood flow is high relative to renal O_2 consumption, and renal blood flow is not tied exclusively to renal metabolic needs. The major metabolic activity in the kidney is the reabsorption of Na^+ filtered at the glomerulus. Consequently, renal O_2 consumption is proportionate to GFR. Because renal blood flow and GFR normally change in parallel, any increase in renal blood flow causes an increase in GFR. The increased renal O_2 consumption (GFR) is offset by an increase in renal oxygen delivery (renal blood flow). This results in a constant arteriovenous O_2 difference across the kidney.

The kidney participates in body carbohydrate and protein balance. The kidney has a powerful gluconeogenesis capacity, second only to the liver, and can synthesize glucose from amino acids. In addition, in some diseases, urine represents a possible loss pathway for glucose or for proteins, representing a major loss of metabolic fuels.

EFFECTS OF NUTRITION

Dietary components can alter renal function at the glomerular and tubular levels. For example, protein ingestion increases renal blood flow and GFR. This postprandial renal hyperemia is due to dilation of the renal afferent arteriole, but the mechanism of this response is not yet determined. The increase in glomerular capillary pressure increases GFR. Protein intake also impairs renal autoregulation.

High protein intake can accelerate the long-term decline in renal function. The dilation of the afferent arteriole and consequent increase in capillary hydrostatic pressure causes progressive damage to glomeruli. This process is augmented by hypertension. Low-protein diets attenuate the age-related decrease in renal function. Patients with impaired renal function are often placed on a low-protein diet to delay the progression of renal deterioration.

TOP 5 TAKE-HOME POINTS

1. Glomerular capillary exchange depends on sympathetic nervous system control of afferent arteriole resistance and on angiotensin II control of efferent arteriole resistance.
2. Inulin clearance allows a noninvasive measure of GFR, as do changes in plasma creatinine concentration.
3. Urinary osmolarity can vary between 50 and 1600 mOsm, based on the hypertonicity of the renal medulla and the circulating levels of ADH.
4. Intrinsic regulation of renal function is accomplished by tubuloglomerular feedback, by which negative feedback control of GFR helps maintain a constant distal tubule NaCl delivery.
5. Extrinsic regulation of urine production is provided by renal sympathetic nerves and the hormones angiotensin II, aldosterone, and ADH and by arterial blood pressure.

Gastrointestinal System 12

Ingested contents pass through mouth, esophagus, stomach, small intestine (duodenum, jejunum, and ileum), and large intestine (colon) before exiting the body at the anus. The gastrointestinal (GI) mucosa provides a barrier through which nutrients must be absorbed. This continuous epithelial cell lining separates luminal contents from the body. Because of the epithelial lining, the GI luminal contents are functionally "outside" the body, and the GI luminal contents can have dramatically different composition (pH, osmolarity, etc.) from other body fluids (Fig. 12-1).

The organs of the GI system receive arterial blood from a variety of arteries, including the esophageal, gastric, celiac, hepatic, and superior mesenteric arteries. Venous drainage is by a variety of veins, all of which empty into the hepatic portal system. The hepatic portal system conducts the blood from the GI organs to the liver. This arrangement allows nutrients and other compounds absorbed into the venous drainage of the intestines to be processed in the liver before entering the general circulation via the hepatic vein. This vascular arrangement assists the hepatic role as a major immunologic and detoxifying system.

In general, the GI tract consists of an inner lumen surrounded by a layer of epithelial cells, secretory cells, muscles, nerves, vasculature, and connective tissue. In the small intestine, the lamina propria contains glands, blood vessels, and lymph nodules. The GI smooth muscle is arranged in an inner circular layer and an outer longitudinal layer. The submucosa has some glands, larger blood vessels, and nerves.

GI function involves motility, secretion, digestion, and absorption (Fig. 12-2). Throughout the GI tract, contraction of the various layers of smooth muscle propels and mixes luminal contents. The movement away from the mouth (aboral) is accomplished by peristaltic contraction of the longitudinal muscle layer. The contraction of circular muscle mixes luminal contents and increases contact with microvilli.

Anatomic or functional sphincters at the upper esophagus, lower esophagus, pylorus and ileocolic junction, and the anus separate regions of the GI tract. Sphincters are tonically contracted with the smooth muscle in a "latch" state that requires little energy to maintain the contraction. Arrival of an aboral peristaltic wave causes the sphincters to relax, allowing GI contents to pass. Distention distal to the sphincter increases contraction of the sphincter, limiting the passage of the luminal contents.

The functional role of the GI secretions is best appreciated by considering the digestion and absorption of carbohydrates, proteins, fats, and other components of the diet. GI secretions lubricate the luminal contents (saliva) and help digest foods. All areas of the GI tract secrete mucus to facilitate movement.

Digestive secretions are limited to the prejejunal GI tract. The mouth secretes salivary amylase. The stomach secretes HCl, intrinsic factor, pepsinogen, and the hormone gastrin. Pancreatic secretions enter the duodenum via the bile duct. Hepatic secretions (bile) also enter via the bile duct.

GI hormones are secreted by cells of the stomach and small intestine (Table 12-1). The presence of chyme in the small intestine is the major stimulus for digestive hormone release. The digestive hormones stimulate secretion of digestive enzymes and thereby promote digestion and absorption.

Absorption occurs in the small and large intestines. The microvilli of the intestinal epithelium contain stem cells located in the crypt. These cells divide and differentiate as they migrate out of the crypt. These epithelia are lost (exfoliated) at the tip of the crypt, with a half-life of 6 days. This high rate of division makes damage to intestinal epithelia a frequent side effect of chemotherapy directed against

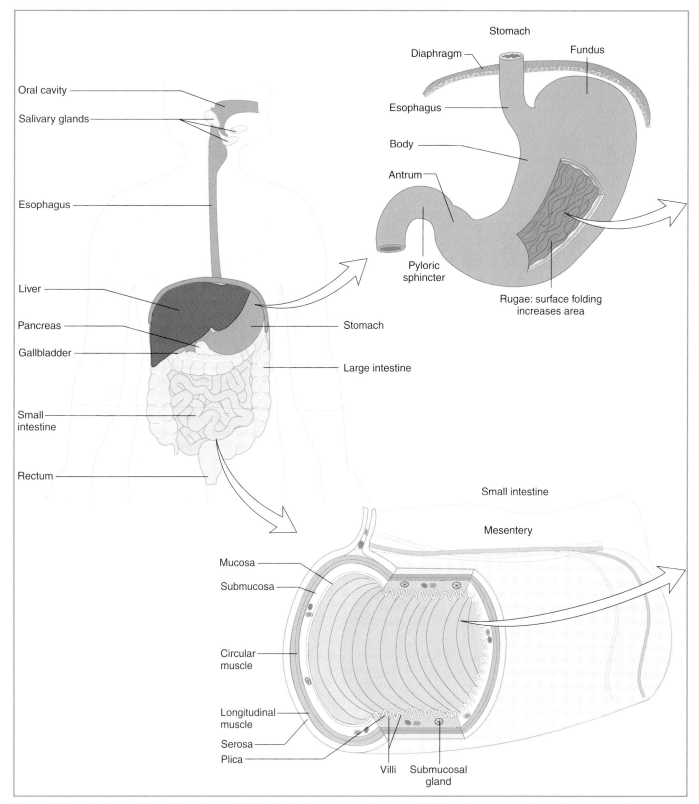

Figure 12-1. Anatomy of the GI system, which includes the organs through which food passes and exocrine organs whose secretions enter the GI tract. Food enters the mouth and passes sequentially through the esophagus, stomach, small intestine, large intestine, and rectum before exiting at the anus. Exocrine glands that empty into the GI lumen include the salivary glands, liver and gallbladder, and pancreas.

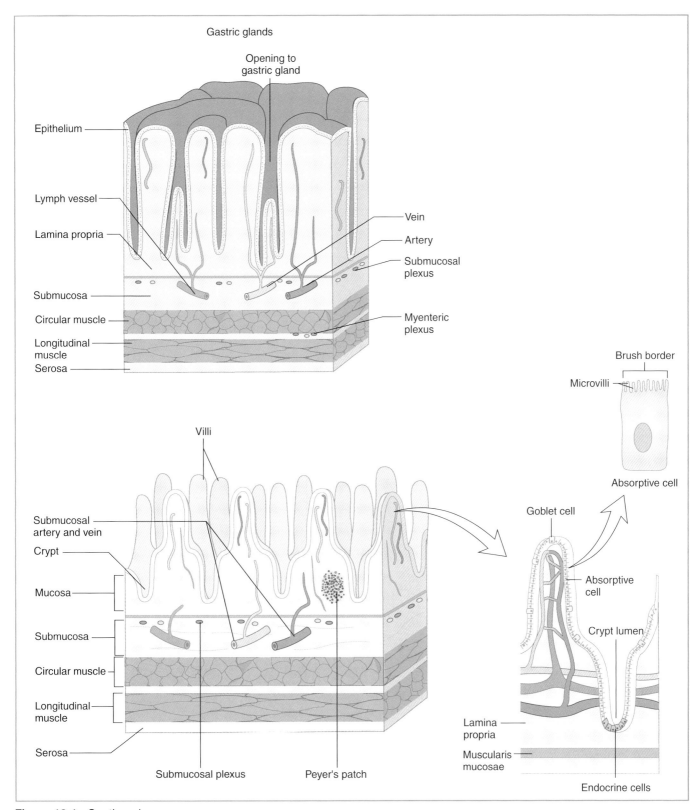

Figure 12-1. *Continued.*

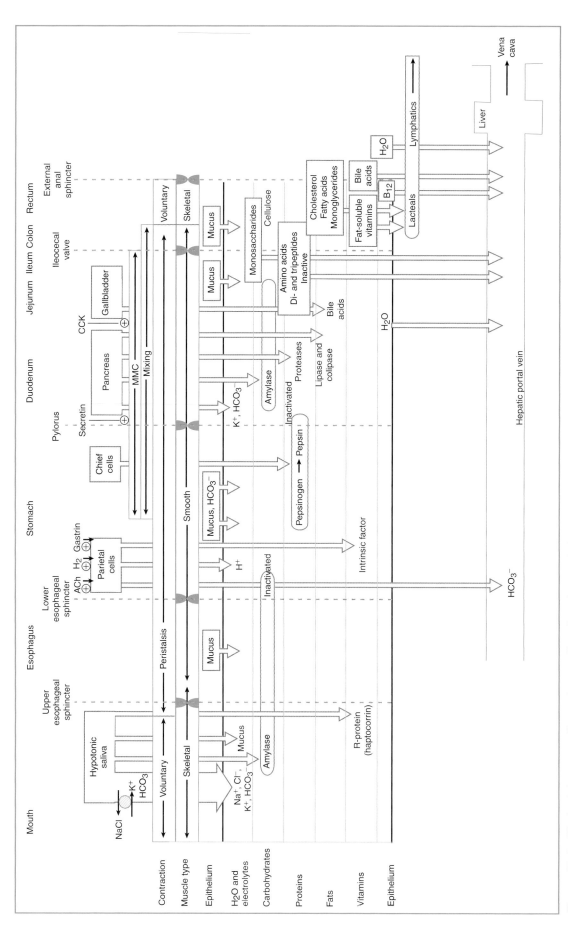

Figure 12-2. GI physiology map illustrating motility, digestion, and absorptive processes. The lumen is indicated by the area between the two epithelial cell layers. The dietary components are identified at left. The top of the diagram shows the anatomic structures with vertical dashed lines marking the sphincters. The top part also shows the main secretions that enter the limit of the GI tract and the locations of skeletal and smooth muscle that propel the diet through the GI tract. Absorption of dietary components into the hepatic portal vein or the lacteals is shown at the bottom.

TABLE 12-1. Major Digestive Hormones

Hormone	Major Actions	Released by	Released from
Gastrin	Gastric H^+ secretion, mucosal hyperplasia	Peptides, amino acids, acetylcholine	Gastric G cells
Cholecystokinin	Pancreatic enzyme secretion, gallbladder contraction, gastric emptying inhibition	Fatty acids	Small intestine
Secretin	Pancreatic HCO_3^- secretion, pepsin release	Luminal acidity	Small intestine
Gastric inhibitory peptide	Insulin release, acid secretion inhibition	Glucose, amino acids, fatty acids	Small intestine
Motilin	Migrating motor complex stimulation	Fasting	Small intestine
Glucagon-like peptide 1	Insulin release, stimulation, glucagon release inhibition	Luminal fats or carbohydrates	Small intestine

rapidly dividing cancer cells. The unabsorbed contents and secretions are lost from the body at the anus as feces.

Intrinsic regulation uses a complex endocrine system and enteric nervous system to integrate motor and secretory activities. GI hormones control and integrate both motility and secretion. The enteric nervous system includes the submucosal plexus (Meissner's plexus), the myenteric plexus (Auerbach's plexus), and a variety of other neurons. Enteric nervous system reflexes do not require interaction with the somatic or autonomic nervous systems. Enteric ganglia receive input from sensory neurons, responding to temperature, chemical agents, and mechanical deformation. Enteric ganglia have effector neurons to smooth muscle, secretory cells, and endocrine and autocrine cells.

The rate of gastric emptying is matched to the duodenal processing ability. The major role of intrinsic regulation is to limit the passage of diet into the duodenum to an amount that can be completely digested and absorbed. The stomach is a storage organ, and the duodenum is the major site of digestion and absorption. The presence of unabsorbed diet components (amino acids, monosaccharides, fats) in the duodenum enhances contraction of the pylorus, limiting further chyme entry from the stomach, as does a highly acidic pH. Neutralization of pH by pancreatic HCO_3^- secretion, or absorption of the diet, relaxes the pylorus and allows further entry of chyme from the stomach.

Extrinsic regulation involves the parasympathetic nervous system, GI hormones, and to a lesser degree, the sympathetic nervous system. The vagus is the major parasympathetic nerve, supplying the GI tract to the level of transverse colon. Pelvic nerves originating from the sacral portion of the spinal cord supply parasympathetic control to the remainder of the colon. Parasympathetic postganglionic neurons are located in the intramural plexus, where they stimulate motor activity, stimulate secretory activity, and stimulate endocrine secretions. Sympathetic nervous system efferent nerves originate in the celiac, superior mesenteric, inferior mesenteric, and hypogastric ganglia. Sympathetics act to inhibit activity in enteric plexuses, constrict GI system blood vessels, and generally decrease glandular secretions. Sympathetics decrease aboral movement by indirectly inhibiting peristalsis and by directly

contracting circular muscle and certain sphincters. Finally, endocrine agents control numerous motility and secretory processes.

GASTROINTESTINAL MOTILITY

The entrance (mouth, upper esophagus) and exit (external anal sphincter) of the GI tract contain skeletal muscle and are partially under voluntary control. The remainder of the GI tract is lined by smooth muscle, which is under involuntary control. The smooth muscle cells are electrically coupled by gap junctions to allow coordinated contractile activity. GI smooth muscle exhibits two different types of electrical activity: slow waves and localized contractions.

The frequency of slow waves varies along the GI tract. Smooth muscle prepotentials, or spontaneous depolarizations, may lead to slow waves and sometimes spike potentials. In the small intestine and colon, depolarization to threshold initiates spike potentials and subsequent contraction. In the stomach, however, smooth muscle contraction is initiated by slow waves without spike potentials. Pacemaker regions in the stomach, small intestine, and colon set the basic electrical rhythm and frequency, which is altered by input from the enteric nervous system and from hormones. For example, norepinephrine and epinephrine lower the amplitude and frequency of the slow waves, and acetylcholine increases the amplitude and frequency of the slow waves.

GI smooth muscle has long, strong contractions. This prolonged time of contraction differs from skeletal and cardiac muscle, which exhibit a twitch contraction. Smooth muscle exhibits a basal tone generating some tension even at rest. This is particularly evident in the GI sphincters, which are characterized by high basal tone. Basal tone in the GI tract is influenced by neurotransmitters, hormones, and drugs. Stretch of GI smooth muscle increases action potential frequency (stress activation), followed by a decrease back toward the original tension (stress relaxation).

Peristalsis is an organized wave of contraction that propels contents aborally. Peristalsis can originate spontaneously, but more commonly it is initiated by distention of GI smooth muscle. This distention elicits a smooth muscle contraction at the site of distention and also of the smooth muscle aboral to the distention. The smooth muscle aboral to the contraction, however, relaxes. Luminal contents are propelled into the relaxed area of the GI tract. This sequence repeats, moving contents for a short distance before the wave of peristalsis diminishes and disappears. A descending wave of peristalsis initiates sphincter relaxation, facilitating aboral movement of the GI contents.

Intrinsic regulation by the enteric nervous system uses interneurons to coordinate smooth muscle activity. Interneurons use both neurotransmitters and neuromodulators, similarly to brain. Intrinsic plexuses act to inhibit basal activity, so action potentials are elicited by one third or one fourth of the slow waves. This coordination is necessary because simultaneous contraction of both circular and longitudinal muscle layers would not generate movement of the chyme. Extrinsic regulation is also complex, since sympathetics and parasympathetics directly innervate smooth muscle, and sympathetics and parasympathetics innervate the enteric nervous system. GI hormones also contribute to the extrinsic regulation of GI motility.

Mouth and Esophageal Motility

Mastication, or chewing, mixes food with salivary mucus. This action subdivides food and exposes ingested starch to salivary amylase to begin the digestive process. Mastication is not essential for normal GI function but facilitates the process.

Swallowing propels food from the mouth into the esophagus. The initiation of swallowing is voluntary, but once started, the process continues involuntarily. During the voluntary oral phase, the tongue positions food against the hard palate. Entrance of the bolus into the pharynx initiates a swallowing reflex. The pharyngeal phase is involuntary. The reflex is initiated by tactile receptors at the entrance to the pharynx. There is integration at the medulla and pons in the "swallowing center." Motor output is via cranial nerves, including the vagus.

During swallowing, the soft palate retracts to close the nasopharynx, and the vocal cords contract. The epiglottis moves to close to the trachea to prevent aspiration. Simultaneously, respiration is inhibited. The upper esophageal sphincter relaxes, and the pharyngeal muscles contract to move the bolus through the pharynx. The peristaltic wave

forces food past the relaxed upper esophageal sphincter and into the esophagus (Fig. 12-3).

The esophagus is a combination of striated and smooth muscle. The upper third of the esophagus is skeletal muscle. Both types of muscle are present in the middle third of the esophagus, and the lower third is only smooth muscle. In the esophagus, the vagus innervates both smooth and skeletal muscle. Sphincters isolate the lumen of the esophagus from the remainder of the GI tract. Contraction of the upper esophageal sphincter prevents entry of tracheal air. Contraction of the lower esophageal sphincter prevents reflux of gastric contents.

The entry of a bolus of food into the esophagus initiates the esophageal phase of swallowing. While the oral phase of swallowing is voluntary, the esophageal phase is involuntary. Contraction of the upper esophageal sphincter isolates the

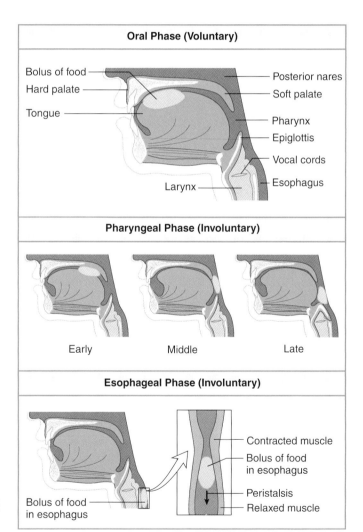

Figure 12-3. Swallowing occurs in three phases. In the voluntary or oral phase, the tongue presses food against the hard palate, forcing it toward the pharynx. In the involuntary or pharyngeal phase, peristalsis forces the bolus between the tonsils. Respirations cease, the airway is covered, and the esophagus is stretched open. In the involuntary esophageal phase, relaxation of the upper esophageal sphincter allows peristalsis to move the bolus down the esophagus.

ANATOMY

Anatomy of the Mouth

The roof of the mouth consists of a bony hard palate and muscular soft palate, with the base formed by a muscular tongue. The mouth is a common pathway for both food and air. The epiglottis helps seal the entry to the trachea, and the cricopharyngeal portion of the inferior pharyngeal constrictor muscle seals the entry to the esophagus.

pharynx from the esophagus. A primary peristaltic wave moves food through the esophagus in 10 seconds. Secondary peristalsis is initiated by esophageal distention via the enteric nervous system, and it propels food still remaining in the esophagus toward the stomach. Relaxation of the lower esophageal sphincter is mediated by the vagus and enteric nerves, using the neurotransmitters nitric oxide (NO) and vasoactive intestinal peptide (VIP) to inhibit smooth muscle contraction.

Abnormalities of the swallowing reflex include disorders of both the esophageal smooth muscle and the muscle tone of the lower esophageal sphincter. A diffuse esophageal spasm results from an inappropriately strong peristaltic contraction. Failure of the lower esophageal sphincter to remain closed allows gastric reflux, causing esophagitis (heartburn). Chronic gastric reflux causes ulceration of the esophagus and can lead to a series of histologic changes known as Barrett's esophagus. Achalasia occurs if the lower esophageal sphincter does not relax sufficiently to allow food to pass.

Gastric Motility

Stomach

The stomach is anatomically and functionally divided into the fundus, body, and antrum. The fundus and body are highly distensible and act as reservoir for the ingested meal. A 1.5 L volume increase causes only a small increase in pressure in the lumen of the stomach. The esophageal swallowing reflex promotes release of NO and VIP in the wall of the stomach, causing relaxation of the fundus and body. This relaxation allows the stomach to accommodate the increased volume.

Food is stored unmixed in the fundus and body of the stomach for up to 1 hour. During this period, there is separation of the ingested food according to density, with fats rising to the surface of the gastric contents. Liquids can flow around the solid food, and they accumulate at the bottom. This separation leads to a sequence of gastric emptying into the duodenum: first liquids, then solids, and finally lipids. The ingested food mixes with gastric secretions, and the luminal contents are now called "chyme" during passage through the GI tract.

Slow waves, which in the stomach do not generate spike potentials, initiate gastric contractions. Slow waves occur at a rate of three per minute and begin at the pacemaker region in the middle of the body of the stomach. Contractions

increase in force and velocity as they approach the antrum. Acetylcholine increases the amplitude and duration of depolarization and therefore contraction. Norepinephrine reduces the amplitude and duration of depolarization.

The antrum has strong contractions, fragmenting the food into smaller particles. The contractions also mix chyme with gastric secretions to initiate digestion. The strength of antral contractions is enhanced when slow waves are augmented by action potentials. The pylorus and terminal end of the antrum contract almost simultaneously; this is called systolic contraction of the antrum. This coordinated contraction allows only a small amount of the antral contents to enter the duodenum before contraction of the pylorus closes the stomach/intestinal opening. Antral contraction continues, but because the pylorus is now closed, the contraction only causes further mixing and grinding of contents (retropulsion).

After a meal, the rate of gastric contractions is equal to the rate of gastric slow waves, about three per minute. During fasting, the antrum is mostly quiescent for 1 to 2 hours, with intervening periods of contraction. The contractions are due to a migrating myoelectric complex, which initiates 10 to 20 minutes of intense contractions against an open pylorus.

The gastric contents empty into the duodenal bulb at a controlled rate, which is modulated by neural reflexes and hormonal reflexes originating in the duodenum (Fig. 12-4). The rate of gastric emptying is modulated by the enteric nervous system and autonomic nervous system. Vagal cholinergics stimulate motility, and sympathetic adrenergics inhibit motility. The enteric nervous system coordinates these external influences and the numerous internal reflexes. The rate of gastric emptying is also under hormonal control. Gastric emptying is increased by gastrin and decreased by secretin. Sensory gastric afferents play a role in satiety, and they are activated by intragastric pressure, gastric distention, and intragastric pH.

Duodenum

When the antrum contracts, the duodenum relaxes, allowing a small volume of gastric chyme to enter the duodenum. The

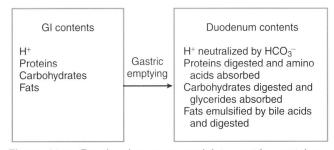

Figure 12-4. Duodenal contents modulate gastric emptying. The stomach is primarily a storage organ and the duodenum the site of digestion and absorption. The rate of gastric emptying is regulated so that the chyme entering the duodenum can be digested and absorbed before more chyme is allowed to enter. Gastric contents appearing in the duodenum will decrease gastric motility and slow the rate of gastric emptying.

pylorus functions as a sphincter, but anatomically it does not qualify, since the muscles across the pylorus are not electrically connected by gap junctions. The rate of gastric emptying is matched to duodenal buffering ability, preventing acid damage to the duodenal mucosa and subsequent duodenal ulcers. The pylorus also prevents regurgitation of duodenal contents back into the stomach, preventing bile damage to the gastric mucosa, which can lead to gastric ulcers.

Negative feedback control balances the rate of chyme entry into the duodenum to the capability of the duodenum to digest and absorb the diet. Gastric chyme is acidic and often hyperosmolar. Within the duodenum, both acidity and hypertonicity initiate reflexes that inhibit gastric motility and therefore the further entry of gastric chyme. This allows the duodenum to process the luminal contents before any new gastric chyme is allowed to enter.

Duodenal acidity (pH < 3.5) decreases the rate of gastric emptying through multiple routes. Acidity initiates a neural reflex that reduces gastric emptying. Duodenal acidity also stimulates secretin release, which increases HCO_3^- buffer secretion from ductal epithelia of the pancreatic and hepatic ducts. HCO_3^- secretion acts to neutralize the chyme present in the duodenum.

Duodenal hypertonicity also decreases the rate of gastric emptying. Chyme becomes more hypertonic as digestion progresses. Duodenal hypertonicity decreases gastric emptying by a neural reflex and an unidentified hormonal component. The duodenal tonicity decreases with time as the digested components of the diet are absorbed across the duodenum. In addition, contraction of the pylorus is increased by unabsorbed products of digestion in the duodenum. Monoglycerides increase contraction of the pylorus and slow gastric emptying. Amino acids, especially tryptophan, and peptides in the duodenum also slow gastric emptying.

Fat content and fatty acids (especially long chain, unsaturated, or both) decrease the rate of gastric emptying. Fats stimulate the release of cholecystokinin (CCK) from the duodenum and jejunum, which contracts the pylorus and relaxes the stomach fundus. Gastric inhibitory peptide (GIP) may also have a role in limiting gastric emptying.

Vomiting

Vomiting is the oral expulsion of gastric (and sometimes duodenal) contents. Retching, whereby gastric contents are forced into the esophagus but not the pharynx, precedes vomiting. The vomiting reflex follows a set pattern: reverse peristalsis is initiated in middle of the small intestine, then the pyloric sphincter and stomach relax to receive the duodenal contents. A forced inspiration against a closed glottis decreases intrathoracic pressure, and a forceful contraction of abdominal muscles increases intra-abdominal pressure. The lower esophageal sphincter relaxes and the pylorus and antrum contract, allowing the gastric contents to enter the esophagus.

Retching occurs when the upper esophageal sphincter remains closed. Vomiting occurs when the gastric contents are forced past the upper esophageal sphincter. The trachea is closed as in normal swallowing to prevent aspiration.

The medulla has a separate vomiting center and a retching center, which normally interact. Afferent inputs arise from stomach and duodenal distention, or from pain in the genitourinary system. Dizziness and tickling the back of throat can also induce vomiting. Emetics are used to induce vomiting. Emetics work by stimulating receptors in the stomach and duodenum (ipecac), or by activating the chemoreceptive trigger zone in the area postrema (opiates).

Small Intestinal Motility

The small intestine is divided into duodenum, jejunum, and ileum, with the duodenum and jejunum being the major site of digestion and absorption. Chyme takes 2 to 4 hours to move through the 5 m of the small intestine. Segmentation, which mixes intestinal contents and enhances contact of the chyme with the intestinal microvilli, is the most frequent type of intestinal contraction. Segmentation can be rhythmic, with adjacent sites alternating contraction and relaxation. Eating increases segmentation.

Peristalsis moves the chyme aborally an average of 10 cm per contraction. Eating actually slows the aboral movement of chyme. An intestinal pacemaker and the enteric nervous system control the frequency of segmentation and short peristalsis. Contractions occur at an intrinsic rate of 11 to 13 per minute in the duodenum, which declines to 8 to 9 per minute by the terminal ileum. This rate is modified by extrinsic neural and hormonal inputs. (Fig. 12-5)

Reflex activity helps coordinate intestinal motility with events elsewhere in the GI system. Distention of one segment of intestine relaxes the remainder of the intestine (intestinointestinal reflex). Distention of the ileum decreases gastric motility (ileogastric reflex). Distention of the stomach increases movement of material out of the ileum (gastroileal reflex) and colon (gastrocolic reflex), a reflex especially evident in the newborn.

Migrating Myoelectric Complex

During fasting, periods of intense electrical activity are followed by long quiescent periods. The electrical activity, called the migrating myoelectric complex, is initiated in the stomach and traverses the entire small intestine. There is evidence for both a vagal and a hormonal (motilin) role in its initiation. The frequency of the migrating myoelectric

---

PHARMACOLOGY

Emetics

Emetics are agents that cause vomiting. There are two general classes of emetics, one acting on the chemoreceptor trigger zone (CTZ) of the medulla and the second acting on the stomach itself. The prototypical central emetic is apomorphine, and the prototypical gastric emetic is ipecac.

complex is altered by substance P, somatostatin, and neurotensin. This contraction sweeps the intestines clean and inhibits the retrograde movement of bacteria from the colon into the small intestine. The electrical and contractile activity require the enteric nervous system for propagation.

Colonic Motility

The colon reabsorbs salts and water. About 1500 mL of fluid enters the colon each day, but only 50 to 100 mL of fluid is excreted in feces. Anatomically, the colon is divided into the cecum, ascending colon, transverse colon, and descending colon. Segmental contraction of the circular smooth muscle divides the colon into numerous haustra (sacculations). There is some retrograde peristalsis, which delays aboral movement of chyme. Mass movement (three per day) is primarily responsible for the aboral movement of the chyme in the colon. During a mass movement, the haustra relax and a peristaltic wave initiates a prolonged contraction of the colon until an entire segment is contracted. After a few minutes, the segment relaxes and haustra reappear. The enteric nerves primarily inhibit colonic smooth muscle contraction. Hirschsprung's disease is characterized by congenital absence of enteric nerves, and the colon is obstructed by a tonic contraction.

Chyme entering from the small intestine is mostly a liquid. There is progressive absorption of water along the length of the large intestine (Fig. 12-6), resulting in the mostly solid

feces being excreted. Enhanced motility decreases the time for water absorption and can cause diarrhea, the excretion of watery feces. Conversely, impaired motility allows time for too much water to be reabsorbed and can cause constipation.

Parasympathetic nerves modulate colonic motility by interacting with the enteric nervous system. Parasympathetic innervation is provided by the vagus for the cecum, ascending colon, and transverse colon, and by parasympathetic nerves originating in the sacral spinal cord for the descending colon. Sympathetic activity inhibits colonic contractions. This reflex control coordinates colonic motility with events in the remainder of the GI system. In the colocolonic reflex, distention causes relaxation in adjacent areas. This is partly mediated by sympathetics. In the gastrocolic reflex, an increase in colonic activity follows stretching of the stomach.

Defecation

The rectum is usually nearly empty, and the anal canal is normally closed by the internal sphincter (involuntary, smooth muscle) and the external sphincter (voluntary, skeletal muscle). The rectum fills following a colonic mass movement. As the rectum fills, the internal anal sphincter relaxes, and the external anal sphincter reflexly contracts. Filling of the rectum also causes an urge to defecate. Voluntary relaxation of the external sphincter and the puborectal muscle allows defecation to proceed. Defecation is facilitated by increased abdominal pressure.

●●● GASTROINTESTINAL SECRETIONS

Most ingested food cannot be directly absorbed but must first be digested. GI secretions digest food to facilitate absorption.

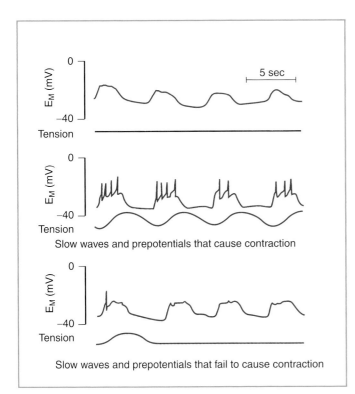

Figure 12-5. Spike potentials precede intestinal smooth muscle contraction. Slow waves occur at regular frequency. Slow waves that give rise to spike potentials will cause contraction of the intestinal smooth muscle.

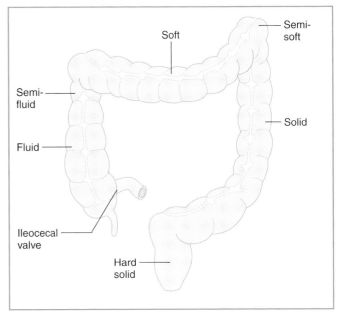

Figure 12-6. Water is absorbed as chyme passes through the large intestine.

Amylases digest carbohydrates, proteases digest proteins, and lipases digest lipids. GI secretions also assist absorption of the diet. Bile is essential for lipid absorption, and intrinsic factor assists vitamin B_{12} absorption. These GI secretions are regulated by a series of hormonal and neural feedbacks.

The cellular composition of the diet is somewhat similar to the cellular composition of the body, including the GI tract. Consequently, GI digestive secretions must be regulated to avoid autodigestion. Gastric acid, secreted in the stomach, can damage the duodenum. Pancreatic HCO_3^- secretion into the duodenum neutralizes gastric acid and protects the duodenal mucosa. Pancreatic proteases can digest the cells of the pancreatic duct and the pancreas itself. This does not occur, because pancreatic enzymes are secreted in an inactive zymogen form and activated only after they reach the lumen of the small intestine. Abrasion from the passing and mixing of chyme can damage the epithelial lining of the GI tract. Mucus secretion along the length of the GI tract prevents mechanical abrasion of the epithelia.

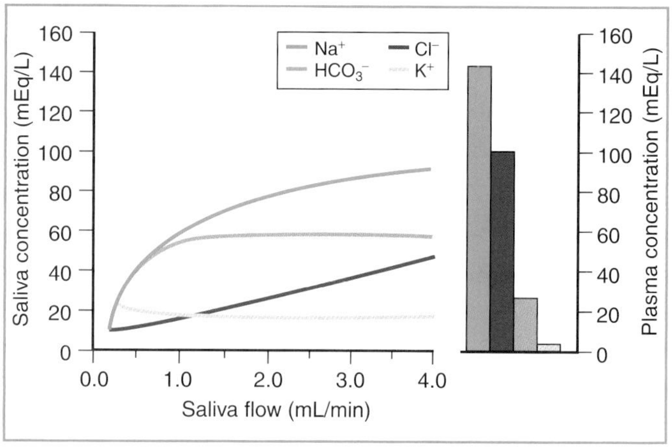

Figure 12-7. Saliva ionic composition varies with flow rate. The ionic composition of saliva is slightly hypotonic to plasma. During low flow rates, Na^+ and Cl^- are reabsorbed, and the saliva becomes even more hypotonic.

Saliva

Saliva is a hypotonic fluid that originates in the acinar region of the salivary glands. The largest salivary glands are the parotids, which produce a serous (watery) secretion. The submaxillary and sublingual glands are mixed serous and mucous glands that produce saliva with some mucins. In all salivary glands, the acinar cell secretions are modified by the epithelial cells of the salivary duct. Salivary glands have a high metabolic rate and blood flow, both of which are proportionate to the rate of saliva formation.

Saliva contains mucins, amylase, and electrolytes in water. Mucins (glycoproteins) lubricate food to facilitate swallowing and facilitate speaking. Salivary amylase initiates the digestion of starch. The absence of salivary amylase does not impair starch absorption, since pancreatic amylase alone can fully digest the starches.

The ionic component of acinar cell secretion is similar to plasma, but the secretion is hypotonic to plasma. Epithelial cells of the ducts process the acinar secretions in a flow-rate-dependent fashion (Fig. 12-7). While passing through the salivary duct, Na^+ and Cl^- are reabsorbed and K^+ and HCO_3^- are secreted. During high flow rates, there is little time for modification of the acinar secretion, and saliva contains mostly Na^+, HCO_3^-, and Cl^- as electrolytes. During low flow rates, saliva is modified to a K^+/HCO_3^--rich secretion, and the net ionic reabsorption by duct cells further decreases the tonicity of the saliva. The salivary duct epithelium is relatively impermeable to water, so water secreted by the acinar cells remains in the salivary duct.

Hormones and nerves regulate the salivary secretion rate and composition. Sympathetic and parasympathetic nerves have similar effects, since both increase the volume of saliva production and enrich the K^+ and HCO_3^- composition, and they also increase salivary amylase secretion. Mucin secretion is increased by parasympathetic nerves but not by sympathetic nerves.

HISTOLOGY

Gastric Glands

The gastric gland is an invagination of the mucosa of the stomach. Each gland contains a variety of cell types. Starting from the middle of the gland, regenerative cells, mucous neck cells, and surface lining cells extend toward the surface. Chief cells, parietal cells, and diffuse neuroendocrine (DNES) cells extend deep into the gland. All the cells are epithelial cells bound together by tight junctions.

Gastric Secretions

HCl, gastrin, pepsinogen, and intrinsic factor are the main gastric secretions. The stomach has specialized secretory regions, all of which secrete mucus, ions, and water. The oxyntic glandular region secretes HCl and intrinsic factor from parietal, or oxyntic, cells, and pepsinogen from chief, or peptic, cells. The pyloric glandular region secretes gastrin from G cells and pepsin from chief cells.

Gastric acid secretion requires the production of H^+ and HCO_3^- from CO_2 and H_2O within the parietal cell, the secretion of H^+ across the apical membrane, and the secretion of HCO_3^- across the basolateral membrane. Hydrogen is secreted across the gastric epithelial cell barrier against an electrochemical gradient. H^+ is exchanged for K^+ by H^+/K^+-ATPase on the luminal surface. Chloride is exchanged for HCO_3^- on the basolateral surface, and crosses the apical surface by facilitated diffusion. Plasma HCO_3^- reabsorption during gastric acid secretion causes a postprandial alkaline tide or an increase in gastric vein pH occurring during the period of acid secretion into the GI lumen.

Intrinsic factor is a glycoprotein secreted by the parietal cells. Intrinsic factor is the only essential gastric secretion, and it facilitates ileal absorption of vitamin B_{12}. Intrinsic factor is released from parietal cells by acetylcholine.

Pepsin is secreted from the chief cells as the inactive proenzyme pepsinogen. Pepsinogen secretion parallels gastric acid secretion. Once pepsinogen reaches the lumen of the stomach, the gastric acidity activates the proenzyme. Pepsins are self-catalytic and also can catalyze further pepsin activation.

Mucous neck cells and surface epithelial cells secrete K^+- and HCO_3^--rich mucus that lines the gastric epithelia. The HCO_3^- comes from metabolic production of CO_2 and carbonic anhydrase. The high HCO_3^- content of mucus helps protect the surface of the stomach from mechanical and chemical destruction by HCl and proteases. Mucous HCO_3^- secretion is stimulated by increased serosal Ca^{++}, acetylcholine, and certain prostaglandins, and inhibited by α-adrenergic agonists. Chronic elevation of adrenal catecholamines or chronic nonsteroidal anti-inflammatory drug (NSAID) ingestion may decrease the buffering ability of the mucous layer and contribute to gastric ulcers.

Gastric secretions initiate protein digestion and protect the gastric epithelium. HCl prevents bacteria growth and catalyzes pepsinogen cleavage to pepsin. Gastric pepsins assist, but are not essential for, protein ingestion. The optimal pH for pepsin function is below 3, and pepsins are inactivated in the duodenum when pH rises. Pepsins may digest up to 20% of dietary protein.

The basal acid secretion rate varies among individuals, as does the number of parietal cells. In addition, basal acid secretion rate varies diurnally and is lowest in the morning. NaCl can be the primary gastric secretory component during the fasting period, when there are low gastric secretory rates. HCl content of the secretion increases as the rate of gastric secretion increases. For example, acid secretion can increase by eightfold following pentagastrin and histamine stimulation.

Gastric acid secretion is stimulated by acetylcholine released from the enteric nerves, gastrin released from the pyloric G cells, and histamine released from the enterochromaffin-like cells. There is powerful synergistic interaction among the three stimulators of gastric acid secretion, with histamine playing a central role. Antagonists directed toward acetylcholine, histamine, or gastrin can inhibit HCl secretion. The powerful synergistic interaction allows blockade of one pathway to greatly diminish acid secretion. HCl secretion can be blocked by cimetidine (a histamine blocker) or atropine (an acetylcholine blocker) (Fig. 12-8).

MICROBIOLOGY

Helicobacter pylori

Helicobacter pylori is a gram-negative bacillus often found in the antrum of the stomach. Although the presence of *H. pylori* is associated with peptic ulcers, most individuals with *H. pylori* do not develop peptic ulcer disease. For individuals who do develop peptic ulcer disease, inhibition of acid secretion provides relief of symptoms, but antibiotic therapy directed against *H. pylori* cures peptic ulcer disease.

There are three distinct phases of gastric acid secretion. The *cephalic phase* is due to the sight, smell, and taste of food, is seen in sham feeding studies, and can account for up to 40% of the maximal acid secretion rate. The cephalic phase is mediated by the vagus, which acts directly on the parietal cells and also induces G-cell gastrin release and enterochromaffin-like cell histamine release. The drop in antral pH acts directly on the parietal cells to limit the effectiveness of the cephalic phase of acid secretion. Consequently, if no food is present, HCl secretion attenuates over time. Decreased cerebral glucose delivery can promote vagal activity and HCl secretion, as can nicotine.

The *gastric phase* of acid secretion results from the increase in luminal pH and distention of the wall of the stomach caused by food ingestion. Food acts as a buffer, neutralizing the normally acidic pH of the stomach. Continued HCl secretion eventually overcomes the buffering ability of food, and luminal pH falls. The fall in luminal pH acts directly on the parietal cells to diminish further acid secretion. Distention from food ingestion activates mechanoreceptors, initiating a vagal reflex. Distention also causes gastrin release from the pyloric G cells. Separately from distention, the presence of amino acids (especially tryptophan and phenylalanine) from protein digestion enhances gastrin release. Calcium ions, caffeine, and alcohol also promote HCl release during the gastric phase.

The *intestinal phase* of gastric acid secretion is determined by the composition of the chyme that enters the duodenum. During the initial phase of digestion, the pH of the chyme in the stomach is less acid because of the buffering capacity of the meal. The entry of this less acidic chyme (pH > 3) into the duodenum stimulates gastrin release and consequently gastric acid secretion. During the later stages of digestion, the chyme in the stomach becomes more acidic (pH < 2) because of continuing gastric acid secretion. The duodenal entry of this very acidic chyme inhibits gastrin release and consequently attenuates further gastric acid secretion. This feedback system ensures that the rate of gastric acid secretion is matched to the need.

The rate of chyme entry into the duodenum is also regulated. Gastric emptying is inhibited when duodenal chyme is too acidic, is too hypertonic, or contains fat products. Hyperacidity inhibits gastric emptying through the release of secretin, bulbogastrone, and local nervous response. Fats in the lumen of the duodenum inhibit gastric emptying by stimulating the release of CCK and GIP. Secretin and bulbogastrone inhibit gastrin release from G cells and also decrease the responsiveness of parietal cells, thereby diminishing gastric acid secretion.

Exocrine Pancreatic Enzymes

Pancreatic enzymes are essential for the normal digestion and absorption of lipids, proteins, and carbohydrates. The exocrine pancreas secretes both a bicarbonate-rich solution and a variety of digestive enzymes, including proteases, lipases, and amylases. Columnar epithelial cells of the pancreatic ducts secrete the aqueous bicarbonate component.

Source	Substance Secreted	Stimulus for Release	Function
Mucous neck cells	Mucus	Tonic secretion; also irritation of mucosa	Physical barrier between lumen and epithelium
	Bicarbonate	Secreted with mucus	Buffers gastric acid to prevent damage to epithelium
Parietal cells	Gastric acid (HCl)	Acetylcholine, gastrin, histamine	Activates pepsin; kills bacteria
	Intrinsic factor		Complexes with vitamin B_{12} to permit absorption
Enterochromaffin-like (ECL) cells	Histamine	Acetylcholine, gastrin	Stimulates gastric acid secretion
Chief cells	Pepsin(ogen)	Acetylcholine, acid, secretin	Digests proteins
	Gastric lipase		Digests fats
D cells	Somatostatin	Acid in the stomach	Inhibits gastric acid secretion
G cells	Gastrin	Acetylcholine, peptides, and amino acids	Stimulates gastric acid secretion

Figure 12-8. Gastric acid secretion is regulated by neural, endocrine, and paracrine agents. Gastric acid secretion by the parietal cell is under complex regulation. The enterochromaffin-like (ECL) cell releases histamine that stimulates acid secretion. Both the hormone gastrin and the neurotransmitter acetylcholine can stimulate the ECL cell to release histamine, and can directly stimulate the parietal cell to secrete acid. Gastrin is released by amino acids or peptides in the lumen of the stomach, and acetylcholine is released by nervous system reflexes. Excess acid in the lumen of the stomach causes D cells to release somatostatin, which inhibits both gastrin release and parietal cell acid secretion.

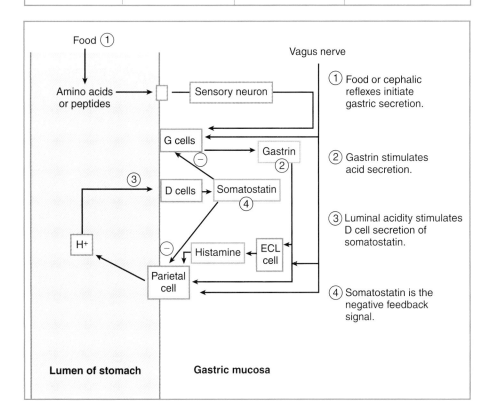

Pancreatic acinar cells secrete the digestive enzymes. Pancreatic secretions are carried to the duodenum by the pancreatic duct. The epithelia of the pancreatic ducts are relatively permeable to water but impermeable to large molecules. Once in the lumen of the duodenum, pancreatic HCO_3^- acts to neutralize duodenal chyme.

Pancreatic proteases are secreted in an inactive zymogen form, along with a trypsin inhibitor, to prevent premature activation. Pancreatic trypsinogen is activated by duodenal enterokinase to become trypsin. Trypsin then acts on zymogens to form more trypsin (autocatalysis), chymotrypsin, and carboxypeptidases. α-Amylase is secreted in an active form, as are lipases, ribonuclease, and deoxyribonuclease.

The water component of pancreatic secretion is produced at a rate of about 1 L/day. The initial ion composition of this fluid is similar to that of plasma except for the higher HCO_3^-

PHARMACOLOGY

Inhibition of Gastric Acid Secretion

Inhibition of gastric acid secretion can be accomplished by blocking the normal stimulation pathways or by directly inhibiting the proton pump. There are three different normal stimulators of gastric acid secretion: histamine, acetylcholine, and gastrin. H_2 antagonists (cimetidine), muscarinic antagonists (atropine), and gastrin receptor CCK-B antagonists can all block gastric acid secretion. Drugs such as omeprazole inactivate the H^+/K^+ proton pump directly and are referred to as proton pump inhibitors.

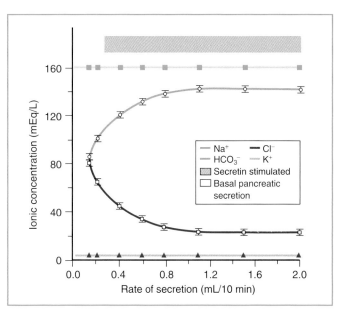

Figure 12-9. Secretin increases the volume of pancreatic secretion. Basal pancreatic secretion is an HCO_3^--enriched Na^+/Cl^- solution. The hormone secretin both increases the volume of pancreatic secretion and further enriches its HCO_3^- composition.

and lower Cl^- content. In the pancreatic duct, some HCO_3^- is exchanged for Cl^- by an apical membrane transporter, so HCO_3^- concentration of pancreatic secretion is low at low flow rates. Secretin stimulates an increase in both HCO_3^- concentration and the volume of pancreatic secretion. Regulation of pancreatic water and bicarbonate secretion is accomplished by both secretin and neural control, primarily in response to the presence of acid and digestive contents in the lumen of the duodenum (Fig. 12-9).

Cholecystokinin, released in response to amino acids and fatty acids in the duodenum, increases secretion of the pancreatic digestive enzymes necessary for digestion of all food groups. There is mutual potentiation of CCK and secretin.

Vagal parasympathetic nerves are necessary for the full pancreatic secretory response. Parasympathetic nerve activity enhances both enzyme and aqueous secretion. Sympathetic nerve activity inhibits pancreatic secretion, perhaps secondary to the decrease in pancreatic blood flow.

Intestinal Secretions

The small intestine secretes 1.5 L/day, and the large intestine secretes an additional 400 mL/day. Intestinal mucus, secreted from goblet cells, lubricates the epithelial surface and prevents physical damage. Pepsins are secreted by Brunner's glands of the duodenum, and the crypts of Lieberkühn of the small intestine secrete an aqueous fluid. The aqueous component of intestinal secretions is rich in HCO_3^- and K^+. Intestinal secretions increase following feeding. Mucous and aqueous secretions are enhanced by parasympathetics and mechanical abrasion.

Hepatic and Biliary Secretions

The exocrine secretion of the liver is bile containing bile acids, water, electrolytes, and proteins. Bile acids, the primary component of bile, are synthesized in the liver from cholesterol. Bile acids are classified as primary bile acids if produced directly by the liver, and as secondary bile acids if produced by bacterial modification of the primary bile acid. Cholic acid and chenodeoxycholic acid are primary bile

HISTOLOGY

Hepatic Acinus

The liver has a complex histologic structure and physiologic function. The hepatic lobule comprises the portal triad of hepatic artery, portal vein, and bile duct. The hepatic artery and portal vein carry blood to the liver, and the central vein carries blood away from the lobules into the hepatic venous drainage. The bile duct also represents an outflow path for the exocrine secretion of the liver, known as bile, to exit the liver.

acids, and the secondary bile acids are deoxycholic acid and lithocholic acid. Proteins similar to plasma proteins enter the initial hepatic secretion, and the protein content of bile is supplemented by some hepatic and duct cell protein secretion. The ionic composition of the hepatic secretion is similar to that of plasma. During transit from the liver, bile duct epithelial cells secrete an HCO_3^--rich fluid in a process similar to that described for pancreatic ducts. A total of 0.25 L to 1.5 L of hepatic secretions enter the duodenum each day.

Bile is stored in the gallbladder, and released into the duodenum after ingestion of a meal. The duodenal bile acids are reabsorbed by both diffusion and active transport in the terminal ileum and returned to liver by the hepatic portal vein. The liver actively extracts bile acids from the portal venous blood and secretes the reabsorbed bile acids into the biliary tree. Hepatocytes actively extract bile components for secretion into the bile ducts. This recovery and re-secretion process is called the enterohepatic circulation.

Bile pigments are formed from hemoglobin breakdown, and hepatocytes extract plasma bilirubin, solubilize it by adding glucuronic acid, and actively secrete it into the bile. Bile acids are normally secreted conjugated to glycine or taurine and, at neutral pH of the small intestine, are salts (bile salts). The ampiphatic nature of bile causes the polar sides of bile acids to congregate in an aqueous solution, forming micelles with the polar surface facing outward and the hydrophobic side facing inward. Cholesterol is localized to the center of micelles. Lecithins (phospholipids) also have the hydrophobic surface localized to the center of micelles and the polar chain extending to the outer surface of the micelle.

Bile secretion is the principal digestive function of the liver. Bile acids assist lipid absorption by emulsifying lipids, forming micelles. In addition, bile plays an essential role in dietary cholesterol absorption. When cholesterol is present in excess, biliary cholesterol is the only pathway for cholesterol excretion.

Bile production is poorly regulated, but nerves can influence gallbladder contraction and therefore bile secretion. Biliary duct epithelial HCO_3^- secretion is stimulated by secretin. The sphincter of Oddi at the junction of bile duct and duodenum normally is contracted, so bile is diverted to and stored in the gallbladder between meals. The epithelia of the gallbladder extract Na^+ from the bile by an active transport process. Anions are absorbed via electroneutrality and water osmotically, resulting in the concentrating of bile.

Cholecystokinin, released by the presence of fats in the duodenum, is the primary stimulus for the gallbladder to contract and expel its contents into the duodenum. Vagal nerves also contract the gallbladder and relax the sphincter of Oddi. In contrast, sympathetics and VIP inhibit emptying of the gallbladder.

Around 5% of the bile acid pool is lost in the feces each day, and this amount is replaced by new synthesis. Bile acids in portal blood (i.e., after a meal) stimulate hepatic secretion of bile acids (choleretic effect). Between meals, new synthesis of bile acids proceeds, but the bile flow rate is low. After a meal, CCK empties the gallbladder and strongly stimulates hepatic secretion of bile acids. Secretin simultaneously increases the duct epithelium HCO_3^- (aqueous) component secretion rate. New bile acid synthesis is increased when hepatic portal venous bile salt delivery to the liver decreases.

Disorders of bile secretions lead to crystal (stone) formation. Gallstones primarily are cholesterol crystals around a bilirubin crystal core. Bile acids and lecithin both retard cholesterol crystal formation. Bile pigment stones can also form from a calcium salt of unconjugated bilirubin. If cholesterol content exceeds the ability of micelles to dissolve, cholesterol crystals can form and act as nucleus for gallstones.

●●● DIGESTION AND ABSORPTION

Digestion reduces complex foods into components that can be absorbed. Carbohydrate digestion breaks large carbohydrates into absorbable monoglycerides. Protein digestion breaks poorly absorbed large proteins into monopeptides, dipeptides, and tripeptides. Pancreatic lipases digest lipids to free fatty acids, which are absorbed via bile acid micelles.

Absorptive capacity is not a rate-limiting step, since the ability to absorb proteins and carbohydrates greatly exceeds normal dietary intake.

Carbohydrates

Ingested carbohydrates range in size from simple sugars to complex starches, but only the simple sugars can be absorbed. Plant starch (amylopectin) is the major dietary source of carbohydrates. Amylose is digested by pancreatic amylases, and to a small degree, salivary amylases. The plant starch cellulose is a source of indigestible dietary fiber because humans lack the ability to dissolve the β-1,4 linkage. Amylases break starches into maltose, maltotriose, branched α limit dextrans, and maltooligosaccharides. Salivary amylase is inactivated by gastric acid and is not required for carbohydrate digestion.

Pancreatic amylase in duodenum is essential for carbohydrate digestion. Final carbohydrate digestion is accomplished by epithelial cell enzymes localized on the apical brush border. Lactase (catalyzes conversion of lactose to glucose and galactose), sucrase (catalyzes conversion of sucrose to fructose and glucose), α-dextrinase (breaks α-1,6 linkages), and glucoamylase (catalyzes conversion of maltooligosaccharides to glucose) all digest complex carbohydrates into monosaccharides.

Absorption of carbohydrates occurs primarily in the duodenum and jejunum. An Na^+-coupled (secondary) active transporter moves glucose and galactose across the epithelial cell apical surface. Facilitated diffusion allows exit of the sugars on basal surface. Glucose and galactose compete for the same transporter site. Fructose is transported by a separate, Na^+-independent, carrier.

Carbohydrate malabsorption and intolerance result from the inability to absorb carbohydrates from the diet. This can be due to deficiency of digestive enzymes or transport proteins. Microflora metabolize any carbohydrates that pass through to the colon, producing gas, increased motility, and diarrhea. Diagnosis of malabsorption is accomplished by an oral sugar tolerance test or histologic examination of jejunal epithelial cells. Treatment involves dietary restriction or supplemental enzyme ingestion.

Proteins

Adults require ingestion of at least 0.5 g/kg/day for normal protein balance and more for growth. Dietary protein intake varies greatly among cultures. Ingestion is not the only source of dietary protein. Proteins contained in digestive secretions add 20 g/day to the luminal protein content, and desquamated epithelial cells add an additional 20 g/day.

Digestion occurs in the stomach and small intestine (Fig. 12-10). Pepsin secreted in the stomach can begin protein digestion, but pepsin is not essential for protein digestion. Pancreatic proteases digest the majority of dietary proteins. Other peptidases are located in the brush border of the small intestine, particularly the proximal jejunum. Digestion breaks large peptides and proteins into amino acids or small

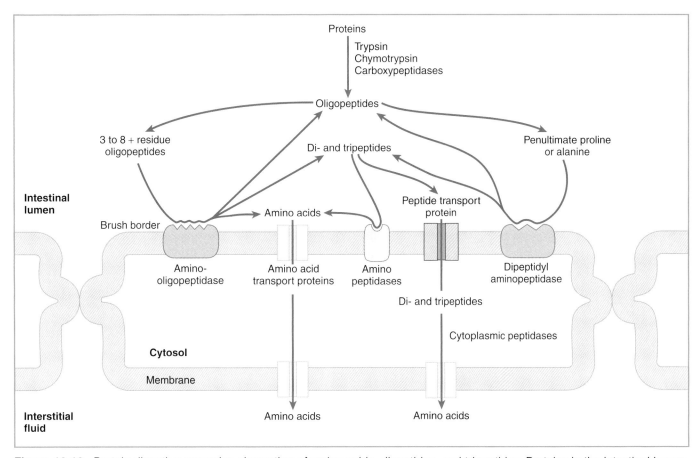

Figure 12-10. Protein digestion precedes absorption of amino acids, dipeptides, and tripeptides. Proteins in the intestinal lumen are digested by multiple enzymes. The apical surface of the epithelial cell has a variety of Na^+-coupled transporters that can transport either individual amino acids or di- and tripeptides. The di- and tripeptides are digested within the epithelial cell by cytoplasmic peptidases. The amino acids exit the basolateral side of the epithelial cell by one of a variety of Na^+-independent amino acid transporters.

peptides. The final digestion of dipeptides and tripeptides occurs within the duodenal and jejunal epithelial cells by cytosolic peptidases. Half of protein digestion occurs in the duodenum and half in the jejunum.

Absorption occurs primarily in the duodenum and jejunum. Large proteins are poorly absorbed. L-Isomers of dipeptides and tripeptides are well absorbed by an Na^+-coupled process. The apical endothelial surface has multiple classes of L–amino acid transporters, similar to those found on the renal proximal tubule. An Na^+-coupled transport absorbs neutral amino acids, proline, hydroxyproline, phenylalanine, and methionine. An Na^+-independent transport process absorbs basic amino acids and most neutral amino acids. Genetic malabsorption and intolerance affect both intestinal and renal transport proteins.

Lipids

Triglycerides are the major component of dietary lipids. Other components include sterols, sterol esters, and phospholipids. Lipids are hydrophobic, so they separate from remainder of chyme as an oily phase in the stomach. Lipids are emulsified in the duodenum by bile acids and digested to form micelles with bile acids. Micelles allow free fatty acid absorption at the intestinal brush border.

Digestion occurs primarily in the small intestine (Fig. 12-11). There is little digestion by water-soluble gastric lipases, since the high gastric acidity promotes phase separation. Lipids are the last component of the meal to enter the small intestine. Gastric emptying is inhibited by fat in the duodenum, restricting the entry of lipids to a quantity that can be processed for absorption.

The duodenum and jejunum are the major site of lipid digestion. Pancreatic lipase, secreted into the duodenum, digests triglycerides. Pancreatic lipase is inactivated by bile salts, and the inactivation is blocked by colipase. A limited amount of cholesterol esterase acts on a variety of substrates. Phospholipase A_2 action yields free fatty acids and lysophosphatides. Bile acids and lecithin emulsify the fats, which increases the available surface area.

Micelles are essential to increase the contact area for absorption in the duodenum and jejunum. Diffusion through the unstirred aqueous layer on the brush border limits the micelle absorption rate. Consequently, cell membrane transporters assist in the reabsorption of free cholesterol. Lipids accumulate in the smooth endoplasmic reticulum,

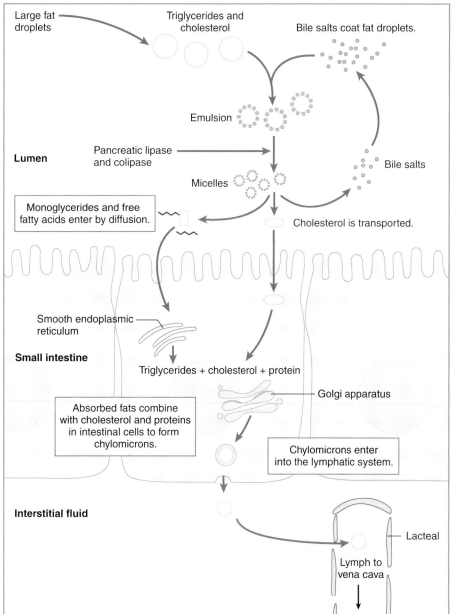

Figure 12-11. Products of lipid digestion are repackaged into chylomicrons in the intestinal epithelium. The combination of hepatic bile salts, pancreatic lipase, and pancreatic colipase digests fats into monoglycerides, free fatty acids, and cholesterol. These digested components enter the intestinal epithelial cells and are transported to the smooth endoplasmic reticulum. The absorbed fats combine with cholesterol and protein to form chylomicrons, which are secreted by exocytosis. The chylomicrons enter the lymphatic lacteals and are transported to the vena cava.

where they are resynthesized to triglycerides, phospholipids, and cholesterol esters and packaged in chylomicrons, along with epithelial cell β-lipoprotein. Chylomicrons are extruded from the cell by exocytosis. After entering the lacteals, chylomicrons pass through the lymphatics to enter the venous circulation at the thoracic duct. This route of absorption bypasses the liver and the portal circulation.

Malabsorption of lipids is tied to impaired digestion or absorption. Complete bile deficiency reduces fatty acid absorption by 50% and impairs absorption of other lipids. Complete absence of pancreatic lipases impairs absorption of all classes of lipids. Impaired absorption can also result from epithelial cell damage due to intestinal mucosal atrophy, tropical sprue, or gluten enteropathy.

Water and Electrolytes

The GI tract absorbs 99% of ingested water and ions. Absorption is determined by transporters and diffusion, with a transcellular pathway across cell membranes or a paracellular pathway through tight junctions. The "tightness" of tight junctions determines water and ion permeability. Tight junctions are loosest in the duodenum and tightest in the colon and stomach.

The GI tract receives 2 L/day from ingestion and 7 L/day from GI secretions. Only 50 to 100 mL/day is lost in feces. The jejunum is the primary site of water absorption. The colon absorbs 400 mL/day, against an apparent osmotic gradient.

The jejunum is also the primary site of Na^+ absorption, secondary to amino acid and carbohydrate absorption. Apical entry occurs by diffusion, and basolateral surface secretion occurs by the primary active transporter Na^+/K^+-ATPase. The colon has active, amiloride-sensitive Na^+ absorption.

Net K^+ balance is determined in the colon. Potassium is reabsorbed in the jejunum and ileum. In these regions, K^+ levels are tied to water movements. Transport in the colon determines final K^+ balance. There is reabsorption if luminal K^+ concentration is high, and secretion if luminal K^+ concentration is low. Aldosterone enhances Na^+/K^+ exchange and causes K^+ secretion. A significant K^+ loss can accompany water loss due to diarrhea.

The intestinal Cl^- load is from ingestion and pancreatic secretions. Cl^- is reabsorbed in the jejunum, ileum, and colon. Transepithelial potential facilitates paracellular reabsorption of Cl^-.

The HCO_3^- intestinal load is primarily from pancreatic secretions. HCO_3^- is absorbed in the jejunum coupled to H^+ secretion into the lumen by an apical Na^+/H^+ exchange. Some HCO_3^- is secreted by HCO_3^-/Cl^- exchange in the ileum and colon. HCO_3^- cannot be secreted against a large gradient. There is net secretion if HCO_3^- levels are high (alkalosis) and net reabsorption if HCO_3^- levels are low (acidosis).

Regulation of Intestinal Ion and Water Balance

Aldosterone provides the major hormonal control of absorption. Just as in the kidney, aldosterone causes colonic K^+ loss and enhances the reabsorption of Na^+ and water. Na^+/Cl^- and water reabsorption are also enhanced by enkephalin (opioid peptides) and somatostatin.

Excessive GI secretion is a clinically important problem and can rapidly lead to dehydration. During cholera, Na^+, Cl^-, and H_2O secretion in small intestine crypts exceeds the absorptive capacity of the remainder of the GI tract. Cholera toxin stimulates crypt cell secretion through the cAMP second messenger system. In pancreatic cholera, a pancreatic tumor secretes VIP, which also increases cAMP and stimulates crypt cell secretion.

Congenital Cl^- diarrhea is caused by defective Cl^-/HCO_3^- exchange. Excessive Cl^- is lost in the feces, and HCO_3^- reabsorption is impaired. This transporter defect results in a metabolic alkalosis.

Impaired nutrient absorption causes an excessive osmotic load on the colon, and water is lost in the feces if the absorptive capacity of the colon is exceeded. Carbohydrate absorption disorders include lactose malabsorption syndrome, congenital lactose intolerance, sucrase-isomaltase deficiency, and glucose-galactose malabsorption syndrome. Fat malabsorption can also increase the colonic osmotic load, since colonic microflora metabolize nutrients that pass into the colon, causing borborygmi and intestinal gas. Hypermotility results in decreased time for absorption and can cause an osmotic load of unabsorbed nutrients to enter the colon as substrate for microflora. In all cases, the water loss is a consequence of the increased amount of osmoles in the lumen of the colon.

Intestinal Divalent Ion Regulation

Calcium is actively absorbed in the duodenum and jejunum as well as in other intestinal segments. Apical absorption occurs by facilitated diffusion, since cytosolic Ca^{++}-binding proteins keep free intracellular Ca^{++} levels low. Basolateral active transport occurs by Ca^{++}-ATPase and an Na^+/Ca^{++} exchanger. Calcium absorption is stimulated by vitamin D, with a small amount of stimulation by parathyroid hormone. Deficiency of vitamin D impairs Ca^{++} absorption, causing hypocalcemia and possibly rickets.

Dietary iron is reabsorbed primarily in the duodenum and jejunum. About 5% to 10% of ingested iron is normally absorbed, but the absorption rate increases to 20% when dietary iron is ingested bound to heme. Heme is digested before free iron is absorbed, and ascorbate binds iron in an absorbable complex.

The epithelial apical surface secretes transferrin to facilitate transcellular iron transport. The iron-transferrin complex is absorbed through receptor-mediated endocytosis. Iron is actively transported across the basolateral surface to the interstitial space. Iron deficiency induces differentiating crypt cells to enhance their iron-absorbing capacity. Conversely, high plasma iron stores increase the ferritin content of epithelial cells. Ferritin binds irreversibly to iron, and iron is lost from the body when epithelial cells desquamate.

Approximately 50% of ingested magnesium is absorbed along the length of the intestine. Phosphate also is absorbed along the length of the intestine, possibly by active transport. Copper is both absorbed and secreted. About 50% of the ingested copper load absorbed, and copper secreted in bile is lost to feces.

Vitamins

Vitamins must be absorbed from a dietary source. Hydrophobicity of vitamins limits the available transport pathways. Water-soluble vitamins can be absorbed by membrane transport proteins. Lipid-soluble vitamins A, D, E, and K are absorbed mostly in micelles.

Folic acid and nicotinic acid are absorbed by diffusion, facilitated diffusion, or both. Diffusion also mediates absorption of pyridoxine and riboflavin, a process enhanced by bile acids. Secondary active transport leads to vitamin C absorption in the ileum, biotin in the upper small intestine, and folic acid and thiamine in the jejunum.

Vitamin B_{12} must be bound to salivary R protein (haptocorrin) in the stomach. The complex is transferred to intrinsic factor (a gastric parietal cell secretion), since R proteins are digested in the duodenum. The intrinsic factor–B_{12} complex binds to the ileal apical membrane, and B_{12} is absorbed. B_{12} crosses the basolateral membrane by a carrier-mediated process. Deficiency in any component of the B_{12} absorption process can lead to pernicious anemia. Pernicious anemia can be due to atrophy of parietal cell gastric mucosa, congenital intrinsic factor deficiency (where other parietal cell secretions are normal), deficiency of pancreatic peptidases (B_{12} stays bound to R proteins and is not absorbed), or deficiency of the ileal B_{12} transporter (congenital B_{12} malabsorption syndrome).

●●● TOP 5 TAKE-HOME POINTS

1. The major function of the GI system is to digest and absorb the diet. A mixed diet contains complex forms of carbohydrates, proteins, and fats, all of which are broken down into components before being absorbed.

2. In general, the pylorus separates the storage components of the GI tract (stomach) from the digestive and absorptive components (small and large intestine).

3. GI luminal contents must be reabsorbed across the epithelial cell layer or they will exit the body in the feces.

4. Intrinsic regulation is accomplished by the enteric nerves and by negative feedback control of the release of a variety of GI hormones.

5. Extrinsic regulation is accomplished primarily by the parasympathetic branch of the autonomic nervous system.

Endocrine System   13

Endocrine hormones are secreted from specialized cells and transported by the blood to a target cell, often a second endocrine cell. The term endocrine describes a secretion that remains within the body, in contrast to exocrine secretions, which cross an epithelial layer (such as pancreatic GI secretions) and are functionally outside the body.

Endocrine organs are distributed throughout the body (Fig. 13-1 and Table 13-1). Organs such as the adrenal gland and pituitary are composed of endocrine secretory cells. Organs such as the pancreas produce both endocrine (insulin, glucagon, somatostatin) and exocrine (pancreatic lipase,

trypsinogen, etc.) secretions. Finally, many organs have an endocrine role that is not usually associated with the other functions of the organ (i.e., renal secretion of erythropoietin).

Endocrine hormone molecular structure falls into one of three classes: peptide/protein, amino acid derivative (catecholamines and thyroid hormone), and steroid. Hormone response characteristics, however, are tied to the location of the receptor (cell membrane surface vs. within the cell).

Peptide and catecholamine hormones first bind to cell membrane receptors and consequently have a rapid onset of response. Some second messenger systems do affect transcription and translation, allowing peptide hormones to also have longer term trophic activities.

Proteins and polypeptides hormones are synthesized in the endoplasmic reticulum (Fig. 13-2). Proteins and polypeptide hormones bind to cell membrane receptors on target tissues. Peptide hormones require second messengers for effects and generally have rapid response times (see Chapter 4).

Steroid hormones are derived from cholesterol. Consequently, steroid hormones are generally poorly soluble in water and, following secretion, are transported bound to plasma-binding proteins. Steroids diffuse across the plasma membrane and bind to a cytoplasmic binding protein. The steroid–binding protein complex diffuses to the nucleus and activates a hormone response element, which initiates DNA transcription and translation. The reliance on DNA transcription and translation means that steroid hormones generally have a long lag time between secretion and effect. Some steroids, like aldosterone and estrogen, can produce acute effects independent of any nuclear effects. This allows such hormones to have both acute and chronic actions.

Catecholamines and thyroid hormone do not share common mechanism of action, even though they are both derived from amino acid precursors. Catecholamines act on cell membrane receptors and work through second messengers similarly to peptide hormones. Thyroid hormones bind cytoplasmic receptors and alter DNA transcription, similarly to steroid hormones.

●●● ENDOCRINE SYSTEM FUNCTION

Endocrine secretions, together with the nervous system, coordinate water and ion balance, metabolism, reproduction, and nutrient absorption. Consequently, most tissues in the body are targets for one or more endocrine hormones.

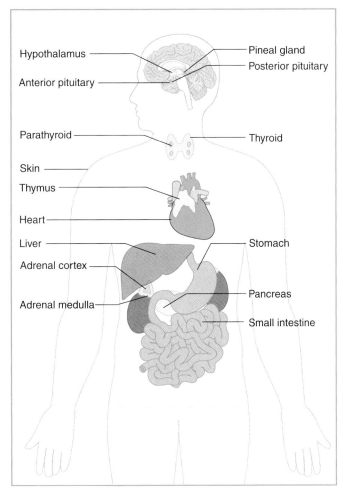

Figure 13-1. Endocrine hormones are secreted from a variety of body tissues and organs. This figure identifies the sites of hormone secretion. See Table 13-1 for their target tissues and actions.

Water and ion balance in the body reflects the complex integration of ingestion, loss, production, and consumption. Hormonal regulation of circulating ion levels also depends on exchange with various storage pools in the body. For example, water balance depends on antidiuretic hormone, renal perfusion pressure, and any system that alters plasma Na^+, with intracellular, interstitial, and plasma water as the buffer pools. Plasma Na^+ is acutely regulated by angiotensin, aldosterone, and atrial natriuretic hormone and long term by antidiuretic hormone, with extracellular fluid Na^+ as the buffer pool. Endocrine regulation of plasma K^+ is by aldosterone, with intracellular fluid K^+ as the buffer pool. Plasma Ca^{++} is tightly regulated by parathyroid hormone and calcitonin, with bone Ca^{++} crystals as the buffer pool. More details of water and electrolyte regulation appear in Chapters 3 and 11.

Plasma glucose is closely regulated by insulin, glucagon, and the metabolic actions of cortisol, growth hormone, and epinephrine, with liver glycogen as the buffer pool. Metabolic regulation also involves shifting consumption between glucose and fats as energy source for mitochondria, based on glucose availability. Metabolic rate is closely regulated by thyroid hormone, with cortisol and epinephrine having some influence, as discussed later in this chapter. The complex interactions among endocrine hormones and target tissues are a recurring theme in physiologic control.

⦿⦿⦿ ENDOCRINE SYSTEM REGULATION

Negative feedback loops provide precise control of endocrine secretions (Fig. 13-3). The controlled component of the negative feedback loop can be ion concentrations, physical parameters (e.g., blood pressure), and hormone concentrations. Stimulators of endocrine gland secretion also have important trophic effects. Stimuli that cause hormone release frequently also cause hypertrophy and hyperplasia of the endocrine organ. This increases the quantity of hormone synthesized and released.

Endocrine control often is integrated with neural function. Sympathetic nerves innervate some endocrine organs, such as the adrenal medulla and pancreas. Nerves in the hypothalamus release factors controlling anterior pituitary secretions. Nervous system function often complements endocrine actions. Hemorrhagic hypotension causes an increase in angiotensin II production and ADH release, as well as an increase in sympathetic nerve activity. Together, these systems promote the renal retention of sodium and water, which helps restore blood volume and blood pressure toward normal. Specific external controls are discussed later in this chapter with the appropriate endocrine hormone.

⦿⦿⦿ HYPOTHALAMUS AND PITUITARY

The pituitary gland (hypophysis) is a small (1 g) structure located on the dorsal surface of the hypothalamus. It is connected to the hypothalamus by the hypophyseal stalk (Fig. 13-4). The pituitary has three histologically distinct sections, two of which secrete hormones in humans. The anterior pituitary (adenohypophysis) contains a variety of secretory cell types. The posterior pituitary (neurohypophysis) contains glia cells and terminal axons from cells of the hypothalamus. The pars intermedia is a vestigial remnant in humans with little physiologic significance and will not be discussed.

The hypophyseal stalk has two distinct pathways leading from the hypothalamus to the pituitary (see Fig. 13-4). The neural stalk contains axons originating in the hypothalamus that terminate in the posterior pituitary. Cell bodies for these neurons are in the supraoptic and paraventricular nuclei. The axons terminate in the posterior pituitary, where the synaptic terminals secrete hormones rather than make a synaptic connection with another neuron.

The hypothalamic hypophyseal portal system provides a vascular connection between the median eminence of the hypothalamus and the anterior pituitary (see Fig. 13-4). Arterial blood enters the capillaries of the hypothalamus, where it picks up hypothalamic-releasing and -inhibiting

TABLE 13-1. Summary of Major Hormones

Location	Hormone	Target	Main Effect
Pineal gland	Melatonin	Unclear in humans	Circadian rhythm; other effects uncertain
Hypothalamus	Trophic hormones (see Table 13-2) Also see posterior pituitary, below	Anterior pituitary	Release or inhibition of pituitary hormones
Posterior pituitary	Oxytocin (OT)	Breast and uterus	Milk ejection; labor and delivery; behavior
	Vasopressin (ADH)	Kidney	Water reabsorption
Anterior pituitary	(See Table 13-2)		
Thyroid	Triiodothyronine and thyroxine (T_3, T_4)	Many tissues	Metabolism, growth and development
	Calcitonin (CT)	Bone	Plasma calcium levels (minimal effect in humans)
Parathyroid	Parathyroid hormone (PTH)	Bone, kidney	Regulation of plasma calcium and phosphate levels
Thymus	Thymosin, thymopoietin	Lymphocytes	Lymphocyte development
Heart	Atrial natriuretic peptide (ANP)	Kidneys	Increased sodium excretion
Liver	Angiotensinogen	Adrenal cortex, blood vessels, brain	Aldosterone secretion, increased blood pressure
	Insulin-like growth factors (IGFs)	Many tissues	Growth
Stomach and small intestine	Gastrin, cholecystokinin (CCK), secretin, others	GI tract and pancreas	Assistance digestion and absorption of nutrients
Pancreas	Insulin, glucagon, somatostatin (SS), pancreatic polypeptide	Many tissues	Metabolism of glucose and other nutrients
Adrenal cortex	Aldosterone	Kidney	Na^+ and K^+ homeostasis
	Cortisol	Many tissues	Stress response
	Androgens	Many tissues	Sexual characteristics
Adrenal medulla	Epinephrine, norepinephrine	Many tissues	Fight-or-flight response
Kidney	Erythropoietin (EPO)	Bone marrow	Red blood cell production
	1,25-dihydroxyvitamin D_3 (calciferol)	Intestine	Increased calcium absorption
	Renin	Angiotensinogen	Angiotensin II production
Skin	Vitamin D	Intermediate form of hormone	Precursor of 1,25-dihydroxyvitamin D_3
Testes (male)	Androgen	Many tissues	Sperm production, secondary sex characteristics
	Inhibin	Anterior pituitary	Inhibition of FSH secretion
Ovaries (female)	Estrogens and progesterone	Many tissues	Egg production, secondary sex characteristics
	Ovarian inhibin	Anterior pituitary	Inhibition of FSH secretion
	Relaxin (pregnancy)	Uterine muscle	Muscle relaxation
Adipose tissue	Leptin	Hypothalamus, other tissues	Food intake; metabolism; reproduction

hormones. This blood then flows through portal vessels in the pituitary stalk. The blood enters a second set of capillaries (sinuses) in the anterior pituitary, where the hypothalamic hormones bind to specific anterior pituitary endocrine cells. This vascular arrangement ensures that releasing and inhibiting hormones secreted in the median eminence remain concentrated until delivered to the target cells of the anterior pituitary. Blood containing the anterior pituitary hormone secretions then exits the anterior pituitary and joins with other venous drainages. Pituitary secretions regulate cell metabolism, regulate salt and water balance, and coordinate secretion of hormones from other endocrine glands.

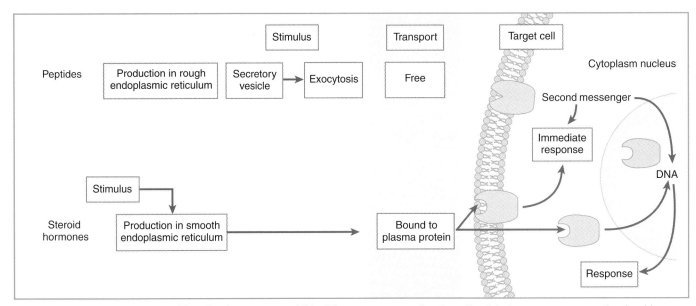

Figure 13-2. Peptide and steroid endocrine agents exhibit different patterns of action. Peptide hormones are synthesized in advance and released by exocytosis following an appropriate stimulus. Once released, they travel within the plasma until binding with a receptor on the cell surface of the target tissue and quickly activating intracellular second messenger systems. In contrast, steroid hormones are synthesized on demand following an appropriate stimulus. Following release, steroid hormones travel bound to plasma protein, enter the cell by diffusion, and bind an intracellular receptor, ultimately affecting DNA transcription and translation.

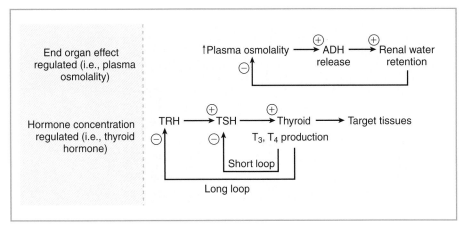

Figure 13-3. Hormone release is regulated by negative feedback loops. The negative feedback signal can be provided by an end organ effect, or the circulating hormone levels themselves may provide the negative feedback signal.

Hypothalamus

The hypothalamus sits dorsal to the pituitary gland and regulates secretion of both anterior and posterior pituitary hormones. Hypothalamic-releasing hormones regulate secretion of five of the six anterior pituitary hormones (Table 13-2). Thyroid hormone–releasing hormone (thyroid-releasing hormone, TRH) controls pituitary output of thyroid-stimulating hormone (TSH). Corticotropin-releasing hormone (CRH) controls pituitary secretion of adrenocorticotropic hormone (ACTH). Gonadotropin-releasing hormone (GnRH) causes release of both pituitary luteinizing hormone (LH) and pituitary follicle-stimulating hormone (FSH). Growth hormone–releasing hormone (GHRH) regulates pituitary secretion of growth hormone (GH).

Two hypothalamic hormones inhibit pituitary secretion (see Table 13-2). Prolactin inhibitory hormone (dopamine) inhibits pituitary release of prolactin. Growth hormone–inhibiting hormone (GHIH, somatostatin) inhibits pituitary release of growth hormone. The anterior pituitary is the end organ for growth hormone and prolactin secretion. Thyroid hormone, ACTH, is discussed in later portions of this chapter, and the hormones FSH and LH are discussed in Chapters 14 and 15.

Anterior Pituitary

The anterior pituitary secretes six hormones, two of which act on the final target tissues and four of which control other endocrine gland secretions. Growth hormone and prolactin act on the final target organs, but growth hormone also uptake and use of glucose, and increases plasma glucose levels. In many tissues, GH exerts its effects through IGF-I and IGF-II.

Insulin has an important permissive role in growth hormone–mediated growth. An increase in blood glucose stimulates insulin release. Insulin enhances entry of both glucose and amino acids into cells. Pancreatectomy abolishes GH effects on growth.

Growth hormone secretion is enhanced by a variety of stressful and normal stimuli (Fig. 13-5). GH is released by starvation or chronic protein deficiency, hypoglycemia, low plasma levels of free fatty acids, exercise, onset of sleep, and following ingestion of arginine-containing foods. Hypothalamic secretion of releasing and inhibitory hormones provides the primary regulation of GH release.

The anterior pituitary is the end organ for prolactin secretion. Hypothalamic control of prolactin is unique in that the normal control of prolactin release is by prolactin inhibitory hormone. Consequently, interruption of the hypothalamic-hypophyseal portal system disrupts the inhibition and as a result increases pituitary prolactin release. Prolactin-releasing hormone is important in the production of milk in nursing mothers (see Chapter 14).

The complex control of some hormone release by tropic hormones means that a variety of abnormalities can cause hyper- or hyposecretion of a hormone. Table 13-3 describes the tropic hormone profile that helps identify whether the initial disorder is in the endocrine tissue or in one of the tropic hormones controlling the endocrine tissue.

Posterior Pituitary

Oxytocin and antidiuretic hormone (ADH, vasopressin) are synthesized in the hypothalamus and transported within axons to the posterior pituitary for secretion. Action potentials arriving at these nerve endings secrete oxytocin or ADH into the blood, much like other nerves release neurotransmitters. In addition to these nerve endings, the posterior pituitary contains glia-like cells, which support and nourish the nerve endings.

Oxytocin is formed primarily in the paraventricular nucleus of the hypothalamus. Oxytocin promotes uterine contraction, thereby assisting labor. Oxytocin also causes milk "let down" following suckling. (This reflex is discussed further in Chapter 14).

ADH is formed primarily in the supraoptic nucleus. ADH release is enhanced by increases in plasma osmolarity, usually tied to changes in plasma Na^+ concentration. Hypotension and hypovolemia have a smaller role in stimulating ADH release, as do stress and trauma. The role of ADH in water and salt balance is discussed in Chapters 3 and 11.

●●● THYROID

Thyroid hormone is a composite of three (T_3) or four (T_4) iodinated tyrosine residues. T_3 and T_4 together are called

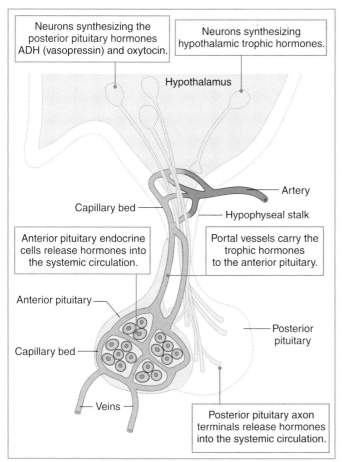

Figure 13-4. The hypothalamus and pituitary have complex neural and endocrine interactions. Neurons in the hypothalamus synthesize oxytocin and antidiuretic hormone. The hormones are transported within axon terminals to the posterior pituitary for release. In contrast, the anterior pituitary is in endocrine gland. Hormone release is controlled by releasing and inhibitory peptides that pass from the hypothalamus to the anterior pituitary by a vascular hypothalamic-hypophyseal portal system.

Within the figure:
- Neurons synthesizing the posterior pituitary hormones ADH (vasopressin) and oxytocin.
- Neurons synthesizing hypothalamic trophic hormones.
- Hypothalamus
- Artery
- Capillary bed
- Hypophyseal stalk
- Anterior pituitary endocrine cells release hormones into the systemic circulation.
- Portal vessels carry the trophic hormones to the anterior pituitary.
- Anterior pituitary
- Capillary bed
- Posterior pituitary
- Veins
- Posterior pituitary axon terminals release hormones into the systemic circulation.

controls secretion of the somatomedins—insulin-like growth factors I and II (IGF-I, IGF-II). The remaining hormones act on endocrine tissues to stimulate the release of another hormone. Corticotropin stimulates adrenocortical secretion of cortisol. TSH stimulates synthesis and release of thyroid hormone. LH promotes female progesterone secretion and conversion of androgens to estrogen, or in the male, testosterone secretion. FSH stimulates estrogen and inhibin secretion in both sexes.

The anterior pituitary is the end organ for growth hormone secretion. GH (somatotropin) stimulates growth in almost all body tissues. It acts on target tissues to increase cell size (hypertrophy) and increase cell number (hyperplasia). Metabolically, GH increases protein synthesis, decreases protein catabolism, and decreases amino acid use in gluconeogenesis. It enhances use of free fatty acids as metabolic substrates, which depletes body fat stores, decreases tissue

TABLE 13-2. Hypothalamic and Anterior Pituitary Hormones

Hypothalamic Hormone	Pituitary Hormone	Intermediate Target	Final Target
Corticotropin-releasing hormone (CHR)	Adrenocorticotropic hormone (ACTH)	Adrenal cortex cortisol	Liver, adipose tissue stress response
Thyroid hormone–releasing hormone (THRH)	Thyroid-stimulating hormone (TSH)	Thyroid hormones T_3 and T_4	Most tissues (metabolism, growth)
Prolactin inhibitory hormone (PIH), dopamine Prolactin-releasing hormone (PRH)	Prolactin	None	Breast milk production
Growth hormone–releasing hormone (GHRH) Growth hormone–inhibiting hormone (GHIH) (somatostatin)	Growth hormone (GH)	Liver, insulin-like growth factors (IGFs)	Most tissues (growth, metabolism)
Gonadotropin-releasing hormone (GnRH)	Follicle-stimulating hormone (FSH)	Female ovary (estrogen) Male testis (estrogen)	Many tissues Secondary sexual characteristics Sertoli cells Sperm maturation
	Luteinizing hormone (LH)	Female corpus luteum (progesterone) Male testis (testosterone)	Many tissues reproduction Many tissues Secondary sexual characteristics

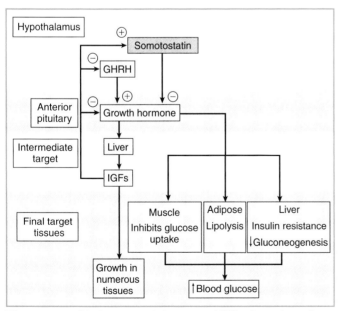

Figure 13-5. Pituitary growth hormone (GH) release is under dual control, stimulated by growth hormone–releasing hormone (GHRH) and inhibited by somatostatin. The hypothalamus regulates GH release. Once released, GH acts directly on tissues to increase blood glucose levels. GH also causes the release of insulin-like growth factors (IGFs) from the liver, and IGFs stimulate growth in numerous tissues.

PATHOLOGY

Dwarfism

Pituitary dwarfism results from a defect in growth hormone synthesis. The absence of growth hormone, and consequently of insulin-like growth factor I, impairs the normal development of bones and cartilage.

thyroid hormone. Thyroid hormone, although derived from an amino acid, acts like a steroid hormone. In the plasma, 99% of thyroid hormone is transported bound to thyroid-binding globulin. Thyroid hormone binds to an intracellular receptor protein and alters DNA transcription and translation. Thyroid hormone effects are chronic. Of the two hormones, the biological effect of T_3 is more rapid and requires 3 days for peak effect. The biological effect of T_4 is slower and requires 11 days for peak effect.

Thyroid hormone increases metabolism. It enhances carbohydrate consumption and increases the size and density of mitochondria. Thyroid hormone promotes growth and is required for normal growth in children. Thyroid hormone also increases mental activity and increases other endocrine secretions.

TABLE 13-3. Independent Changes in Extracellular Fluid Osmolality and Body Fluid Volume

Tropic Hormon Concentration	Target Gland Hormone Concentration		
	Low	Normal	High
Low	Tropic hormone source failure		Autonomous secretion of hormone (cancer)
Normal		Normal	
High	Failure of target tissue		Autonomous secretion of tropic hormone (cancer)

Thyroid hormone assists in acclimatization to cold environments by increasing the metabolic rate. Cold stimulates thyroid hormone release, and the basal metabolic rate is increased, generating heat as a by-product of metabolism.

Regulation of Thyroid Hormone Synthesis and Release

Of the two biologically active forms, T_4 is produced in greater amount and represents 90% of thyroid gland output. T_3 is more stable than T_4, and T_3 has greater potency than T_4. Consequently, T_3 is generally considered the active intracellular form of thyroid hormone (Fig. 13-6).

Thyroid hormone is formed in epithelium-lined follicles. These follicles contain the glycoprotein thyroglobulin. Iodine is oxidized within the follicles and binds to a tyrosine residue of thyroglobulin (monoiodinated tyrosine, MIT). Iodinated tyrosines are coupled while still part of the thyroglobulin molecule, forming diiodinated tyrosine (DIT) and finally T_3 and T_4. Mature hormone is released by the proteolysis of thyroglobulin, with recycling of unused iodine, MIT, and DIT. The thyroid gland stores sufficient thyroid hormone for a few months.

Dietary iodine is required for thyroid hormone synthesis. Natural iodine is available in (saltwater) coastal areas but in decreasing amounts inland. In the United States, iodine is added to salt to prevent iodine deficiency. Dietary iodine is absorbed by the GI tract, and circulating iodine is absorbed by the thyroid gland or cleared by the kidneys.

Feedback regulation is primarily by T_4 inhibition of thyroid-stimulating hormone at the anterior pituitary (Fig. 13-7). TSH stimulates proteolysis of thyroglobulin, releasing T_3 and T_4. TSH stimulates iodine uptake by thyroid for new thyroid hormone synthesis, increases activity of thyroid gland cells, and increases thyroid hormone synthesis. TSH release is controlled by hypothalamic tripeptide thyrotropin-releasing hormone. Cold exposure is a potent stimulus for thyrotropin-releasing hormone release, but the feedback loop for the effect of temperature on this hormone is not yet established.

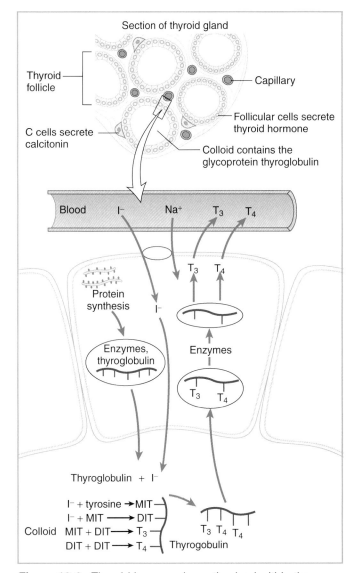

Figure 13-6. Thyroid hormone is synthesized within the colloid of thyroid follicles. The thyroid follicular cells actively transport iodide (I⁻) into the follicle, where it combines with the tyrosine residues attached to the protein thyroglobulin to make T_3 and T_4. The T_3 and T_4 are separated from the protein and secreted into the blood. MIT, monoiodinated tyrosine; DIT, diiodinated tyrosine.

PATHOLOGY

Goiter

Goiter is enlargement of the thyroid gland and is found in both hyperthyroid and hypothyroid states. Goiter can result from excessive activation of TSH receptors on the thyroid cells. In hypothyroid states, the elevated TSH may be the result of normal negative feedback control, impaired synthesis of thyroid hormone (i.e., from iodine deficiency), or lack of response at the tissue level. In hyperthyroid states, goiter can result from excessive production of TSH, or in Graves' disease, from activation of TSH receptors by circulating antibodies.

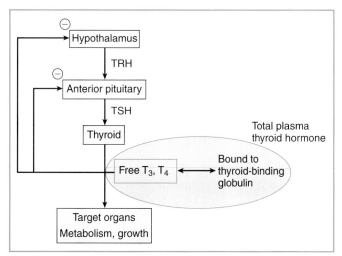

Figure 13-7. Free T_3 and T_4 provide feedback control for pituitary thyroid-stimulating hormone (TSH) release. Most circulating thyroid hormone is bound to thyroid-binding globulin. Free thyroid hormone levels produce both the biological effects and the negative feedback signal regulating TSH release. TRH, thyroid-releasing hormone.

●●● PARATHYROID HORMONE AND CALCITONIN

Plasma calcium levels are regulated by the polypeptides parathyroid hormone and calcitonin. Parathyroid hormone, secreted by the parathyroid glands embedded in the thyroid, acts to increase plasma calcium levels. Parathyroid hormone also decreases plasma PO_4. Calcitonin, secreted from the parafollicular cells of the thyroid, acts to decrease plasma Ca^{++}. Of the two hormones, parathyroid hormone is the more biologically powerful regulator of plasma Ca^{++}, and calcitonin has only a minor role.

Actions of Parathyroid Hormone

Parathyroid hormone (PTH) increases free plasma Ca^{++} (Fig. 13-8). PTH-stimulated bone reabsorption acutely

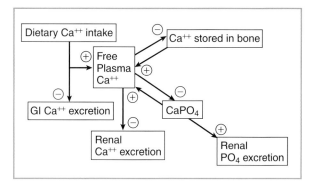

Figure 13-8. Parathyroid hormone increases free plasma Ca^{++}. Free plasma Ca^{++} represents the balance between dietary Ca^{++} uptake, exchange with the bone Ca^{++} storage pool, binding to PO_4, and renal Ca^{++} loss. Parathyroid hormone increases dietary Ca^{++} uptake by increasing vitamin D synthesis, increases osteoclast activity to release Ca^{++} stored in the bone, increases renal PO_4 excretion, and decreases renal Ca^{++} excretion. All these actions increase free plasma Ca^{++} levels.

increases absorption of recently deposited Ca^{++} salts, and chronically increases osteoclast number and activity. PTH increases renal activation of vitamin D_3, which increases GI absorption of dietary Ca^{++}. PTH decreases renal Ca^{++} excretion by increasing Ca^{++} reabsorption in the renal distal tubule and collecting duct.

PTH decreases plasma PO_4 and body PO_4 stores. PTH significantly enhances renal excretion of PO_4. The decrease in plasma PO_4 occurs because the magnitude of the increased renal PO_4 excretion is greater than the increase in plasma PO_4 from bone reabsorption. The increased dietary absorption of PO_4 from vitamin D_3 activation also is insufficient to overcome the enhanced renal PO_4 loss. The decrease in plasma PO_4 increases the percentage of plasma Ca^{++} that circulates in the free, or unbound, state.

Free plasma Ca^{++} is the primary determinant of PTH release. Hypocalcemia increases PTH synthesis and release. Hypocalcemia can occur during pregnancy and lactation. Prolonged hypocalcemia causes excessive PTH-mediated bone reabsorption and can cause osteoporosis and rickets. Stimuli that increase the release of PTH also cause hypertrophy of the parathyroid gland. Hypercalcemia decreases PTH synthesis and release.

Actions of Calcitonin

Calcitonin decreases plasma Ca^{++} concentration by enhancing Ca^{++} crystal deposition in bone, transiently increasing osteoblast activity, and chronically stimulating the formation of new osteoblast cells. Calcitonin effects are more pronounced in children, who have a more labile bone Ca^{++} storage pool, and calcitonin is of limited importance in adults. Calcitonin responds more rapidly than PTH but is a less powerful regulator of Ca^{++} balance. No disease states are associated with calcitonin deficiency or calcitonin excess.

Integrated Calcium Balance

Plasma Ca^{++} is tightly regulated, around 9.4 mg/dL, with a normal range of 9 to 10 mg/dL. Forty percent of plasma Ca^{++} is tightly bound to plasma proteins, 10% is combined in un-ionized salts with citrate and PO_4, and 50% is free, about 5 mg/dL.

Bone contains cells, Ca^{++} and PO_4 hydroxyapatite crystals, and an organic matrix. Osteocytes are the primary bone cells, formed when hydroxyapatite crystals surround osteoblasts. Osteoblasts promote growth or formation of new bone. Osteoclasts promote reabsorption of bone, returning Ca^{++} and PO_4 to the circulation. Bone is constantly remodeled in response to mechanical stress and endocrine regulation of plasma Ca^{++}. In bone, newly deposited Ca^{++} salts are more easily reabsorbed than are hydroxyapatite crystals.

Dietary absorption of Ca^{++} requires activated vitamin D_3. Vitamin D is absorbed from the diet or through ultraviolet (sunlight) action on 7-dehydrocholesterol. Vitamin D is then converted successively in liver and kidney to 1,25-dihydroxycholecalciferol. Renal vitamin D activation requires PTH. Vitamin D stimulates intestinal epithelial cell synthesis of Ca^{++}-binding protein, which enhances apical transport of Ca^{++} into the cells. End-product inhibition by 1,25-vitamin D_3 provides hepatic regulation of vitamin D activation.

Hypercalcemia decreases parathyroid hormone secretion. This results in a decrease in vitamin D activation, reduced dietary Ca^{++} absorption, increased osteoblast activity and bone growth, and enhanced urinary loss of Ca^{++}.

Hypocalcemia increases neuronal excitability. Motor neurons exhibit spontaneous depolarizations, leading to tetanic muscular contractions. The muscles of the hand are particularly susceptible, and the tetany is called carpopedal spasm. Spontaneous depolarization of sensory neurons gives rise to paresthesias. In contrast, hypercalcemia depresses neuronal and muscle activity.

Phosphate Metabolism

Plasma PO_4 exists in two forms: HPO_4^{--} and $H_2PO_4^{-}$. Plasma HPO_4^{--} (1.0 mmol/L) is about fourfold higher than plasma $H_2PO_4^{-}$ (0.26 mmol/L). Total inorganic plasma phosphorus is the sum of these two ions, normally about 4 mg/dL. Plasma PO_4 is not tightly regulated and can vary up to threefold without significant physiologic effects.

HISTOLOGY

Bone

Bone consists of an extracellular matrix of proteins and calcium hydroxyapatite crystals [$Ca_{12}(PO_4)_6(OH)_2$]. Osteocytes are cells that are surrounded by this extracellular matrix and occupy spaces known as lacunae. The active portion of bone represents an area of bone synthesis by osteoblasts and bone reabsorption by osteoclasts.

ADRENAL GLAND

The adrenal glands are paired endocrine organs situated at the superior pole of the kidneys. Each adrenal gland is divided into an outer cortex and an inner medulla. The cortex has three zones. The outermost is the zona glomerulosa, which secretes the mineralocorticoid aldosterone. The next is the zona fasciculata, which secretes the glucocorticoids cortisol and corticosterone. Next is the zona reticularis, which secretes the androgen sex hormone dihydrotestosterone. Corticosterone and deoxycorticosterone are secreted in small amounts and have both glucocorticoid and mineralocorticoid effects. The innermost adrenal layer is the adrenal medulla, which secretes the catecholamines epinephrine and norepinephrine (Fig. 13-9).

The adrenocortical hormones are steroids formed from a cholesterol nucleus. The distribution of the synthetic enzymes varies by zone, which is why specific hormones are associated with regions of the adrenal cortex. Stimuli enhancing adrenocortical secretions also cause hypertrophy of the appropriate cortical zones.

Adrenal Medulla

The adrenal medulla secretes the catecholamines epinephrine and norepinephrine. The proportion of epinephrine release can vary, but at rest, 80% of adrenal medullary secretion is epinephrine. Epinephrine and norepinephrine actions mimic those of the sympathetic nervous system but have a longer duration. Actions include vascular smooth muscle contraction, increased heart rate, and inhibition of GI smooth muscle activity. Epinephrine has strong β-adrenergic effects and consequently is a more potent stimulator of heart rate but a less potent stimulator of vascular smooth muscle contraction than norepinephrine is. Epinephrine has strong metabolic effects, increasing the metabolic rate by up to 100% and increasing plasma glucose by stimulating hepatic and muscle glycogenolysis and adipocyte lipolysis.

Adrenal Cortex

Aldosterone is the primary mineralocorticoid secreted by the adrenal cortex. Half of aldosterone circulates free in the plasma; the remaining half is bound to plasma proteins. Aldosterone is degraded in the liver and excreted in urine and feces as a glucuronide or sulfate.

Aldosterone causes a drop in plasma K^+. It stimulates renal reabsorption of Na^+ and excretion of K^+ in the distal tubule segment and collecting duct (see Chapter 11). The reabsorption of Na^+ causes water retention and can lead to mild hypertension. Aldosterone also promotes K^+ loss from sweat and enhances Na^+ reabsorption from the intestines by a similar mechanism (Fig. 13-10).

As a steroid hormone, aldosterone crosses the cell membrane, binds to a cytoplasmic receptor protein, and acts on the nucleus to effect DNA transcription and translation.

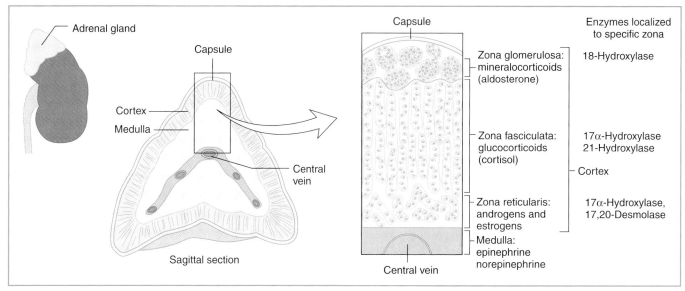

Figure 13-9. A, The adrenal gland has an inner medulla and an outer cortex consisting of three main zones. The adrenal medulla consists of chromaffin tissue that synthesizes epinephrine and to a lesser extent norepinephrine and dopamine. The location of specific enzymes in the zones of the adrenal cortex allows regional synthesis of a variety of steroid hormones. The zona glomerulosa has the enzyme 18-hydroxylase and can synthesize the mineralocorticoid aldosterone. The zona fasciculata has the enzyme 17α-hydroxylase and can synthesize the glucocorticoid cortisol. The zona reticularis has the additional enzyme 17,20-desmolase and can synthesize androgens and estrogens.

HISTOLOGY

Adrenal Cortex

The adrenal cortex has three concentric layers. The layer of cells immediately beneath the connective tissue capsule is the zona glomerulosa, which represents 13% of the volume of the adrenal gland. The next layer of cells is the zona fasciculata, representing up to 80% of the total volume of the adrenal gland. The innermost layer of cortex is the zona reticularis, representing only 7% of the total volume of the adrenal gland.

PHARMACOLOGY

Adrenergic Receptors

Adrenergic receptors are named for their response to pharmacologic agents, not for their function. α-Adrenergic receptors are blocked by phentolamine, and β-adrenergic receptors are blocked by propranolol. There are two broad subtypes of α-adrenergic receptors, and three broad subtypes of β-adrenergic receptors, and there are drugs that can discriminate among the various subtypes.

BIOCHEMISTRY

Cholesterol and Steroid Hormones

Cholesterol is a 27-carbon steroid that is the precursor of all steroid hormones. The four rings of cholesterol remain intact, and the modifications occur at C_{19} through C_{27}. Steroid hormones can be classified by the number of remaining carbon atoms. C_{21} steroids include cortisol and aldosterone; C_{19} steroids include testosterone, androstenedione, and dehydroepiandrosterone (DHEA); and C_{18} steroids include estrone and estradiol.

Aldosterone may acutely stimulate activity of the Na^+/K^+-ATPase through a nongenomic effect.

Plasma K^+ concentration is the primary regulator of aldosterone release. Increases in plasma K^+ enhance aldosterone release. Other stimuli also can increase aldosterone production and release. Angiotensin II, formed following renin release from the kidney, stimulates adrenal aldosterone secretion. Prolonged Na^+ depletion causes aldosterone release. Finally, ACTH has a permissive role in aldosterone production and secretion.

Cortisol is the primary glucocorticoid secreted by the adrenal cortex. Following secretion, 94% of cortisol is bound in the plasma to transcortin, a cortisol-binding globulin, and 6% is free. Cortisol is degraded in the liver and excreted in urine and feces as a glucuronide or sulfate.

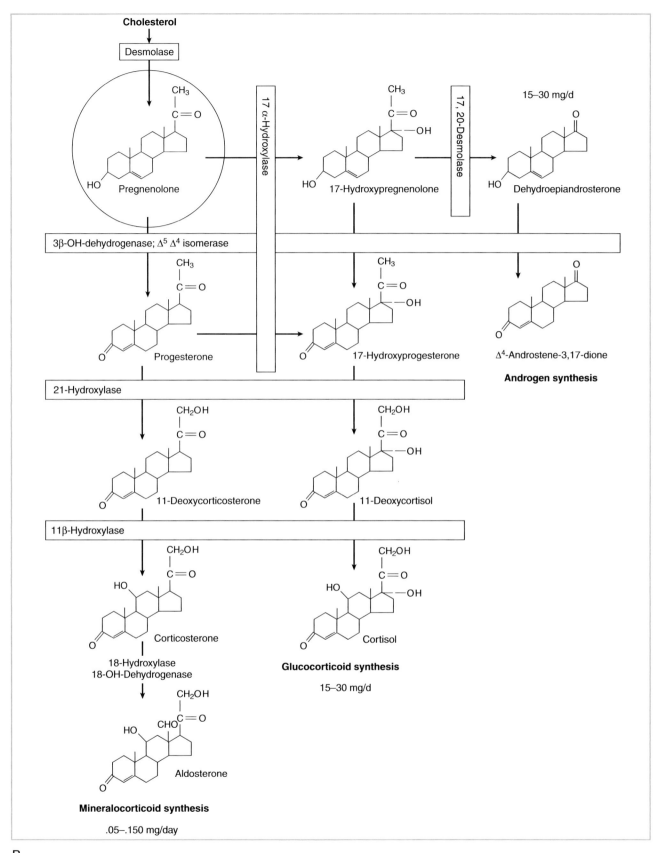

B

Figure 13-9. *Continued.* **B**, The pathways of adrenal steroid biosynthesis show the sites of enzymatic action. A congenital deficiency in any of the adrenal enzymes will diminish the synthesis of some hormones and inappropriately increase the synthesis of other hormones. For example, a 21-hydroxylase deficiency inhibits both glucocorticoid and mineralocorticoid production but results in increased adrenal androgen production.

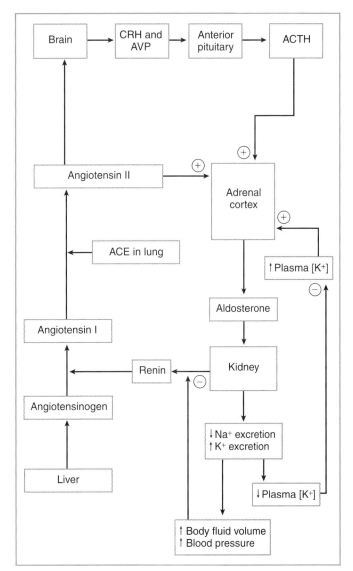

Figure 13-10. Aldosterone release is stimulated by increases in plasma potassium, angiotensin II, and ACTH. The normal release of aldosterone is tied to plasma potassium and angiotensin II, with a minor role for ACTH. This multiple control reflects the actions of aldosterone to increase renal potassium excretion and to decrease renal sodium excretion. AVP, vasopressin; CRH, corticotropin-releasing hormone.

Cortisol is a potent metabolic regulatory hormone. It increases plasma glucose and promotes use of alternative metabolic substrates for energy. For example, cortisol stimulates muscle protein breakdown to support hepatic gluconeogenesis and hepatic glycogen storage. Cortisol decreases cellular absorption and use of glucose, and it mobilizes amino acid stores from extrahepatic tissues. Amino acid mobilization increases both hepatic protein stores and hepatic synthesis of plasma proteins. Cortisol mobilizes fatty acids from peripheral adipose tissue and stimulates appetite. Sustained high cortisol levels lead to central deposition of fat in some adipose tissues in spite of fat use from peripheral

tissues. These metabolic changes are characteristic of the transition from glucose to fatty acids as a metabolic substrate during starvation.

Adrenal cortisol secretion is controlled by the hypothalamus and pituitary (Fig. 13-11). The hypothalamus secretes corticotropin-releasing hormone (CRH). The hypothalamic-hypophyseal portal system carries CRH to the anterior pituitary, where it stimulates ACTH release. ACTH travels in the blood to the adrenal, where it promotes conversion of cholesterol to pregnenolone, the rate-limiting step in adrenal glucocorticoid and androgen secretion. Glucocorticoid secretion exhibits a strong diurnal rhythm—high in the early morning and low in the late evening.

Cortisol release is enhanced by a variety of stresses, possibly supporting the need of damaged tissues for amino acids. Painful stimuli promote release of CRH from the hypothalamus. Emotional stress generated in the limbic system also promotes hypothalamic release of CRH. Cortisol has significant anti-inflammatory effects, retarding the development and enhancing the resolution of the inflammatory response.

Pituitary ACTH also stimulates adrenal androgen production, particularly dehydroepiandrosterone. Androgens, from either the adrenal or the male testes, are converted to dehydroepiandrosterone in postpubescent males and females, and they may contribute to genital and axillary hair growth.

ACTH release coincides with the release of three other compounds formed from the same preprohormone. These include epidermal cell pigment-producing melanocyte-stimulating hormone; β-lipotropin, which may stimulate aldosterone release; and the opiate β-endorphin, described later this chapter.

●●● ENDOCRINE PANCREAS

The pancreatic islets of Langerhans are composed of three distinct types of cells, each of which secretes a different hormone regulating blood glucose. α-Cells secrete the polypeptide glucagon, β-cells are the most numerous and secrete insulin, and δ-cells secrete somatostatin, identical to the growth hormone–inhibitory hormone secreted by the hypothalamus. Islet cell secretions interact with the other islet cells in a paracrine fashion. Insulin inhibits glucagon release, and somatostatin inhibits both insulin and glucagon release.

Insulin

Insulin is a small protein derived successively from a preprohormone and a prohormone, with C peptide being the remainder of the prohormone. In individuals taking exogenous insulin to supplement a defect in endogenous insulin release, C-peptide concentration can be used to quantitate the endogenous insulin production. Insulin circulates as a free hormone and has a short plasma half-life ($t_{(1/2)}$) of 6 minutes. Insulin is cleared from the plasma primarily by the liver and kidneys. Insulin binds to receptors on the surface of target tissues and enhances glucose uptake into the cells.

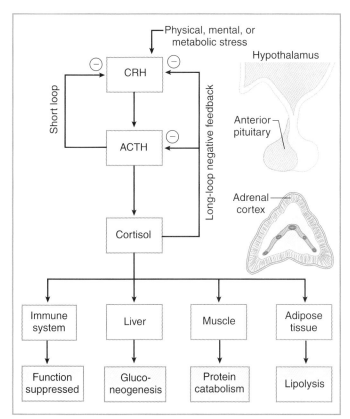

Figure 13-11. Cortisol is released in response to physical, mental, and metabolic stress. Cortisol increases the plasma glucose level through a variety of mechanisms (shown in Fig. 13-14D) and suppresses the action of the immune system. Circulating cortisol levels provide the normal feedback signal inhibiting CRH and ACTH.

PATHOLOGY

Cushing's Syndrome

Cushing's syndrome results from chronic exposure to an excess of circulating levels of glucocorticoids. Cushing's syndrome results in a moon-face appearance with truncal obesity from the redistribution of body fat, and thin extremities from protein depletion. When caused by ectopic ACTH secretion, patients can also exhibit hyperpigmentation due to melanocyte-stimulating hormone secretion.

Insulin decreases blood glucose by enhancing uptake, use, and storage of glucose in hepatic, muscle, and adipose tissues (Fig. 13-12). Insulin promotes skeletal muscle (see Fig. 13-12A) and hepatic glycogen formation and inhibits hepatic glycogenolysis (see Fig. 13-12C). Glucose stored as hepatic glycogen can be mobilized by glycolysis to restore plasma glucose levels when plasma glucose levels fall (see Fig. 13-12D). In contrast, glucose stored as muscle glycogen is used to support muscle metabolism but cannot be mobilized and returned to the plasma. Insulin enhances glucose transport into muscle cells by increasing the number of functional GLUT4 transport proteins. Insulin also promotes hepatic formation of fatty acids from glucose and inhibits gluconeogenesis.

Glucose uptake by the brain occurs via an insulin-independent mechanism. The brain glucose transporter has a much higher glucose affinity than the GLUT4 transporter. Neuronal glucose uptake can occur when blood glucose falls below 80 mg/dL, when GLUT4 transport no longer works. This enhanced glucose uptake affinity ensures that the brain is supplied with glucose even when other organs are not. This is important, because neurons cannot effectively utilize fatty acids as a metabolic substrate. Brain cells need a constant supply of glucose, and severe drops in blood glucose (<60 mg/dL) can lead to depressed cognitive function and hypoglycemic shock.

Insulin enhances fat deposition in adipose tissue. After liver glycogen storage is saturated, additional glucose entering the liver is converted to fatty acids. Hepatic cells release both fatty acids and triglycerides into the plasma. Glucose, fatty acids, and fatty acids derived from lipase action on plasma triglycerides are all absorbed into the adipose cells and used for fat storage.

Insulin enhances amino acid transport into cells and supports cell hypertrophy and hyperplasia. In this effect, insulin acts synergistically with growth hormone. Insulin directly increases protein formation and inhibits protein catabolism. Insulin decreases hepatic gluconeogenesis, again preserving amino acid stores.

Insulin is released following ingestion of a carbohydrate meal (Fig. 13-13) during the cephalic, gastric, and intestinal phases of digestion. Parasympathetic nerves stimulate insulin release during the cephalic phase, and the GI hormones cholecystokinin and gastrointestinal inhibitory peptide release insulin during the gastric and intestinal phases. Glucose absorbed from the meal is the most powerful stimulus for insulin release.

The initial phase of insulin secretion is due to the release of stored insulin and peaks in 5 minutes. This is followed by a delayed phase, secretion from synthesis of new insulin, that persists until blood glucose returns to fasting levels. Simultaneous protein absorption potentiates insulin release by glucose. In addition, glucagon, growth hormone, and cortisol all potentiate the release of insulin by glucose.

Lack of insulin decreases metabolic glucose consumption and enhances the use of fats as a metabolic substrate. The brain still uses only glucose, and the liver absorbs some of the fatty acids and stores them as triglycerides. β-Oxidation of fatty acids becomes the primary metabolic pathway and yields acetyl-CoA, which is condensed to form the ketones acetone, acetoacetic acid, and β-hydroxybutyrate. Lack of insulin leads to excess plasma ketone concentration (ketosis), which can lead to metabolic acidosis and diabetic coma. Lack of insulin elevates blood glucose, causing the osmotic diuresis characteristic of diabetes mellitus. Lack of insulin also promotes protein catabolism and inhibits growth.

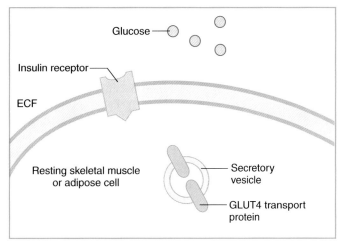

A. In the absence of insulin, glucose cannot enter the cell.

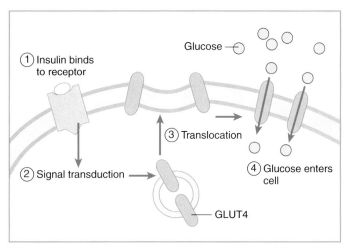

B. Insulin signals the cell to insert GLUT-4 transporters into the membrane, allowing glucose to enter the cell.

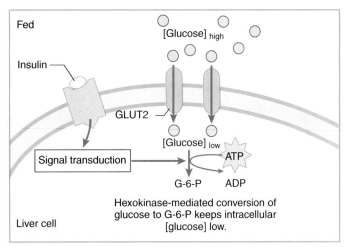

C. Hepatocyte. In the fed state, the liver cell takes up glucose and forms glycogen and fatty acids.

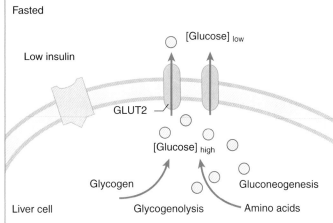

D. Hepatocyte. In the fasted state, the liver cell makes glucose from glycogen or amino acids and transports it to the blood.

Figure 13-12. Insulin entry by the GLUT4 transporter requires the action of insulin. In skeletal muscle and adipose tissue, glucose enters or requires insulin binding to a cell membrane receptor (**A**) and translocation of the vesicular GLUT4 transporters into the cell membrane (**B**). In contrast, glucose entry into hepatocytes (**C, D**) or neurons uses different GLUT transporters, which do not require insulin for activity.

Glucagon

Glucagon is an extremely potent hormone released by drops in blood glucose. Glucagon acts on the liver to elevate plasma glucose, an action opposite to that of insulin. Glucagon promotes hepatic glycogenolysis and increases hepatic gluconeogenesis. cAMP is the second messenger for glucagon, and this allows high glucagon levels to have nonmetabolic effects on other tissues. These actions include enhancing cardiac contractility, enhancing bile secretion, and inhibiting gastric acid secretion.

Protein ingestion enhances glucagon release as well as insulin release. The simultaneous secretion of insulin and glucagon allows cells to use and store glucose without severely dropping plasma glucose levels. Glucagon is released during exercise and helps prevent hypoglycemia in spite of enhanced glucose use by muscle.

Somatostatin

Somatostatin is a small polypeptide with a short (2-minute) half-life that has many inhibitory actions. Somatostatin is released following ingestion of a meal. Somatostatin release is stimulated by increased plasma amino acids, fatty acids, and glucose. Somatostatin release is also stimulated by GI hormones.

Somatostatin inhibits the release of both insulin and glucagon, and it decreases activity and secretion by the GI tract. The net action of somatostatin is to delay nutrient absorption by the GI tract and thus prolong the duration of intestinal food absorption after a meal.

Integrated Regulation of Carbohydrate Metabolism

Mitochondria can metabolize both glucose and fatty acids to synthesize ATP. Glucose is the preferred metabolic substrate

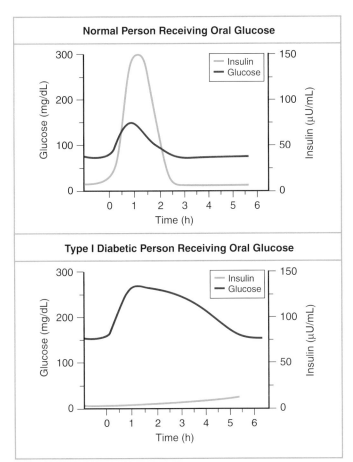

Figure 13-13. The glucose tolerance test causes parallel increases in plasma concentrations of glucose and insulin. Ingestion of glucose causes an increase in plasma glucose concentration, which stimulates insulin release. Insulin promotes glucose movement into storage pools (see also Figure 13-14B), returning plasma glucose to normal levels. An individual with type 1 diabetes caused by the lack of insulin production has a higher resting glucose level and does not show the expected hyperinsulinemic response to feeding. Consequently, plasma glucose levels remain elevated for a much longer period.

PATHOLOGY

Diabetes

Type 1 diabetes mellitus is caused by selective T lymphocyte–mediated autoimmune destruction of β-cells of the pancreatic islets. The decreased insulin production prevents the use of glucose as a metabolic fuel by skeletal muscle and results in greatly elevated plasma glucose levels. Free fatty acid oxidation is incomplete, and free fatty acids are metabolized by the liver into ketone bodies.

when insulin is present, such as following carbohydrate ingestion. Fasting blood glucose averages 85 mg/dL and is tightly regulated. Hepatic glycogen stores and gluconeogenic ability provide an important mechanism to replace glucose consumed by cells. Hyperglycemia stimulates insulin release and enhances glucose uptake, utilization, and storage.

Hypoglycemia stimulates glucagon release, which inhibits glucose uptake, storage, and utilization and increases glucose formation from glycogen and amino acid stores (Fig. 13-14).

Plasma glucose levels are buffered via a variety of storage pools, shown on the left side of Figure 13-14. Hepatic and skeletal muscle glycogen represent a storage area that can be mobilized to replenish plasma glucose levels. Amino acids represent a source of glucose through gluconeogenesis, but excess glucose cannot be converted to amino acids. Adipose tissue is a storage form for excess glucose, but glucose cannot be recovered directly from adipose tissue.

Glucose consumption is shown on the right side of Figure 13-14. Glucose uptake by the brain and liver is not insulin dependent. Glucose uptake by skeletal muscle and other tissues is insulin dependent. Adipose tissue can provide free fatty acids as a metabolic substrate for mitochondria, diminishing the metabolic use of glucose.

Insulin decreases plasma glucose (see Fig. 13-14B). Insulin moves glucose into storage, enhancing glycogen synthesis, adipose synthesis, and in the presence of growth hormone, protein synthesis. Insulin also enhances the uptake of glucose by skeletal muscle and by a variety of other tissues.

Glucagon makes glucose available for cells (see Fig. 13-14C). Glucagon removes glucose from storage by promoting the breakdown of glycogen and gluconeogenesis as well as triglyceride oxidation. Glucagon does not interfere with cellular uptake and metabolic use of glucose.

Cortisol and other glucocorticoids increase glycogen stores (see Fig. 13-14D).

Glycogen synthesis requires excess plasma glucose. Cortisol increases plasma glucose through protein breakdown and gluconeogenesis. Cortisol also mobilizes fatty acids from peripheral adipose tissue and consequently diminishes metabolic use of glucose. Through an unknown mechanism, cortisol enhances fat accumulation in central adipose tissue.

Epinephrine increases plasma glucose levels (see Fig. 13-14E). Epinephrine mobilizes glucose from storage by stimulating glycogenolysis and gluconeogenesis. Additionally, epinephrine diminishes the metabolic use of glucose and through lipolysis promotes the use of free fatty acids as an alternative metabolic substrate.

Growth hormone protects amino acid stores (see Fig. 13-14F). GH increases plasma glucose through breakdown of glycogen, and it diminishes the metabolic use of glucose by stimulating lipolysis. If insulin also is present, growth hormone promotes amino acid storage as protein.

Ingestion of a meal promotes anabolic activities (see Fig. 13-14G). Ingestion of a mixed meal containing fats, proteins, and carbohydrates shifts metabolic regulation to anabolic storage activities. The simultaneous elevation of insulin and growth hormone increases protein synthesis, and the elevation in plasma glucose increases glycogen synthesis. Glucose is used by mitochondria as the preferred metabolic substrate.

During prolonged fasting, metabolism shifts to a catabolic state (see Fig. 13-14H). In the absence of food, plasma glucose is maintained by mobilizing glucose stores. Glycogen

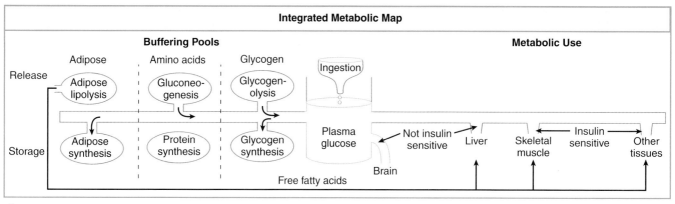

A

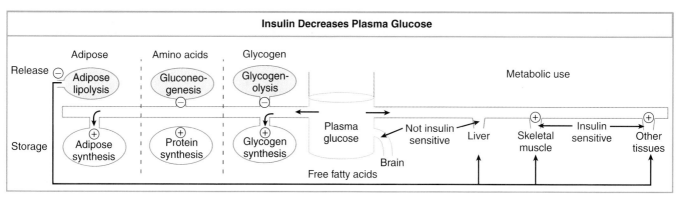

B

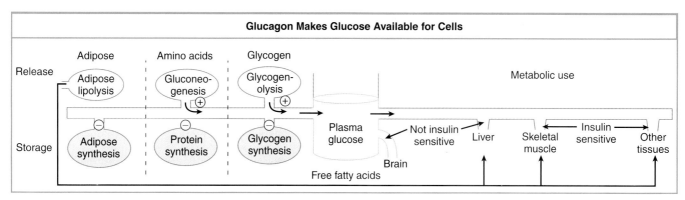

C

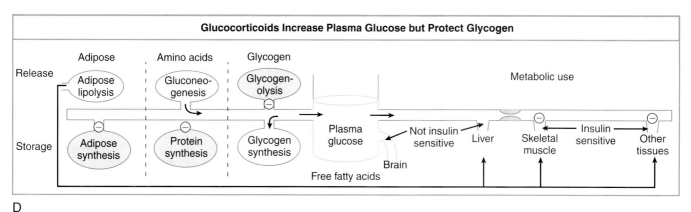

D

Figure 13-14. Plasma glucose levels represent the balance between GI glucose absorption, movement into and out of storage pools, and metabolism by mitochondria.

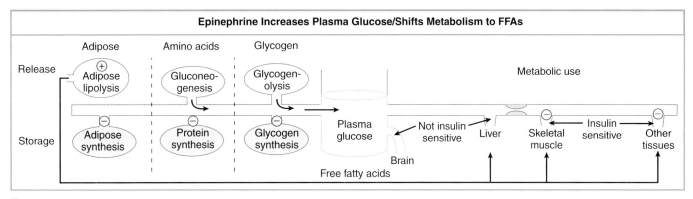

E

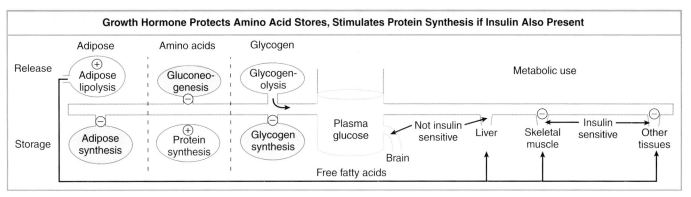

F

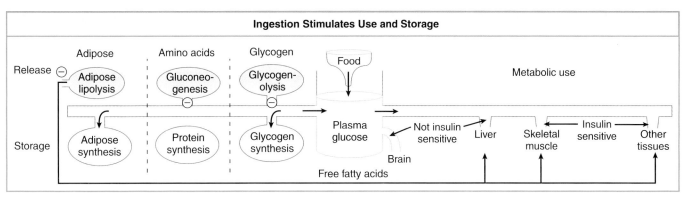

G

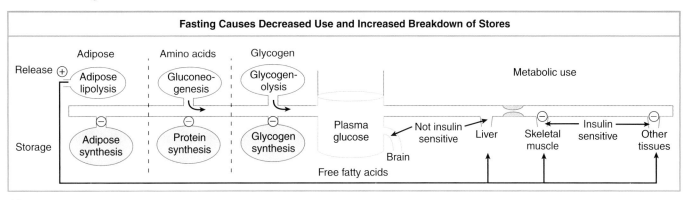

H

Figure 13-14. *Continued.*

is broken down, and protein is broken down to provide substrates for gluconeogenesis. Metabolic use of glucose is diminished, and free fatty acids become the preferred metabolic substrate. Fatty acids are the preferred metabolic substrate when cortisol and growth hormone are elevated. Cortisol is released by stress and starvation. GH is secreted during prolonged hypoglycemia also. Epinephrine increases both fatty acids and glucose but generally promotes use of fatty acids as the metabolic substrate.

Even in starvation, plasma glucose must be maintained above 50 mg/dL to support brain metabolism. The shift from glucose to fatty acids as a metabolic substrate in insulin-sensitive tissues helps preserve the small remaining amount of glucose to support brain metabolic needs.

●●● RENIN-ANGIOTENSIN SYSTEM AND ATRIAL NATRIURETIC PEPTIDES

Angiotensin and atrial natriuretic peptides generally act to oppose each other. Angiotensin II has strong acute vascular effects and is an important mediator of renal Na$^+$ retention. Atrial natriuretic peptides are released from the atria of the heart by distention and enhance renal Na$^+$ excretion. Angiotensin works through the cAMP second messenger, and atrial natriuretic peptides works through cGMP.

The enzyme renin is synthesized and stored in the juxtaglomerular cells of the renal afferent arteriole. Renin is released by a variety of stimuli including decreased Na$^+$ delivery to the macula densa, decreased renal perfusion pressure, increased sympathetic nerve activity secondary to arterial hypotension, and β-adrenergic agonists, such as epinephrine (Fig. 13-15).

Renin acts on the plasma protein angiotensinogen (renin substrate) to form angiotensin I. Angiotensin I is hydrolyzed to angiotensin II by angiotensin-converting enzyme (ACE), found in high concentrations in the pulmonary epithelium. Angiotensin is rapidly degraded by peptidases collectively called angiotensinases. Angiotensin II can also be formed locally in the brain and in the kidney, independently of the plasma conversion process.

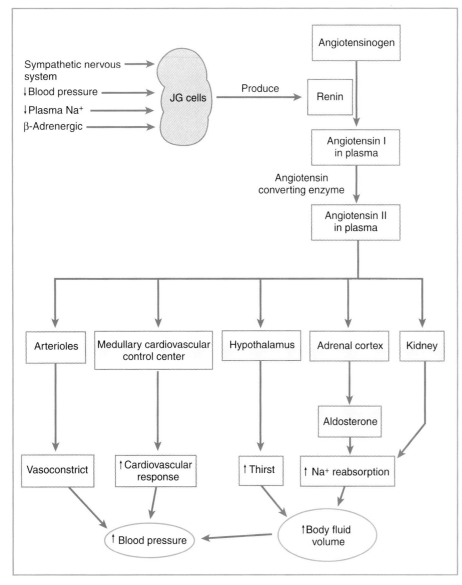

Figure 13-15. Renin release is the first step in the pathway leading to angiotensin II formation and aldosterone release. Renin is released by four stimuli: a decrease in blood pressure, renal sympathetic nerves, a drop in plasma Na$^+$, and β-adrenergic stimulation. Renin acts on the plasma protein angiotensinogen to form angiotensin I, which is converted by angiotensin-converting enzyme to angiotensin II. Angiotensin II has a variety of actions, including stimulating aldosterone released from the adrenal cortex. More renal actions of angiotensin II are described in Chapter 11.

Acutely, angiotensin is a potent constrictor of vascular smooth muscle. Consequently, angiotensin II increases total peripheral resistance and therefore arterial blood pressure. Angiotensin II also causes venoconstriction, which enhances cardiac output.

Angiotensin promotes renal retention of Na^+ and water. Efferent arteriolar constriction acts to increase GFR but also increases peritubular fluid reabsorption. Angiotensin II also enhances proximal tubule Na^+ reabsorption and acutely increases aldosterone release, which augments renal Na^+ reabsorption. Angiotensin stimulates ADH release from the posterior pituitary and acts in the central nervous system to increase thirst.

Atrial myocytes synthesize and store a class of peptides collectively called atrial natriuretic peptides. Stretch of the myocytes, as occurs with volume overloading, stimulates secretion of atrial natriuretic peptides.

The physiologic importance of atrial natriuretic peptides is not yet established. Acutely, atrial natriuretic hormone acts to increase renal Na^+ excretion. Atrial natriuretic peptides dilate renal afferent and efferent arterioles and increase glomerular filtration rate. Atrial natriuretic peptides decrease renin release, inhibit antidiuretic hormone secretion, and decrease Na^+ reabsorption in the renal collecting duct. The natriuresis caused by atrial natriuretic peptides decreases plasma volume.

Prostaglandins and Other Eicosanoids

Prostaglandins (PGs), thromboxanes, and leukotrienes arc three classes of arachidonic acid derivatives collectively called eicosanoids. The primary prostaglandins of biological interest are prostaglandin E_2 and $F_{2\alpha}$. Arachidonic acid for the synthesis of these two eicosanoids is obtained from the plasma membrane (Fig. 13-16).

Cyclooxygenase converts arachidonic acid to prostaglandins G_2 and H_2. Thromboxane synthase converts PGH_2 to thromboxanes A_2 and A_3. Prostacyclin synthase converts PGH_2 to PGI_2. Prostaglandins E_1 and E_3 are derived from precursors similar, but not identical, to arachidonic acid. Lipoxygenase converts arachidonic acid to leukotrienes.

Actions of Prostaglandins

Prostaglandins have diverse intracellular, local, and endocrine effects. Thromboxane A_2, prostaglandin $F_{2\alpha}$, and leukotrienes

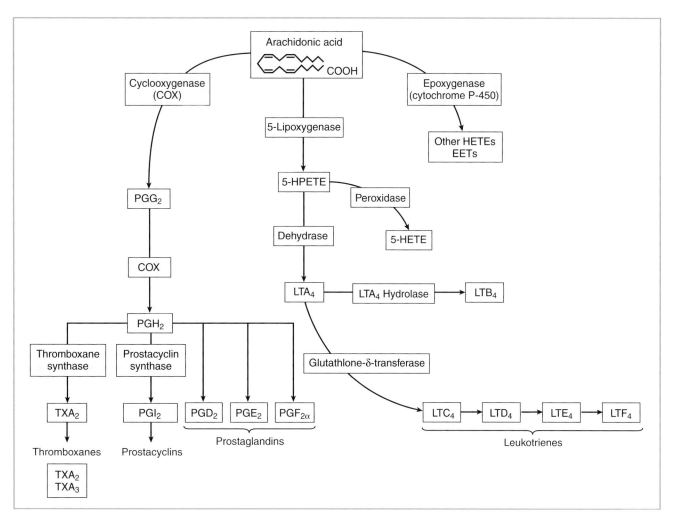

Figure 13-16. Prostaglandins, prostacyclins, thromboxanes, and leukotrienes are all synthesized from arachidonic acid.

Cyclooxygenase

Cyclooxygenase (COX) first oxidizes arachidonic acid to prostaglandin G_2 and then peroxidizes it to prostaglandin H_2. COX exists as two isoforms: COX-1, which is constitutively active, and COX-2, which can be induced and mediates the inflammatory response. Aspirin and other nonsteroidal anti-inflammatory drugs (NSAIDs) inhibit both COX isoforms and therefore block either or both prostaglandin production and inflammation. Inhibition of COX-1 can lead to gastric distress, and selective COX-2 inhibitors such as celecoxib have been introduced for analgesia without producing gastric distress.

C_4 and D_4 constrict pulmonary airway smooth muscle, and prostaglandin E_2 dilates airway smooth muscle. Platelet aggregation is enhanced by thromboxane A_2 but inhibited by prostacyclin. Thromboxane A_2 is the primary pulmonary vasoconstrictor, and prostacyclin (prostaglandin I_2) is a pulmonary vasodilator. Hemorrhage (sympathetics and angiotensin II) causes renal formation of vasodilator prostaglandins PGE_2 and PGI_2.

Endorphins and Enkephalins

Endorphins, enkephalins, and dynorphin are powerful peptide or polypeptide analgesics. Their analgesic action requires binding to opiate receptors on nerve cells. Naloxone antagonizes the action of these opiate agonists.

The prohormone containing endorphin also contains ACTH and melanocyte-stimulating hormone. Enkephalins are small peptides that can serve as neurotransmitters in the brain. Enkephalins act to attenuate substance P release in the dorsal horn of the spinal cord and inhibit afferent pain fibers. Opiates inhibit transmission at sympathetic and locus caeruleus synapses. Dynorphins and other endorphins contain an enkephalin sequence on the amino terminal end of the peptide.

⬤⬤⬤ TOP 5 TAKE-HOME POINTS

1. Endocrine agents allow complex regulation of homeostasis, metabolism, and growth.
2. Extracellular fluid osmolality is controlled by ADH; plasma Na^+, K^+, and Ca^{++} are regulated by angiotensin II, aldosterone, and parathyroid hormone, respectively.
3. Plasma glucose regulation is perhaps the most complex, with one hormone (insulin) causing decreases in plasma glucose and at least four hormones causing increases in plasma glucose. This metabolic diversity allows the body to shift to anabolic metabolism during periods of excess substrate and to a catabolic state when substrates are limited.
4. Hormone levels are controlled by negative feedback loops, tied either to plasma hormone concentration or to a biological action of the hormone.
5. Extrinsic regulation of hormone is accomplished by higher nervous system control of hypothalamic releasing hormones.

Female Reproductive System   14

CONTENTS

The human reproductive system is specialized for the production and joining of germ cells—ovum or egg (female) and sperm (male). The female reproductive system is also specialized to nurture and protect the fertilized ovum during the 9-month gestation period. Gonadal development begins in utero, but maturation of the reproductive system, which occurs at puberty, is delayed until adolescence. At 45 to 60 years of age, female fertility gradually decreases, ending at menopause, the permanent cessation of menstruation. Following menopause, decreases in estrogen and progesterone secretion have significant health effects.

The ovaries, which secrete the female sex steroids estrogen and progesterone, are the gonads of the female. Their primary function is to form germ cells, which have half the normal number of chromosomes. During the period between puberty and menopause, the ovaries release mature ova at a rate of about once each month (Fig. 14-1).

This chapter is organized along developmental lines. It begins with sexual determination in utero and follows the growth and maturation of the female reproductive system. Pregnancy and fetal development are discussed in Chapter 16.

●●●● SEXUAL DIFFERENTIATION IN UTERO

Human somatic cells have 46 chromosomes: 22 pairs of somatic chromosomes and one pair of sex chromosomes. The sex chromosomes are identified as X or Y, with the female genotype being XX and the male genotype XY. The ovary contributes one X chromosome, and the sperm contributes either an X or a Y chromosome, to the fertilized ovum.

Both male and female reproductive systems develop and begin to mature in utero. The undifferentiated gonads are medial to two parallel duct systems, the mesonephric (wolffian) duct, and the paramesonephric (müllerian) duct. Development of a female reproductive system is genetically programmed and occurs in the absence of fetal testosterone secretion.

Gonadal development begins during the fifth week of fetal life, and gonadal differentiation occurs in the seventh and eighth weeks of gestation. In XX embryos, the gonads differentiate into the ovaries. The female germinal epithelia develop into follicles, containing oocytes surrounded by a layer of granulosa cells. Meiotic division in the female is completed in utero, and the ovaries contain 300,000 to 400,000 immature follicles at birth.

In utero, ovarian release of estradiol and progesterone is stimulated by placental human chorionic gonadotropin (hCG), supplemented by gonadotropin-releasing hormone (GnRH) from the fetus. In females, the wolffian ducts regress and the müllerian ducts develop into fallopian tubes, uterus, and upper vagina. Formation of the external genitalia—clitoris, labia majora, and labia minora—is complete by 11 weeks of gestation. The sexual differentiation of males and females is contrasted Chapter 15 (see Fig. 15-2).

Following birth, luteinizing hormone (LH) and follicle-stimulating hormone (FSH) secretions are diminished, and sexual development is halted at an immature stage. There is little sexual development during childhood. Maturation of the reproductive system, or puberty, is delayed until adolescence (Fig. 14-2).

●●●● PUBERTY

Some time after the age of 8 years, hypothalamic production of GnRH resumes, and the gender-specific development of reproductive systems resumes for a 2- to 4½-year period.

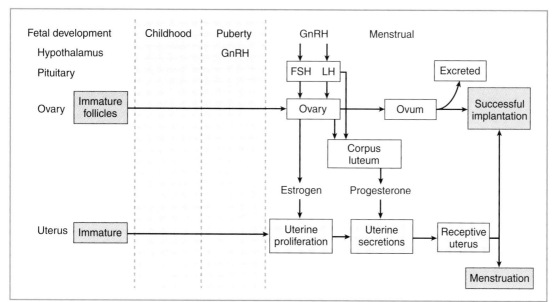

Figure 14-1. Female reproduction prepares an ovum for fertilization and successful implantation.

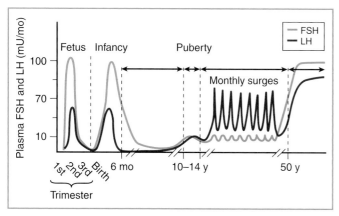

Figure 14-2. Plasma FSH and LH levels show peaks in utero and during infancy, monthly cycling during the reproductive years, and sustained elevation following menopause. In utero, FSH and LH secretion is stimulated by human chorionic gonadotropin. Following puberty, FSH and LH secretion is stimulated by GnRH and inhibited by estrogen and progesterone. Following menopause, impaired secretion of ovarian estrogen and progesterone results in elevated FSH and LH levels.

Resumption of GnRH production depends on maturation of the amygdala or some other component of the limbic system. Nutritional and environmental factors also play a role in the onset of puberty, as the average age of female puberty has gradually decreased in the United States during the last century. Onset of puberty is likely tied to appropriate body fat stores, since severe obesity, heavy exercise, and severe malnutrition all delay the onset of puberty.

During puberty, GnRH begins a pulsatile pattern of secretion, especially during REM sleep at night. This pulsatile pattern eventually leads to an LH surge that marks the onset of the first menstrual cycle. Early menstrual cycles are irregular but gradually settle into an adult "monthly" ovulatory cycle.

The increase in GnRH appears to be due to diminished sensitivity of the hypothalamus to the negative feedback signals from circulating estrogens. The increased GnRH leads to increased FSH and LH secretion from the anterior pituitary and consequent increased production of estradiol and progestin by the granulosa cells of the ovaries. Under the influence of estradiol and other estrogens, the development of female sexual characteristics resumes.

Estradiol stimulates development of secondary female sexual characteristics. These include an increase in size of external genitalia and internal reproductive organs, toughening of the vaginal epithelium, growth of ciliated epithelia in the fallopian tubes, appearance of pubic hair around the labia majora, enlargement of breasts, and development of secretory ducts. Body changes include increased osteoblast activity and closure of the epiphyseal plates, increased metabolic rate and protein growth, and a female pattern of fat deposition in the breasts, buttocks, and thighs. Puberty also causes the skin to become thicker, smoother, and more vascular. This period of pubertal growth generally occurs earlier in females than in males.

Progesterone has few effects on secondary sexual characteristics. Progesterone does promote secretion by the uterine endometrium and fallopian tubes in preparation for implantation, and it causes growth of breast alveoli in preparation for milk secretion. Progesterone promotes fluid retention and increases the body temperature by 0.5°C.

●●● ADULT FEMALE REPRODUCTIVE STRUCTURES

External Structures

External female reproductive organ structures are collectively termed the vulva or pudendum (Fig. 14-3). The vulva plays a role in sexual stimulation and provides a barrier to protect

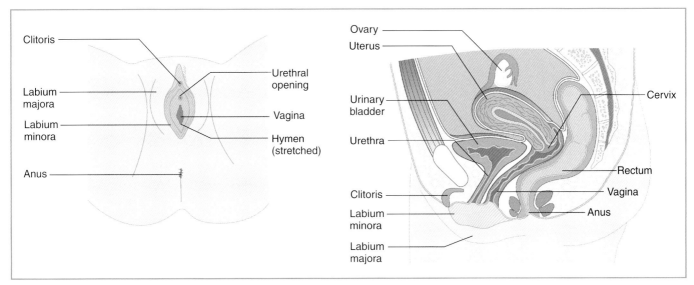

A

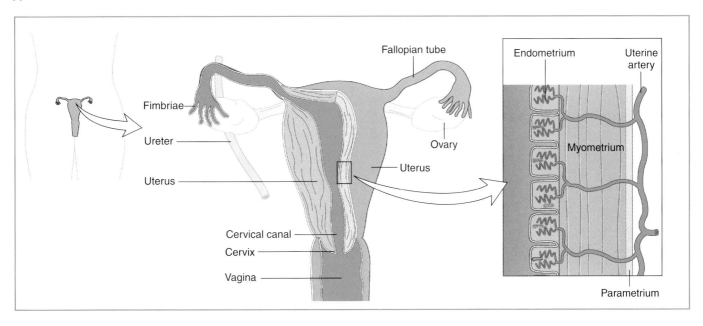

B

Figure 14-3. Gross anatomy of the female reproductive organs and histology of the uterus.

the body from foreign materials. The vulva includes the mons pubis, labia majora, labia minora, clitoris, vestibular bulbs, and vestibule. The perineum is the region posterior to the vestibule.

Internal Structures

The internal female genital structures are the ovaries, fallopian tubes, uterus, and vagina. They function to produce and release ova, transport ova to the potential site of fertilization, provide a route for sperm access and movement, and provide an appropriate physical and endocrine environment for the implantation, growth, and delivery of the fetus.

The ovaries are the female reproductive organs. The ovaries produce both the female ovum and the female sex steroids

estrogen and progesterone. The paired ovaries are located in the pelvis, lateral to the uterus and below the fallopian tubes.

The primary structure in the ovary is the ovarian follicle. Ovarian follicles consist of ova, in various stages of development, and associated endocrine tissue. Each follicle contains a developing ovum, a nutritive stromal cell layer, and an abundant blood and lymphatic supply. A mature follicle is an endocrine gland secreting estrogen. At birth, several hundred thousand follicles, each containing an oocyte or end-stage ovum, are present. The number of follicles decreases as puberty approaches, and they gradually disappear completely around menopause.

The corpus luteum is a glandular body that forms from the remnants of the graafian follicle after ovulation. It is the source of the hormones progesterone and estrogen during the second half of the ovulatory cycle. In young females, ovarian surfaces are smooth; with age, they become pitted from the remnants of graafian follicles.

The ovum released from the ovary is captured by the fimbria of the fallopian tube and transported by ciliary action toward the uterus. Each fallopian tube is about 10 cm long, and the fallopian tubes are the usual site of fertilization.

The uterus sits slightly below and between the fallopian tubes and has three functional layers (see Fig. 14-3B). The outer parametrium is the thin peritoneal and fascial covering of the uterus. The bulk of the uterine mass is the myometrium, a muscular layer composed of three layers of smooth muscle. The interior of the uterus is lined with an endometrium. The endometrium is shed and regrows each month in response to the changes in estrogen and progesterone levels during the ovarian cycle. If fertilized, the ovum normally implants in the endometrium. An ovum implanting in any other region is termed an ectopic pregnancy. When the ovum is not fertilized, the endometrial lining is shed during menstruation.

The vaginal canal connects the uterus with the external genitalia. The mucosa of the inner vaginal wall folds in small ridges (rugae) that add to the vagina's elasticity, making it highly distensible. The outer layer of the vagina is smooth muscle. The vagina's smooth rugal pattern and elasticity diminish during the menopausal and postmenopausal years.

Pelvic Blood Supply

The internal iliac (hypogastric) artery is the major blood vessel supplying the external genitalia. In addition, this artery branches to supply the pelvic floor, pelvic walls, and pelvic

viscera. The internal genitalia are supplied by the uterine arteries, a branch of the internal iliac artery, or the ovarian artery, which branches directly from the aorta. As the names suggest, the uterine artery supplies the uterus and its branches, and the vaginal arteries supply the vagina. The ovarian artery supplies blood to the ovaries, fallopian tubes, and body of the uterus. Venous drainage for all of these structures parallels the arterial supply. The pelvic lymphatics also roughly parallel the blood supply.

Innervation

Both sympathetic and parasympathetic nerves innervate the female reproductive organs. Sexual arousal is controlled by the parasympathetic dilation of blood vessels in the vestibular bulbs and clitoris. The uterine myometrium, however, is innervated only by sympathetic nerve fibers.

BREASTS

Breasts are a secondary sexual characteristic; that is, reproduction can occur without them. The physiologic function of female breasts is secretion of milk to feed infants. An average nonlactating breast weighs between 150 and 250 grams, and a lactating breast weighs 400 to 500 grams.

The parenchyma of a breast is complex, consisting of ductular, lobular, and acinar epithelial structures. The stroma of a breast is primarily composed of fibrous and fatty tissue. A breast consists of up to 20 lobes, subdivided into lobules and made up of acini. Breast lobes are arranged like the spokes of a wheel around the nipple. The duct that drains each lobe opens independently on the surface of the nipple. The upper lateral quadrant of the breast, which is mostly glandular, is the most common site of tumor occurrence.

The nipple is located at the fourth intercostal space. Surrounding the nipple is a circular pigmented area called the areola. Estrogen increases pigmentation of the areola. The areola epithelium contains some small hairs and sebaceous glands, sweat glands, and accessory mammary glands. The sebaceous glands enlarge to lubricate the nipple during pregnancy and lactation.

The lateral mammary artery and the lateral thoracic artery provide the majority of the blood supply to the breast. These arteries form an extensive interconnecting network. The main veins and the large lymphatics both parallel the arteries. There are three types of lymphatic drainage of the breast: cutaneous lymphatic drainage, areola lymphatic drainage, and glandular lymphatic drainage from deep glandular tissue (Fig. 14-4). Lymphatic drainage pathways and lymph nodes are important in the prognosis and treatment of breast cancer. The nerve supply derives from the anterior and lateral branches of the fourth to sixth intercostal nerves.

The physiologic changes that affect the breast are growth and development, the menstrual cycle, and pregnancy and lactation. Breast development and function require the action

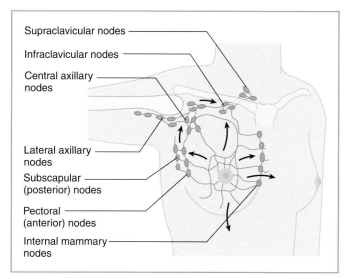

Supraclavicular nodes

Infraclavicular nodes

Central axillary
nodes

Lateral axillary
nodes

Subscapular
(posterior) nodes

Pectoral
(anterior) nodes

Internal mammary
nodes

Figure 14-4. Surface anatomy and lymphatic drainage of the breast.

PATHOLOGY

Breast Cancer

Breast cancers are malignant tumors that typically begin in the ductal-lobular epithelial cells of the breast and are spread by the lymphatic system to axillary lymph nodes. Once past the lymph node, the tumor may metastasize to different regions of the body. The finding of breast cancer in the axillary lymph nodes is an indicator of a tumor's capacity for potential distant metastasis. Most primary breast cancers are adeno-carcinomas, with about 50% being located in the upper lateral quadrant of the breast.

of multiple hormones, including estrogen, progesterone, prolactin, and corticotropin. Breast development usually occurs between 9 and 16 years of age and takes 4 to 5 years. Estrogen is responsible for the growth of the breast and periductal stroma. Progesterone promotes the development of lobular and acinar structures.

After menopause, the ovaries stop producing estrogen and progesterone. The adrenal gland represents the remaining source of estrogen after menopause. Loss of the trophic stimulation from estrogen results in an involution of the breast with loss of glandular elements and tissue atrophy.

Increases in breast size, vascularity, and duct development occur during pregnancy in response to the increases in estrogen, progesterone, and pituitary hormones. When pregnancy ends, prolactin initiates lactation, and continuing lactation also requires corticotropin. The expression of milk is a complex response involving a mother's subjective response and the mechanical stimulation of suckling. Suckling releases the pituitary hormone oxytocin into the circulation. This causes the mammary acini to contract and release milk into the duct system.

●●● FEMALE REPRODUCTION

Role of Hormones

Under control of the hypothalamic GnRH and anterior pituitary FSH and LH, the ovaries manufacture estrogens and progesterones. The hypothalamic-pituitary-ovarian axis mediates the events of the ovulatory cycle, including follicular development, ovulation, corpus luteum formation, and menstruation. In addition, the estrogens and progesterone stimulate sexual desire and exert additional effects throughout in the body.

Progesterone and the estrogens are synthesized from a 27-carbon cholesterol precursor (Fig. 14-5). Progesterone has 21 carbons and is structurally most like cholesterol. The three estrogens have 18 carbons and are formed from the action of the enzyme aromatase on the "male" sex steroids testosterone and androstenedione.

Estrogens

Estrogens produce cyclic changes in the uterine endothelium and vaginal epithelium. Estrogens are steroids that are secreted in both males and females by the adrenal cortex and in females by the ovary (main source) and placenta. Natural estrogens include estradiol, estrone, and estriol. Estrogens in low doses may be used therapeutically as replacement hormone during menopause.

At puberty, estrogen stimulates breast growth (fatty tissue deposition, pigmentation), fat deposition in the vulva, bony pelvis growth and broadening, closure of the epiphyseal plates of long bones, vaginal epithelial changes, and general growth. The role of estrogen in the menstrual cycle is discussed later.

Progesterone

Progesterone is a steroid hormone that helps prepare the endometrium to receive and implant the fertilized ovum; it also promotes development of the placenta (a spongy structure in the uterus that provides nourishment for a developing fetus) and the mammary glands.

Progesterone is used therapeutically to treat threatened spontaneous abortion and such menstrual problems as dysmenorrhea or amenorrhea. It is secreted from the placenta and the corpus luteum under control of LH from the anterior pituitary. Progesterone plays a minor role in Na^+ and water balance. It also influences nitrogen balance, breast function, and body temperature during the menstrual cycle, raising body temperature by 0.5°C in the postovulatory phase of the cycle.

Menarche

Menarche is the onset of menstruation. The average age for menarche in the United States is now 12.8 years. Menarche is preceded by puberty-induced body changes that occur between ages 9 and 16 years.

The age at which menarche occurs is affected by genetic and environmental factors. Menarche may be delayed by poor nutrition, high levels of exercise (athletes or dancers), and several medical conditions, such as diabetes mellitus,

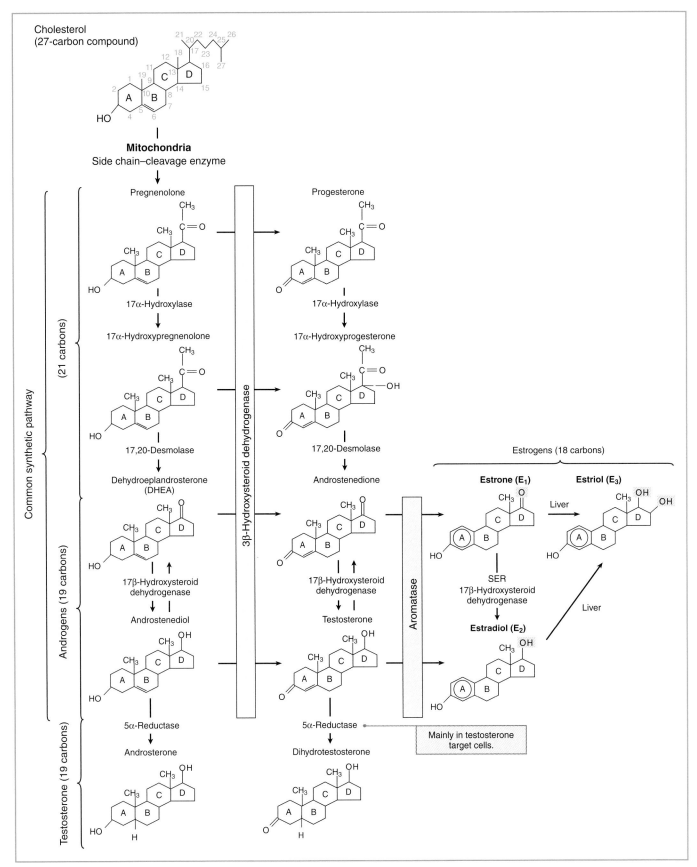

Figure 14-5. Biosynthetic pathways of the ovarian sex steroids. Estrogens and progesterone both derive from cholesterol. There are three major estrogens: estrone, estradiol, and estriol. Estrogen synthesis first requires that cholesterol be transformed to androgens and then converted to estrogen by the action of aromatase.

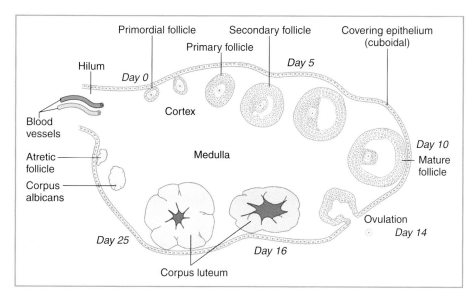

Figure 14-6. Ovarian ovulatory cycle. FSH stimulates the development of a primordial follicle during menstruation, which gradually matures over a 10-day period. The mature follicle ruptures on day 14, releasing the ova. The remnants of the follicle form the corpus luteum, which persists until day 25. Involution of the corpus luteum diminishes progesterone secretion, which initiates menstruation.

congenital heart disease, and ulcerative colitis. Early menarche may occur with other conditions, such as hypothyroidism, CNS tumors, and head trauma. Girls usually show an increase in height of only 2 to 3 inches after the onset of menstruation.

Early menstrual cycles are often irregular and anovulatory (not preceded by ovulation and discharge of an ovum). Although menstrual cycles may not be regular for several years, the woman is still potentially fertile.

Menstrual (Ovulatory) Cycle

The menstrual cycle is a complex set of recurrent changes in the uterus, ovaries, cervix, and vagina. The cycle can generally be divided into a preovulatory phase (including menstruation), ovulation, and a postovulatory phase.

The length of the menstrual cycle is calculated from the first day of menstrual flow. Variations in the length of the preovulatory phase (which ends with ovulation) typically cause a change in the length of the entire cycle. Ovulation occurs 12 to 15 days before the onset of the next menstrual period. The cycle generally runs about 25 to 32 days but can vary from month to month. The menstrual cycle depends on interactions between the CNS, anterior pituitary, ovaries, and uterus. Environmental influences, climatic changes, emotionally traumatic experiences, stress, and acute or chronic illness also may affect the menstrual cycle.

The complexities of the menstrual cycle are best illustrated by separately examining the ovarian, uterine, and endocrine changes that occur during the cycle, and then integrating the events from a functional perspective.

Ovarian Changes During the Menstrual Cycle

The onset of menstrual flow signals the beginning of the ovarian preovulatory phase of the menstrual cycle. FSH stimulates the maturation of numerous follicles. One follicle from this group becomes the primary, or dominant, follicle and matures into a graafian follicle, surrounded by theca cells that produce androgens and granulosa cells that produce estrogens and progesterones. The remainder of the follicles from the group degenerate in a process called atresia. About 2 days before ovulation, a graafian follicle reaches full maturity (Fig. 14-6).

A spike in LH secretion causes the theca and granulosa cells lining the follicle to hypertrophy and proliferate. Ovulation occurs when the graafian follicle migrates to the ovary's cortex. Proteolysis of the follicular capsule and swelling allow the mature follicle to rupture through the ovarian wall. The ovum is released into the abdominal cavity. The granulosa cells remain in the ovary. Some hemorrhage occurs into the center of the ruptured follicle, where a clot quickly forms. Ovulation may produce a transient abdominal pain (called mittelschmerz). Following ovulation, the ovarian follicle collapses and estrogen production temporarily drops.

The postovulatory phase involves the movement of the ovum through the fallopian tube and uterus, and the formation of the corpus luteum by the granulosa cells remaining in the ovary. The fallopian tube is lined with ciliated epithelia that move fluid from the abdominal cavity toward the uterus. Once in the abdominal cavity, the ovum is usually picked up by the fimbriated ends of the fallopian tube and slowly transported to the uterus. Unless it is fertilized, the ovum eventually passes out of the body with the menstrual flow.

In the ovary after ovulation, the corpus luteum (yellow body) develops within the ruptured ovarian follicle. First, the clot that developed in response to follicular hemorrhage is replaced with yellowish luteal cells containing lipids. These cells eventually form the corpus luteum, an endocrine body that secretes progesterone and some estrogen. Full maturity of the corpus luteum occurs about 9 days after ovulation. If implantation of a fertilized ovum (pregnancy) does not occur, then the corpus luteum begins to degenerate. Degeneration (involution) of the corpus luteum occurs about 2 to 4 days before menstruation.

Uterine and Vaginal Changes During the Menstrual Cycle

Menstruation, commonly called a "period" or menses, results from the withdrawal of estrogen and progesterone. Menstruation is preceded by a period of uterine endometrial retraction and degeneration. The premenstrual phase ends as the constricted arteries open. Small patches of necrotic endometrium separate from the endometrial wall, and menstrual flow begins. Menstrual flow is assisted by contractions of the uterine myometrium. The superficial layers of the uterine endometrium are lost over the initial 48 hours (Fig. 14-7).

Menstrual flow consists of blood, mucus, endometrial tissue fragments, and vaginal epithelial cells. Menstrual flow is usually dark red and contains 60 to 150 mL of fluid. This fluid is 50% to 75% blood with few, if any, small clots present. Menstruation usually lasts about 4 to 5 days until the endometrium is reepithelialized, but from 1 to 10 days may be normal for some women.

At the end of a menstrual flow, the uterine endometrium (containing surface epithelium, glands, connective tissue, spaces, and blood vessels) is very thin because much of it has sloughed off during menstrual flow. Estrogen from the developing follicle stimulates creation of a new endometrial surface layer and uterine epithelium. It stimulates growth of glands and stroma. The epithelium becomes thicker (up to 4 mm) and more vascular. Endometrial proliferation peaks about 2 days before ovulation.

The cervix also undergoes changes during the menstrual cycle. Most important, secretion of mucus, a clear fluid that is receptive to sperm, greatly increases just before ovulation. Vaginal changes during this phase include proliferation and thickening of the vaginal epithelium due to estrogen. This change is greatest at the time of ovulation.

Ovulation is followed by the uterine secretory phase, lasting 10 to 14 days. Progesterone and estrogen promote marked changes in the endometrium. Connective tissue hypertrophies, and the arteries coil and become tortuous. The glands become larger and more tortuous and abundantly secrete glycogen. The endometrium becomes edematous, compact, and thickened. Development peaks 7 to 8 days after ovulation. This is the most favorable time for implantation of a fertilized ovum.

During the premenstrual phase, a drop in progesterone and estrogen production causes endometrial retraction and degeneration. Leukocytes infiltrate the endometrium. The

PATHOLOGY

Endometriosis

Endometriosis is an abnormal condition in which the uterine endometrium is located in internal sites other than the uterus. The most common sites are the ovary and the dependent portion of the pelvic peritoneum. The endometrial tissue responds to hormonal stimulation and undergoes changes typical of uterine endometrial tissue. Pain is the most common clinical manifestation, and infertility is the most common major complication of this disorder.

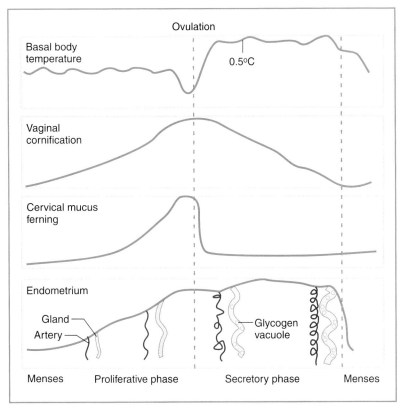

Figure 14-7. Uterine and vaginal changes during the menstrual cycle. Following menstruation, the uterine endometrium increases in size, and vaginal cornification and secretions provide a nutritive environment for sperm. Following ovulation, the uterine endometrium enters the secretory phase, providing a suitable environment for implantation of a fertilized ovum.

coiled arteries constrict, and ischemia results. The endometrium shrinks. At the same time, cervical mucus decreases, becoming more opaque and somewhat resistant to sperm. The premenstrual phase ends as menstrual flow begins.

Endocrine Events During the Menstrual Cycle

Two separate systems regulate female hormone production: the GnRH-FSH-estrogen system and the GnRH-LH-progesterone system (Fig. 14-8). As with the other hypothalamic-pituitary hormones, estrogen inhibits both GnRH and FSH release, and progesterone inhibits both LH and GnRH release. In addition, the ovaries release inhibin, which can inhibit FSH release.

Following puberty, GnRH secretion by the hypothalamus follows a cyclical rhythm. In the preovulatory phase, FSH causes growth of the ovarian follicles, only one of which matures to a graafian follicle. The growing follicles secrete estrogen. LH acts synergistically to enhance follicular growth and estrogen secretion. Estrogen secreted by the developing follicles increases the sensitivity of that follicle to FSH, setting

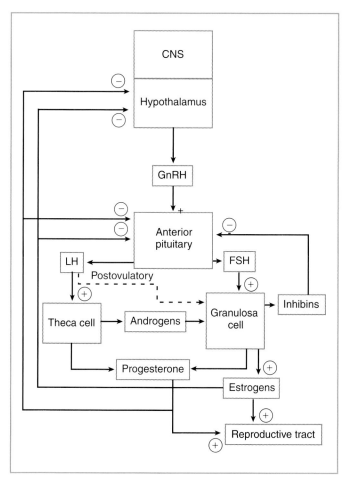

Figure 14-8. Complex regulation of estrogen and progesterone production. FSH stimulates estrogen secretion by ovarian granulosa cells, and LH stimulates progesterone secretion by the ovary. Complex negative feedback loops inhibit both hypothalamic and anterior pituitary hormone secretion. –, Negative feedback; +, positive feedback.

up a positive feedback loop promoting further estrogen secretion. The increasing levels of estrogens inhibit pituitary production of FSH, but LH release is not inhibited. As estrogen secretion increases rapidly, estrogen serves as a positive feedback to promote a surge of LH release (Fig. 14-9).

Over a 24-hour period, this process causes the theca and granulosa cells lining the follicle to hypertrophy and proliferate. LH becomes dominant, stimulating maturation of the follicle. LH decreases estrogen secretion and initiates progesterone secretion by the developing follicle. Pituitary LH release peaks 18 hours before ovulation.

After ovulation, LH stimulates follicular granulosa cells to form a corpus luteum, which secretes progesterone. Estrogen is also secreted from the corpus luteum in the postovulatory phase. Secretion of progesterone, estrogen, and inhibin by the corpus luteum decreases FSH and LH secretion by the anterior pituitary. The corpus luteum degenerates 12 days after ovulation, greatly decreasing progesterone and estrogen secretion. The degeneration of the corpus luteum releases the feedback inhibition of FSH and LH, allowing the pituitary secretion of these hormones to resume.

Integrated Menstrual Cycle

The menstrual cycle is organized around the cyclic release of an ovum and the preparation of a suitable environment for the fertilization and subsequent implantation in the uterus (see Fig. 14-9).

During the preovulatory phase, FSH stimulates the development of an ovum-containing follicle, which also secretes estrogen. Estrogen promotes the further maturation of the ovarian follicle. Estrogen also promotes growth and vascularization of the uterine endometrium.

Ovulation follows a marked increase in LH, which causes the maturing follicle to rupture and release an ovum. The released ovum moves to the fallopian tube, where over the next 6 days, the ciliated epithelia of the fallopian tube move the ovum toward the uterus.

The postovulatory phase is dominated by progesterone action on the uterine endometrium. LH stimulates the ovarian corpus luteum to secrete progesterone. Progesterone initiates secretion in the uterine endometrium, preparing the uterus for implantation of the fertilized ovum. The postovulatory phase lasts for a relatively fixed duration and ends approximately 14 days after ovulation as the corpus luteum degenerates. The postovulatory phase ends with menstruation, unless the fertilized ovum secretes hCG to maintain corpus luteum viability and progesterone secretion.

Menopause

Menopause is the permanent cessation of menstruation. Menopause usually occurs between the ages of 48 and 54, but it may occur as early as age 35. The average age at menopause appears to be increasing in industrialized countries.

Menstrual cessation may be abrupt, but usually it occurs over 1 to 2 years. Cyclic menstrual flow volume gradually lessens, occurs less frequently, and becomes irregular.

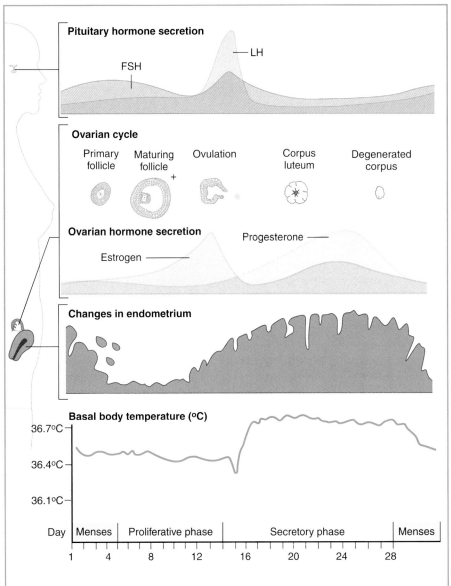

Figure 14-9. Hormone changes during the menstrual cycle. The dominant endocrine event during the first half of the menstrual cycle is FSH stimulation of estrogen secretion. The middle of the cycle is characterized by a drop in estrogen secretion and a surge in LH secretion. The second half of the cycle is dominated by LH stimulation of progesterone secretion.

PHARMACOLOGY

Estrogen Replacement Therapy

Replacement therapy involves administration of estrogen to diminish the symptoms of menopause. Estrogen replacement therapy can be used to reduce the risk of osteoporosis and to increase the psychological sense of well-being. A disadvantage is an increased tendency for blood clot formation.

Anovulatory cycles are common, and occasional episodes of profuse bleeding may be interspersed with episodes of scant bleeding. Menopause is said to have occurred when there have been no menstrual periods for 12 consecutive months.

As menopause approaches, there is gradual decrease in the number of maturing ovarian follicles and a parallel decline in the production of ovarian estrogen. The decline in estrogen production removes the normal inhibition on the hypothalamus and anterior pituitary, and FSH and LH production increases. The ovaries, however, become unresponsive to pituitary hormones, and they atrophy. Other changes associated with menopause, such as hot flashes and vaginal atrophy, are related to decreased estrogen production.

●●● TOP 5 TAKE-HOME POINTS

1. The immature female reproductive system forms in utero and matures during puberty.
2. The mature female reproductive system undergoes extensive cyclic changes centered on monthly ovulation and menstruation.
3. Estrogen dominates the first half of the menstrual cycle, as the ovary prepares for ovulation and the uterus recovers

from menstruation. Ovulation, induced by an LH surge, marks the midpoint of the menstrual cycle.

4. Progesterone dominates the second half of the menstrual cycle, preparing the uterus to receive a fertilized ovum. If implantation does not occur, progesterone production ceases, and the uterine endothelium is lost during menstruation.

5. The monthly menstrual cycle continues until menopause, when the ovaries are no longer able to produce sufficient estrogen to support the cycle.

Male Reproductive System 15

CONTENTS

Most organ systems assist the survival of an individual and maintain a baseline homeostasis and the ability to adapt to a changing environment. The reproductive system is unique in that it is centered on survival of the species, using sexual reproduction to ensure genetic variability across the generations. The DNA in a mature human cell is packaged in 46 chromosomes, and the cell reproduces exact copies of itself by mitosis. In organisms that propagate by sexual reproduction, germ cells are formed by meiosis that contain half the normal DNA complement—23 chromosomes. The reproductive system is specialized for the production and joining of germ cells—the ovum (female) and sperm (male). Mature sperm contain the 23 chromosomes, a tail for movement, and hyaluronic acid and proteolytic enzymes for penetrating the ovum. The union of two germ cells (fertilization) creates a new cell with a full complement of 46 chromosomes. This new cell contains the genetic template for the individual.

The male contribution to reproduction centers on the production of sperm and ejaculation of functional sperm during sexual intercourse (Fig. 15-1). Male sexual differentiation begins in utero with the development of primary sexual characteristics, resumes again at puberty with the development of adult secondary sexual characteristics, and continues through adult life. This chapter is organized along developmental lines. It begins with the sexual determination in utero and follows the growth and maturation of the male reproductive system.

●●● SEXUAL DIFFERENTIATION IN UTERO

Sexual identity is established in utero. The fertilized ovum has 46 chromosomes, grouped as 22 pairs of somatic chromosomes, and one pair of sex chromosomes. Somatic chromosomes form an X-shaped structure, with four arms extending outward from a central acrosome. The sex chromosomes are classified according to structure as X or Y, with the Y chromosome containing only three of the four arms that make up the normal X appearance. The female genotype is XX, and the male genotype is XY.

Both male and female reproductive systems develop and begin to mature in utero. The undifferentiated gonads are medial to two parallel duct systems, the mesonephric (wolffian) duct and the paramesonephric (müllerian) duct.

Development of a male reproductive system occurs only when testosterone is secreted by the developing fetus. In XY males, the gonads differentiate into testes. Placental human chorionic gonadotropin (hCG) and later fetal luteinizing hormone (LH) release stimulate Leydig cells to synthesize and release androgens, including testosterone. Male testosterone secretion stimulates maturation of the wolffian duct into the vas deferens (Fig. 15-2). The Sertoli cells of the testes produce antimüllerian hormone, which causes the müllerian ducts to degenerate. Development of the male external genitalia requires dihydrotestosterone, which is formed in the target tissues from testosterone.

At birth, the normal male reproductive structures all are formed but not yet mature. During the final month of gestation, the testes descend into the scrotum. This descent allows the testes to be at a temperature lower than the body core temperature, which is important for optimal function of the testes. Following birth, LH and follicle-stimulating hormone (FSH) stimulation is lost, and further sexual development is retarded. There is little sexual development during childhood. Maturation of the reproductive systems, or puberty, is delayed until adolescence.

Androgen Biosynthesis

Testosterone is the primary androgen produced in the male. It is formed from the sequential action of enzymes on a cholesterol precursor (see Fig. 15-4). Other steroids in the

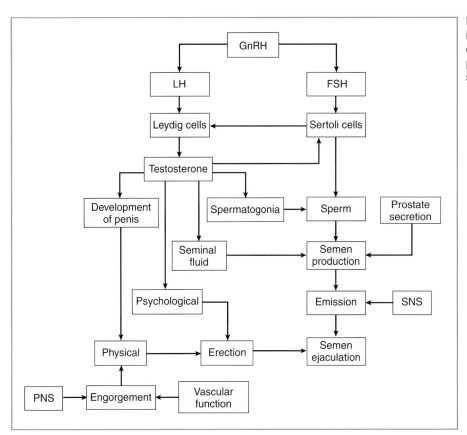

Figure 15-1. Male reproductive map illustrates factors contributing to ejaculation of functional sperm. PNS, parasympathetic nervous system; SNS, sympathetic nervous system.

synthetic pathway can have significant androgenic effects. At the tissues, some testosterone is converted by 5α-reductase to dihydrotestosterone, the compound that produces many of the male secondary sexual characteristics.

● ● ● PUBERTY

Some time after the age of 9 years, hypothalamic production of GnRH resumes, and the gender-specific development of reproductive systems resumes for a 2- to 4½-year period. Resumption of GnRH production depends on maturation of the amygdala or some other component of the limbic system.

As in utero, testosterone is the primary male sex steroid during puberty. Testosterone is converted to dihydrotestosterone within the target tissue cells and activates DNA transcription and translation. During this time, androstenedione and estradiol are secreted by Leydig cells. Under this combined hormonal influence, the development of primary and secondary sexual characteristics resumes.

Enlargement of the penis and testes are the primary sexual characteristic changes of puberty. In later stages of puberty, the testes begin production of mature sperm. Secondary sexual characteristics also develop during puberty. These include the appearance of body hair, especially on the face and the genital regions, deepening of the voice due to growth of the larynx and vocal cords, toughening of the skin, increased secretion of sebaceous glands, growth of muscle mass, and

closure of the epiphyseal plates. The pubertal growth spurt occurs late in puberty and is due to both testosterone and growth hormone (GH).

● ● ● ADULT MALE REPRODUCTIVE STRUCTURES

The adult male reproductive organs are the testicles, epididymis, seminal ducts, spermatic cords, seminal vesicles, ejaculatory ducts, bulbourethral (Cowper's) glands, prostate gland, and penis. The scrotum, which contains the testes, and penis are external, visible genitalia. The remaining structures are internal (Fig. 15-3).

Penis and Related Structures

The penis is an organ of urination and, after puberty, an organ of copulation. This cylindrical, pendulous structure suspends from its attachment to the pubic arch. The skin of the penis is dark, hairless, thin, and loose, permitting considerable distention during the erectile response. The shaft of the penis is the portion of the penis between its end and its attachment to the pubic bone. The urethra's external opening, or meatus, is in the glans penis, the cone-shaped end of the penis. The glans is an expansion of the corpus spongiosum. The flap of movable foreskin or prepuce that normally covers the penis is removed if male circumcision is performed.

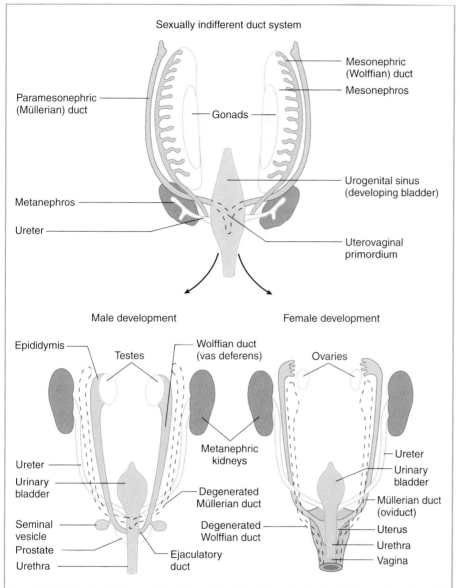

Figure 15-2. Both male and female genitalia are present early in fetal development. The development of the testes in the male genitalia is driven by the testis-determining factor on the short arm of the Y chromosome. Differentiation of the fetal gonad to the testis allows production of testosterone and the antimüllerian hormone, leading to development of the male phenotype.

PATHOLOGY

Turner's Syndrome

Turner's syndrome is a genetic abnormality in which the second sex chromosome is absent (genotype 45,XO). Individuals with Turner's syndrome have female internal and external genitalia, but the genitalia are usually small and poorly developed.

The penis is homologous to the female clitoris and shares a common mechanism for erection during sexual excitement. Usually, the penis is flaccid, but it becomes rigid when physically stimulated or during sexual excitement. An erection occurs when the corpora cavernosa become engorged with blood. Following orgasm and ejaculation, blood leaves and the penis again becomes flaccid.

Scrotum and Testes

The scrotum is a pouch suspended from the root of the penis. It is separated into halves internally by the tunica dartos (dartos muscle) and externally by a ridge that runs over the scrotum from the root of the penis to the anus. Each half of the scrotum contains a testicle with its epididymis and a part of a spermatic cord. The vas deferens is a continuation of the epididymis that conveys sperm from the testicle to the prostatic urethra. Sperm joins with other semen components and is conveyed to the urethra by the ejaculatory duct.

The testicles are both an endocrine organ and the source of sperm. The testicle is divided into many lobules, separated by septa. Each lobule contains seminiferous tubules, the site of sperm production. Seminiferous tubules make up 90% of the weight of a mature testis. Leydig cells, the source of testosterone, are situated between the seminiferous tubules. Sertoli cells of the testis are joined by tight junctions, creating

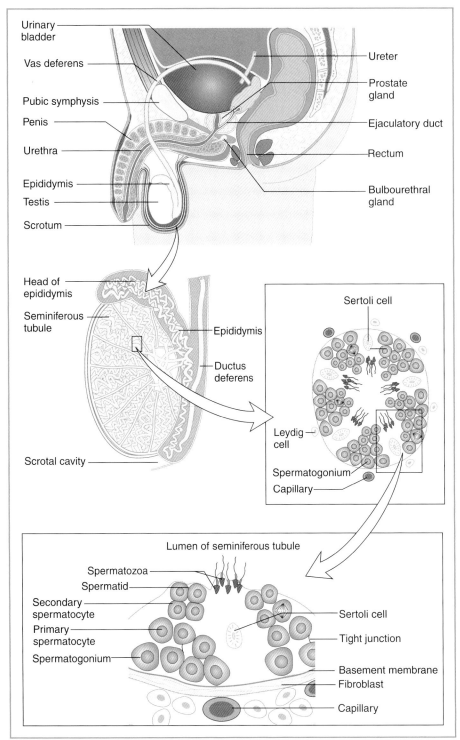

Figure 15-3. Gross and microscopic anatomy of the male reproductive system. The male reproductive system consists of the external penis, testis, and scrotum and the internal vas deferens, prostate gland, and bulbourethral gland. The histology of the testis is complex, revealing that maturation of the spermatozoa is supported by the Sertoli cells.

a blood-testis barrier analogous to the blood-brain barrier. This means that the interior of the testis is an immuno-protected site and that water-soluble drugs have difficulty in reaching the developing spermatogonia.

The epididymis rests on and beside the posterior surface of the testicle. It originates in the upper end of the testicle and joins the testis with the vas deferens. The vas deferens joins other vessels to form the spermatic cord.

Prostate Gland and Related Structures

The prostate gland is a partly muscular, partly glandular structure that surrounds the neck of the male urinary bladder and urethra. In childhood the prostate is small, but it grows along with the other reproductive structures during puberty. The prostate is enclosed by a firm, fibrous capsule. The bladder is on the basal surface of the prostate. The posterior surface of the prostate is in close contact with the rectal wall, and this surface can be palpated by digital examination. The prostatic urethra is the portion of the urethra that passes through the prostate. Prostatic muscle fibers encircle the urethra and separate the glandular tissue of the prostate. Prostatic secretions contribute to the liquefaction of semen following ejaculation.

The seminal vesicles are a pair of 5-cm-long sac-like structures that connect to the vas deferens. Seminal secretions are a component of semen that contribute to sperm nutrition and activation.

Testicular function is regulated by a negative feedback loop in an anterior pituitary–hypothalamus–testicular axis. The hypothalamus secretes gonadotropin-releasing hormone (GnRH) in a pulsatile fashion. The single hypothalamic releasing factor GnRH stimulates the anterior pituitary gland to produce both LH and FSH. LH stimulates testicular Leydig cells to produce testosterone, which modulates the secretion of GnRH and therefore LH through negative feedback to the hypothalamus and pituitary gland. FSH and testosterone stimulate testicular Sertoli cells and germ cells to start and complete spermatogenesis. Inhibin, released from Sertoli cells, provides negative feedback to FSH release by the anterior pituitary (Fig. 15-4).

Sperm

Sperm are mature male germ cells that develop after puberty. Sperm are produced in the seminiferous tubules of the testicles. Sperm develop in great quantities from spermatids and are stored in the vas deferens. Sperm propel themselves through motion of their thin tails. A normal sperm has a flattened, broad, oval head with a nucleus. During fertilization, the sperm's head pierces an ovum, and the sperm DNA joins with the ovum DNA.

Spermatogenesis

Spermatogenesis is the process of sperm production and development. Primordial germ cells migrate to the testes during fetal development but remain immature until adolescence. At puberty, sperm production is initiated following an increase in pituitary FSH and LH secretion. Spermatogonia are the germinal epithelial cells. The spermatogonia divide and migrate toward the Sertoli cells during the first stage of

spermatogenesis. The spermatogonia penetrate the membranes of Sertoli cells and become enveloped within the cytoplasm of these cells. This close proximity allows Sertoli cells to nourish the spermatogonia throughout their development.

After 24 days of contact with Sertoli cells, the spermatogonium matures into a primary spermatocyte. After this development, the spermatocyte undergoes meiosis and splits into two secondary spermatocytes, each with only 23 chromosomes. After 2 to 3 days, the spermatocytes undergo a second meiotic division to form four spermatids, each again with 23 chromosomes.

Spermatogenesis takes about 74 days. As spermatogonia develop, the cells lose some cytoplasm and the chromatin material reorganizes to form a compact head. The remaining cytoplasm contractile proteins and cell membranes collect at the other end of the cell to form the tail of the sperm.

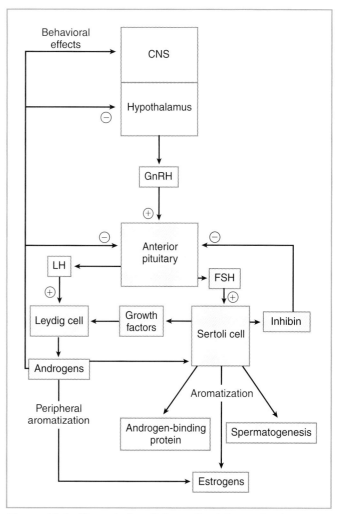

Figure 15-4. The anterior pituitary stimulates endocrine secretions of the testis. LH from the anterior pituitary stimulates antigen production by the testicular Leydig cells, with androgens providing a negative feedback inhibition at the level of both hypothalamus and anterior pituitary. FSH stimulates Sertoli sell secretions, including the hormone inhibin, which provides a negative feedback signal diminishing FSH released by the anterior pituitary. –, Negative feedback; +, positive feedback.

ANATOMY

Prostate Gland

The adult prostate gland lies like a flattened cone in the pelvis, about 2 cm posterior to the symphysis pubis. In a normal adult man, the prostate weighs 15 to 20 g and is 4 to 6 cm long. The prostate is inverted, so that its apex is inferior, and it is suspended from the sphincter urethrae muscle and the perineal membrane. The base of the prostate is superior and at the bladder neck, anterior to the rectum.

Hormones are essential to the growth and division of the germinal cells and the formation of sperm. LH stimulates Leydig cells to secrete testosterone. FSH stimulates Sertoli cells to promote spermatogenesis. Estrogens, formed from testosterone when Sertoli cells are stimulated by FSH, are required for spermatogenesis.

Sperm spend several days passing through the epididymis. After about 24 hours, they become motile and capable of fertilization. The majority of sperm are stored in the vas deferens and the ampulla of the vas deferens, with a small amount stored in the epididymis. Sperm can maintain their motility and fertility for up to a month, but when sexual activity is frequent, sperm may be stored for only a few days.

Semen

Semen is a viscid, thick, opalescent secretion discharged by males through the urethra at the climax of sexual excitement or orgasm. It contains sperm, clotting proteins, fibrinolytic proteins, and other secretions. About 60% of semen is a fructose, prostaglandin, and fibrinogen-rich fluid from the seminal vesicles. Thirty percent is composed of prostatic fluid and small amounts of mucoid secretion from the bulbourethral glands. The remaining 10% of the semen is composed of sperm and fluid from the vas deferens.

The prostate gland produces a thin, milky secretion containing Ca^{++}, clotting enzymes, and profibrinolysin. Prostatic secretions are manufactured in a network of branching glands embedded in muscle within the prostate. This muscle contracts during ejaculation, and prostatic secretions are ejected through the ejaculatory ducts into the urethra.

The clotting enzymes of the prostatic secretion interacts with the fibrinogen of the seminal vesicle fluid to form a weak coagulum following ejaculation. This coagulum holds the semen near the uterine cervix. The coagulum dissolves in about 15 to 30 minutes, at which time the sperm become highly motile. The sperm can live within the vagina for 24 to 48 hours after ejaculation.

●●● INTERCOURSE AND ORGASM

Intercourse deposits sperm in the vagina to allow fertilization of the ovum. Preparation for intercourse involves an often complex set of physical and psychic stimulation and is influenced by social values. Sensory inputs are primarily from the glans penis but also from the adjacent genital areas and the perineal region (Fig. 15-5).

Sympathetic, parasympathetic, and somatic nerves contribute to the male sexual response. Erection is mediated by the pelvic parasympathetic nerves. The initiation of an erection depends on the NANC (nonadrenergic, noncholinergic) branch of parasympathetic nerves. Both NANC and acetylcholine (ACh) neurotransmitters stimulate nitric oxide (NO) release. ACh activates NO synthase, causing a cGMP-mediated smooth muscle relaxation. The relaxation of the corpora cavernosa and corpus spongiosum vascular smooth muscle allows an increase in blood flow and engorgement of the tissue.

Parasympathetic activation results from a spinal reflex due to sensory stimulation and can be modified (enhanced or blunted) by descending autonomic control. At the same time, penile sympathetic activity (which normally vasoconstricts) is diminished. Penetration and friction increase sensory input.

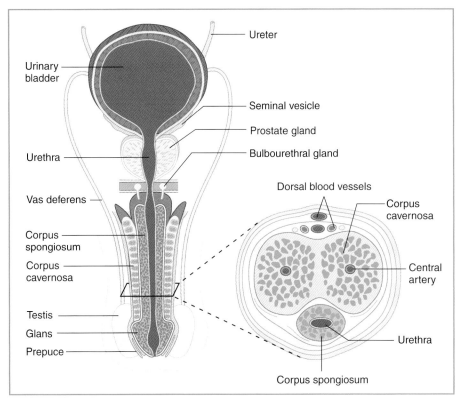

Figure 15-5. The paired corpora cavernosa provide most of the volume of the penis. Dilation of the blood vessels supplying the corpora cavernosa allows them to become engorged with blood, causing the penis to become erect and rigid.

PHARMACOLOGY

Treatment for Erectile Dysfunction

Sildenafil is a phosphodiesterase-5 inhibitor used to treat erectile dysfunction (ED). The dilation of vascular smooth muscle required to achieve an erection is mediated by NO and the intracellular second messenger cGMP. cGMP is broken down by phosphodiesterase. Consequently, inhibition of phosphodiesterase allows endogenous NO to produce a more pronounced vasodilation.

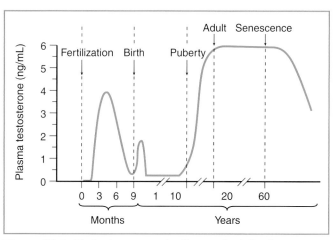

Figure 15-6. Testosterone production peaks following puberty and remains elevated until late adulthood. In utero, testosterone production is stimulated by hCG and fetal LH. During childhood, testosterone production remains low until the onset of puberty, when the increase in LH stimulates testicular production of testosterone.

Continuing stimulation leads to emission, the movement of sperm from the vas deferens and into the urethra. Prostate and seminal gland secretions are also moved into the urethra. Emission is under sympathetic control, and sympathetic activity also contracts the internal bladder sphincter, isolating the bladder from the urethra.

Continued stimulation leads to a climax, with male ejaculation. Sympathetics mediate ejaculation, with successive contraction of the vas deferens and ampulla, the prostate, and finally the seminal vesicles. Ejaculation is supplemented by contraction of abdominal muscles. Climax is followed by a period of resolution, with reversal of the events that preceded intercourse.

Testosterone is necessary for sexual function. Plasma testosterone levels increase at puberty, coinciding with the onset of male sexual potency. Plasma testosterone levels remain elevated beyond the sixth decade of life, and because sperm production continues at a reduced rate, it is possible for males to become fathers in the late adult years (Fig. 15-6).

The term andropause describes a state of lower androgen levels. Although not as abrupt as menopause, andropause is associated with a decrease in the changes that accompany puberty: a loss of energy, decreased libido, and erectile dysfunction.

●●● TOP 5 TAKE-HOME POINTS

1. Development of male reproductive structures requires the stimulation of testosterone production in utero.
2. LH stimulates the Leydig cells to produce testosterone, and FSH stimulates the Sertoli cells to produce spermatozoa.
3. Many biological actions of testosterone first require the conversion to 5-dihydrotestosterone in the cells of the target tissues.
4. Semen is a viscous fluid with components produced by the testes, the prostate gland, and the seminal vesicles.
5. Testosterone production peaks in the early adult years and declines gradually after the age of 50 years.

Life Span

16

CONTENTS

The human life span proceeds through a series of functional stages beginning at conception and ending with the elderly years. Each stage requires a significant physiologic adaptation to ensure continued survival.

This chapter begins with conception. Intercourse deposits sperm in the vagina. The sperm migrate and ideally encounter the ovum in the fallopian tube. If the ovum is successfully fertilized, the developing embryo can implant in the uterine endometrium, and pregnancy ensues. The mother is an active participant in gestation and experiences numerous physiologic changes to allow for successful nurturing of the embryo through development.

The human gestational period is a 40-week period during which the fetus develops in utero. The gestational period is actually calculated from the first day of the mother's last menstrual cycle. Within the gestational period, significant development events are identified by the week in which they occur, or in one of the three "trimesters," each of which lasts 13 weeks. The gestational period ends with birth.

Birth is a significant physiologic challenge and represents the transition from a dependent existence in utero to an independent existence. Dramatic cardiac and respiratory adaptations to enable this change must occur in the first minutes following birth.

The neonatal period is the first 28 days of life. The postnatal stages progress through a continuum, but a person can be identified as an infant, a juvenile, an adolescent, a young adult, a mature adult, and an elderly person. Each of these life stages requires unique physiologic challenges and adaptations (Fig. 16-1).

●●● PREGNANCY

Female fertility requires the release of one ovum, which normally occurs once a month from the onset of menstruation through menopause. Ovum viability is generally less than 24 hours after release from the ovary. To achieve pregnancy, intercourse must be timed to allow simultaneous presence of sperm and ovum in the fallopian tube. Fertilization results in the joining of 23 chromosomes from the sperm with the 23 chromosomes of the ovum to achieve the haploid 46 chromosome complement of normal somatic cells.

The fertilized ovum travels through the fallopian tube for 3 to 5 days before reaching the uterus. During this time, the fertilized ovum continues mitotic divisions and becomes a zygote. The zygote is nourished by uterine secretions until implantation (Fig. 16-2).

Early in pregnancy, the fertilized ovum produces chorionic gonadotropin, a hormone that maintains progesterone and estrogen secretion by the corpus luteum. This is essential, since continued progesterone production prevents menstruation.

One week after ovulation, the ovum implants in the uterine endometrium, which is in the secretory phase of the ovulatory cycle. The zygote differentiates into two structures. One becomes the fetus, and the other becomes the placenta (Fig. 16-3).

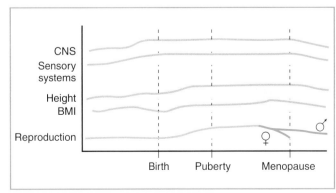

Figure 16-1. Map of the life stages illustrates the age related change in organ system function.

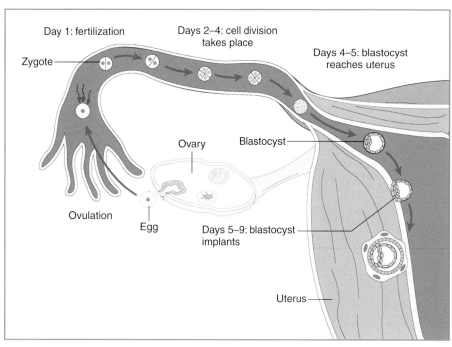

Figure 16-2. Fertilization in the fallopian tube and implantation in the uterus occur during normal pregnancy. Conception occurs when sperm and ovum unite in the fallopian tube. The fertilized ovum begins a series of mitotic cell divisions and reaches the zygote stage before implanting in the uterus.

The placenta is an important endocrine and circulatory structure. The highly vascular placenta exchanges nutrients and wastes between the maternal and fetal circulations. In the XY zygote, placental gonadotropin stimulates testosterone production, allowing the development of male sexual organs.

During implantation, the cells destined to become the placenta digest the uterine endometrium for nutrition. By 12 weeks of gestation, the placenta is developed and becomes the major source of fetal nutrients. Fetal blood enters the placenta by the placental artery and exits by the placental vein. Maternal blood enters the placenta by the uterine artery and exits by the uterine vein.

Chorionic gonadotropin secretion decreases as the placenta assumes the role of estrogen and progesterone production for the second and third trimesters. The corpus luteum involutes and becomes nonfunctional about 18 weeks after ovulation. In the placenta, estrogen is produced from conversion of fetal adrenal steroids rather than by de novo synthesis.

In the mother, placental estrogens increase the growth of the uterus, breasts, and external genitalia and relax pelvic ligaments. Placental progesterone prepares breasts for lactation. The placenta secretes human somatomammotropin, a hormone that decreases maternal insulin sensitivity and causes an increase in maternal circulating glucose levels. Somatomammotropin additionally has some growth hormone–like effects, especially on the breasts.

The placenta is the primary site of nutrient and waste exchange between the maternal and fetal circulations. The higher maternal glucose levels enhance glucose diffusion to the fetus. In addition, facilitated diffusion enhances glucose transport across the placenta. The placenta absorbs amino acids, Ca^{++}, inorganic phosphate, and ascorbic acid from the maternal blood for delivery to the fetus.

Fetal hemoglobin is specialized to extract O_2 from maternal blood. The fetal isoform of hemoglobin has a higher O_2 affinity than does adult hemoglobin. Fetal hematocrit is higher than maternal hematocrit, further enhancing fetal blood O_2-carrying capacity. In addition, movement of CO_2 from fetal to maternal plasma enhances the O_2-carrying capacity of fetal hemoglobin. CO_2 and other fetal metabolic wastes cross the placenta primarily by diffusion.

The maternal adjustments to pregnancy are intended to meet the metabolic and nutritional needs of the developing fetus. Maternal blood volume increases during gestation, expanding by 20% by the third trimester. Maternal cardiac

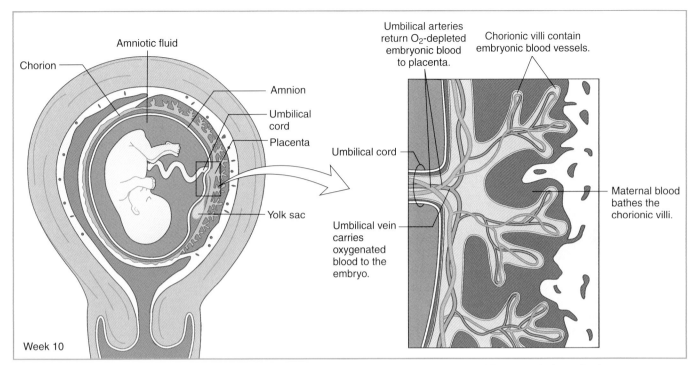

Figure 16-3. An extensive capillary network facilitates exchange between the maternal and fetal circulations. During pregnancy, the uterine vascular supply increases dramatically. As the placenta grows, the placental blood vessels intertwine with the maternal uterine capillaries. This highly vascular structure facilitates the diffusional exchange of nutrients and wastes.

BIOCHEMISTRY

Placental Estrogen Synthesis

The fetus can produce cholesterol and pregnenolone, but it cannot synthesize estrogens because it lacks the enzymes 3β-hydroxysteroid dehydrogenase and aromatase. The placenta lacks the enzymes 17α-hydroxylase, 16α-hydroxylase, and 17,20-desmolase. The placenta acts on fetal adrenal steroids to convert them to estrogens.

---

output increases during the gestational period to support the increased maternal blood flow to the placenta. Maternal alveolar ventilation is increased, which causes a drop in maternal plasma CO_2 levels in spite of the additional CO_2 load caused by the fetal metabolism.

The maternal pituitary endocrine secretions are altered by pregnancy. Pituitary ACTH stimulates adrenal glucocorticoid and aldosterone production. The glucocorticoids mobilize maternal amino acids for gluconeogenesis. Aldosterone enhances maternal sodium and water retention. Pituitary TSH stimulates thyroid hormone production, and increases metabolic rate. Pituitary prolactin stimulates growth of the breasts in preparation for milk production.

Maternal parathyroid hormone production increases, stimulating vitamin D formation and consequently intestinal Ca^{++} absorption. The increase in parathyroid hormone mobilizes maternal bone Ca^{++} if dietary Ca^{++} restricted. The

elevation in parathyroid hormone is maintained during lactation to maintain production of Ca^{++}-enriched milk.

Growth-stimulating effects of estrogen and progesterone target organs such as the uterus and breasts. Weight gain during pregnancy averages 24 pounds, 11 pounds of which is the fetus, amniotic fluid, and placenta. The uterus grows by 2 pounds, and breasts grow by 2 pounds. Fluid expansion accounts for an additional 6 pounds from the enhanced renal sodium and fluid retention. There is a maternal shift to fatty acid rather than glucose for substrate. Maternal insulin resistance increases maternal glucose levels and can lead to gestational diabetes. Glucocorticoids support the maternal use of free fatty acids as metabolic substrates.

Fetal Development

A fetus develops from a single fertilized ovum over a 9-month period, adapting for life in utero and for the transition to an independent life following birth.

The cardiovascular system develops as the increase in fetal size limits the diffusion of nutrients to cells in the interior. The fetal circulation develops to assist fetal transport of nutrients and wastes, with the placenta serving as the site for exchange of nutrients and wastes with the maternal circulation. This exchange occurs at the maternal sinus–fetal umbilical capillary interface. The fetal umbilical artery carries blood to the placenta, and the umbilical vein carries blood from the placenta back to the fetus. Maternal blood passes from the uterine arteries to maternal sinuses in the placenta. Maternal blood leaves the placenta via the uterine veins. The maternal and fetal blood systems remain separate.

Fetal blood cell formation begins in week 3 of fetal development. Blood cells are formed initially in the yolk sac and placental mesothelium. Blood formation then shifts to the blood vessel endothelium, liver, spleen, and other lymphoid tissues. During the final 3 months of gestation, blood cell formation shifts to the bone marrow, which remains the site of blood cell formation throughout adult life. The fetal heart begins contracting at the fourth week after fertilization, and the heart rate increases to 140 beats per minute by term.

The fetal cardiovascular system has three adaptations to allow gas exchange at the placenta rather than the lungs: (1) ductus arteriosus, (2) umbilical artery, and (3) umbilical vein/ductus venosus. The fetus has an additional adaptation to allow oxygenated blood to perfuse the brain and heart—the foramen ovale. Fetal circulation supplies the developing heart and brain with high-O_2 blood (Figs. 16-4 and 16-5).

Oxygenated blood returns to the fetus by the umbilical vein, which passes through the fetal liver as the ductus venosus before flowing into the fetal vena cava. Within the vena cava, there is a flow of two streams of blood—the O_2-rich blood from the umbilical vein and the O_2-depleted blood returning from the lower half of the fetal body. There is little mixing of these two streams because of the laminar flow pattern in the vena cava. Both streams enter the right atrium, but the O_2-enriched blood flows through the foramen ovale in the interatrial septum and enters the left atrium. This blood then flows through the left ventricle and into the aorta. The O_2-enriched blood flows to the coronary, carotid artery, and cerebral arteries that originate from the aorta proximal to the ductus arteriosus. This allows the brain, heart, and upper part of the fetal body to receive well-oxygenated blood.

The O_2-depleted blood traveling in the vena cava passes into the right atrium and continues through the right ventricle and into the pulmonary artery. Hypoxia at the ductus arteriosus stimulates the production of the vasodilator prostaglandin E, and the ductus arteriosus remains open. Hypoxia also causes constriction of the pulmonary arteries, reducing blood flow through the lung. Most O_2-depleted blood entering the pulmonary artery flows through the ductus arteriosus and into the arch of the aorta, where it mixes with the O_2-enriched blood ejected from the left ventricle. Only about 10% of the output of the right ventricle enters the pulmonary circulation.

PATHOLOGY

Gestational Diabetes

Gestational diabetes mellitus is diagnosed when the diabetes or impaired glucose tolerance first appears during pregnancy. The diabetes is due to a decrease in sensitivity to insulin and thus resembles type II diabetes mellitus. Gestational diabetes develops in up to 5% of all pregnant women and disappears following delivery.

HISTOLOGY

Placenta

The placenta is a temporary organ facilitating exchange between the fetus and the mother. The fetal part of the placenta consists of a chorionic plate and the chorionic villi. The maternal part of the placenta is the decidua basalis. The chorionic villi containing fetal blood are surrounded by maternal blood, facilitating exchange of nutrients and wastes. This exchange takes place without commingling of fetal and maternal blood.

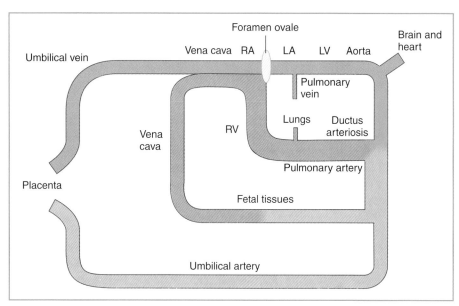

Figure 16-4. Fetal circulation directs the oxygenated blood from the umbilical vein to the blood vessels supplying the heart and brain. The O_2-rich blood from the umbilical vein is directed through the foramen ovale into the left atrium (LA), left ventricle (LV), and out the aorta. The O_2-depleted blood from the superior and inferior vena cava flows through the right atrium (RA), right ventricle (RV), and out the pulmonary artery before passing through the ductus arteriosus and joining the fetal systemic circulation.

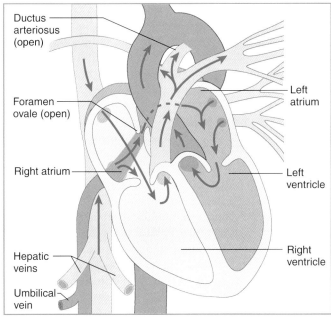

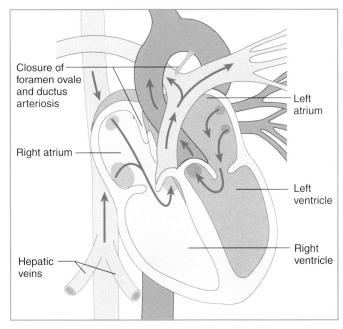

Figure 16-5. Cardiovascular adjustments to birth.
A, In utero, oxygenated blood flows from the inferior vena cava to the right atrium and through the foramen ovale into the left atrium. This oxygenated blood is pumped by the left ventricle into the aorta and supplies the myocardium, brain, and upper body. In utero, the oxygen-depleted blood then enters the right atrium and passes through the right ventricle into the pulmonary artery. About 10% of the pulmonary artery blood flow goes through the fetal lungs, and about 90% of the pulmonary artery blood flow bypasses the lungs and enters the aorta through the ductus arteriosus. **B**, At birth, the closure of the ductus arteriosus and the foramen ovale ensure that all of the blood that enters the right atrium passes through the lungs of the neonate.

Fetal pulmonary artery pressure is higher than fetal aortic pressure. Fetal pulmonary vascular resistance is high because of hypoxic pulmonary vasoconstriction. Fetal aortic pressure is low because of the decrease in peripheral resistance due to the placental artery. About 50% of the fetal cardiac output flows through the placental artery for gas exchange. This is in contrast to the 100% of adult cardiac output that passes through the lungs for gas exchange.

Embryologic development of the GI tract is apparent by 4 weeks of gestation, and by 6 weeks, anatomical divisions become apparent. The esophagus begins as a common tubular structure that develops into the esophagus, pharynx, trachea, and bronchi. Anatomically, the stomach is developed by 5 weeks of gestation, but the development of gastric function begins in the second trimester. Gastric acid production does not begin until the third trimester and increases rapidly following birth.

Anatomic development of the small intestines is completed during the first 10 weeks of gestation. Small-intestinal functional development begins during the second trimester, and the small intestine remains a plastic organ throughout life. The ability to digest disaccharides develops during the second and third trimesters, but significant lactase activity develops only after birth.

The lumen of the GI tract fills with a dark green mixture of shed intestinal epithelial cells, bile, and the solid elements of swallowed amniotic fluid, called meconium. Normally, meconium is excreted shortly after birth. Intrauterine distress, however, can stimulate in utero excretion of meconium into the amniotic fluid.

Fetal lungs are filled with fluid and do not participate in gas exchange. In utero the fluid in the fetal lungs is continuous with amniotic fluid. The inhibition of fetal respiratory movements prevents the inspiration of any meconium that was discharged into the amniotic fluid from the fetal GI tract. In addition, the continuous secretions of the alveolar epithelium help prevent entry of meconium into the alveoli.

Fetal surfactant secretion increases in the final trimester and signals the ability to survive ex utero. Insufficient surfactant production in the preterm neonate can lead to the development of infant respiratory distress syndrome.

The fetal renal system function is similar to that of the neonate. Amniotic fluid is swallowed by the developing fetus

BIOCHEMISTRY

Fetal Hemoglobin

Hemoglobin is an O_2 transport protein composed of two pairs of unlike chains. Fetal hemoglobin has two α-chains and two γ-chains. The γ-chain allows fetal hemoglobin to have a higher affinity for O_2 than does adult hemoglobin. This facilitates O_2 transfer from the maternal blood to the fetal blood across the placental barrier.

and absorbed across the fetal GI tract, providing fluid intake to the fetus. The fetal kidneys provide a mechanism for excretion of this fluid load. Although renal excretion occurs in utero, regulatory processes are poorly developed until after birth.

Parturition

At term, maternal uterine contractions cause the fetus to be forced from the uterus, a process called parturition. Uterine contractions generally begin at the top of the uterine fundus and spread down toward the cervix. Uterine contractions during the final trimester increase the strength of the uterine muscle. Called Braxton-Hicks contractions, these are slow, rhythmic contractions of the uterine myometrium.

Oxytocin dramatically increases the strength and frequency of uterine contractions and can be used to initiate labor if labor does not begin spontaneously. During natural labor, uterine contractions increase in intensity and force the fetus into the birth canal. Stretch of the cervix causes the reflex release of additional oxytocin from the posterior pituitary, further increasing the strength of uterine contractions in a positive feedback cycle. In addition, stretch of the cervix can directly increase the strength of uterine contractions (Fig. 16-6).

During labor, uterine smooth muscle contractions increase in strength and frequency until the fetus is expelled. Expulsion is facilitated by abdominal muscle contraction. Estrogens, and the hormone relaxin, secreted during the final stages of pregnancy, loosen the ligaments and connective tissue of the birth canal. Expulsion of the fetus removes the stimulus for labor, and the uterine smooth muscle contractions

now compress the size of the uterus. Uterine contractions in the 10 to 45 minutes after birth dislodge the placenta. Uterine contraction also compresses the uterine blood vessels, limiting maternal blood loss after placental detachment. At parturition, only 0.5 L of maternal blood is lost, with the remaining excess volume lost gradually.

Strong uterine contractions compress uterine blood vessels, preventing a continuous hemorrhage at childbirth.

Birth

The first breath initiates a transition from a fetal circulatory pattern to that of a neonate (and an adult). Vasospasm of the umbilical cord occludes the umbilical artery and vein. The loss of the umbilical blood flow causes a 50% increase in systemic vascular resistance and an increase in systemic arterial blood pressure and pressures on the left atrium and ventricle. Inspiration brings O_2 into the neonatal lungs, removing the hypoxic pulmonary vasoconstriction. The 90% decrease in pulmonary vascular resistance causes pulmonary arterial blood to flow through the lungs rather than the ductus arteriosus (Fig. 16-7).

The fetal circulatory adjustments are now inoperative. Vasoconstriction occludes the umbilical vessels. The increase in left atrial pressure causes closure of the foramen ovale flap valve. Oxygenated blood from the now high-pressure aorta flows backward through the ductus arteriosus into the pulmonary artery. The presence of oxygenated blood in the ductus arteriosus decreases production of the vasodilator prostaglandin E, and consequently the ductus arteriosus constricts and, over a few days to weeks, closes. The right (pulmonary) and left (systemic) circulations are now separate.

The onset of respiration is essential for survival. Gas can no longer be exchanged at the placenta, but the fetal lungs are filled with fluid from epithelial cell secretions. At birth, the first inspiration is stimulated by sensory input from the cooling of the skin and the release of compression caused by birth. Respiration is further stimulated by hypoxia and hypercapnia, a reflection of the respiratory control system that continues to function through adult life. Fluid in lungs opposes entry of air at inspiration. Consequently, the first breath requires up to –60 mm Hg intrapleural pressure. Subsequent breaths require less force, since fluid is reabsorbed across the epithelia. Inspiration creates an air-water interface with high surface tension in the lung. Neonatal lungs require surfactant to reduce alveolar surface tension. Lack of surfactant causes infant respiratory distress syndrome (IRDS, or "hyaline membrane disease"). Surfactant is produced in the second trimester, so premature babies are at particular risk for IRDS.

After birth, all gas exchange must occur at the lungs. Inflation of the fetal lungs at birth allows O_2 exchange. Lung inflation increases alveolar oxygenation and relieves the hypoxic pulmonary constriction. The decreased pulmonary vascular resistance allows pulmonary artery flow to pass through the lungs. Ventilation/perfusion matching occurs within the first seconds of life.

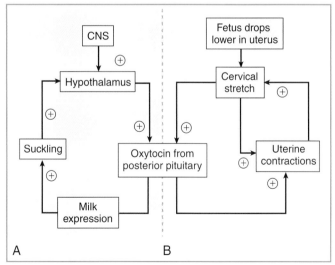

Figure 16-6. Oxytocin is released by neural reflux and stimulates labor and milk expression. **A**, Suckling activity in the nipple stimulates the reflex release of oxytocin, which increases the expression of milk in a lactating mother.
B, During labor, increased pressure on the head of the cervix stimulates the reflex release of oxytocin, which enhances uterine contractile activity.

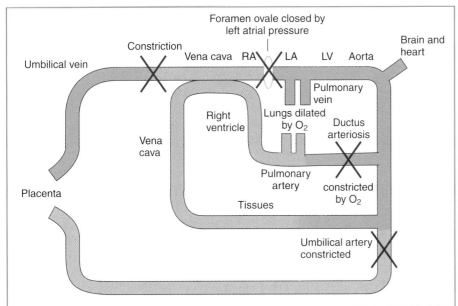

Figure 16-7. Fetal cardiovascular adjustments at birth stop blood flow to the placenta and increase blood flow to the lung. Constriction of the umbilical artery and vein isolate the placenta from the fetal vascular system. Inspiration causes a drop in neonatal pulmonary vascular resistance and an increase in pulmonary blood flow. These vascular changes combine to increase pressures in the left side of the heart. The increase in left atrial pressure causes closure of the foramen ovale. The presence of oxygenated blood causes constriction of the ductus arteriosus.

PATHOLOGY

Infant Respiratory Distress Syndrome (IRDS)

Surfactant production is not sufficient to support life before the twenty-sixth week of gestation. Alveoli of preterm infants with insufficient surfactant have very high surface tension and consequently do not open sufficiently to allow adequate oxygen exchange.

Lactation

Maternal breasts enlarge during pregnancy and transform into a secretory organ following delivery. Estrogen, growth hormone, prolactin, and glucocorticoids all work synergistically to stimulate breast growth during pregnancy. Progesterone causes growth of lobules and stimulates the duct epithelia to become secretory. Estrogen and progesterone support breast growth but inhibit actual lactation during pregnancy. Prolactin and somatomammotropin cause small amounts of colostrum to be formed during the later stages of pregnancy. Colostrum lacks fat, but contains lactose and milk proteins.

Expulsion of the placenta (a source of estrogen during pregnancy) at birth diminishes maternal estrogen and progesterone levels and allows prolactin to stimulate milk production. Growth hormone, cortisol, and parathyroid hormone have permissive roles.

Maternal lactation is established by 48 hours after delivery. Oxytocin stimulates the expression of milk, or "let down." Suckling at the nipple activates sensory afferents to the hypothalamus, releasing oxytocin from the posterior pituitary (see Fig. 16-6). The oxytocin contracts myoepithelial cells of the breast alveoli, expressing milk into the alveolar ducts. Oxytocin can also be released as a conditioned response to infant crying. There is an emotional influence on lactation, as oxytocin release is enhanced in quiet, undisturbed environments.

Prolactin production is stimulated by nursing, so milk production continues to match nursing activity. Milk production gradually diminishes after 9 months. Lactation places a significant demand on maternal energy and Ca^{++} stores, and maternal intake of nutrients needs to be increased to support lactation.

NEONATAL PHYSIOLOGY

In utero, the mother provided a stable environment for growth. The placenta was the major source for nutrient delivery and gas exchange. Thermoregulation was controlled by the mother. Maternal and placental hormonal production provided the major tropic stimulation of growth.

At term, the neonate must assume independent existence. Gas exchange now must occur at the neonatal lungs. Neonatal nutrients must be derived from internal stores until maternal milk production begins. Neonatal thermoregulation processes become functional over the first few days. In addition, the reproductive endocrine environment changes as the absence of maternal FSH and LH suspends maturation of genitalia until puberty.

Fetal dependence on maternal glucose ends at birth. Following birth, fetal blood glucose drops to 50% of values in utero. Capacity for gluconeogenesis is limited and consequently provides only a limited amount of glucose. Fetal glycogen stores are limited, so stored fats and proteins are used for energy for the first 2 days. The low volume of maternal milk, combined with the continuing neonatal metabolism of energy stores, causes a drop in fetal fluid volume and weight for 2 days after birth. Maternal milk protein and fat content, as well as volume, increases by the second day after birth to restore adequate nutritional intake.

Hepatic function is poorly developed in the neonate. Immediately after birth, bilirubin accumulates in the plasma, often causing jaundice. In addition, the concentration of the plasma proteins synthesized by the liver, including clotting factors, drops. After a few days, glucuronyl transferase activity increases, and bilirubin is eliminated in the feces. Renal function is initially poor, leading to potential problems of dehydration, acidosis, and if fluid intake is too high, possibly overhydration. Renal function gradually increases during the neonatal period.

Neonatal thermoregulation is poorly developed. The high neonatal metabolic rate produces heat, and neonatal metabolism of brown fat by adrenergic activity generates additional heat. In spite of these heat production mechanisms, neonatal body temperature falls at birth. The thermoregulatory systems stabilize after a few days.

Higher nervous system functions are poorly developed in utero. Central nervous system function develops gradually during the neonatal period, and the CNS continues to mature during infancy and childhood.

●●● GROWTH

Growth is a complex process and is assessed by age-dependent changes in height, weight, and body mass index. Growth regulation is complex because growth is controlled by genetic factors, a variety of hormones, and local factors (Fig. 16-8).

The endocrine control of growth varies by life stage. Insulin is important during gestation and throughout life. Insulin-like growth factor (IGF) II is important early in gestation, and IGF I becomes more important later in gestation. Following birth, growth hormone (through IGF I) and thyroid hormone begin to exert significant influence. During puberty, androgens and estrogens contribute to a growth surge. Disorders in any of these hormones will have an impact on growth and development.

The fastest rate of growth is observed in embryonic and fetal life. During the 40 weeks of gestation, the fetus progresses from a single fertilized ovum to a neonate weighing 3 kg. During the first trimester, growth is due primarily to hyperplasia. The indices of growth (increases in weight, head circumference, and length) occur proportionately. In contrast, growth during the last trimester is due primarily to hypertrophy, with a greater increase in weight than length.

The rate of growth slows during the last weeks of gestation, due in part to limited nutrient absorption across the placenta. Following birth, there can be a 5% drop in body weight due mostly to a loss of extracellular fluid and limited neonatal nutritional intake. After a few days, maternal lactation and neonatal feeding patterns result in the resumption of growth.

When measured as height, the rate of growth is high in first year of life but declines to a plateau by age 4 (Fig. 16-9). There is a brief growth spurt at puberty, and then growth diminishes to zero by age 20. The earlier onset of puberty in females leads to an earlier growth spurt, which ends around age 15. The male pubertal growth spurt ends around age 17, with

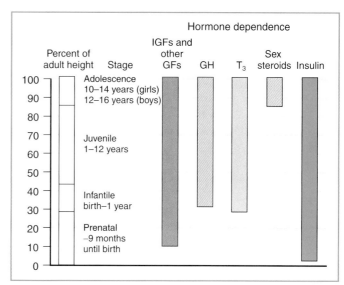

Figure 16-8. Hormonal support of growth differs based on the life stage. In utero, insulin and insulin-like growth factors (IGFs) are the major regulators of growth. At birth, thyroid hormone (T_3) and growth hormone (GH) are added to the growth regulators. During puberty, estrogens and testosterone contribute to the final growth spurt and maturation of the reproductive organs.

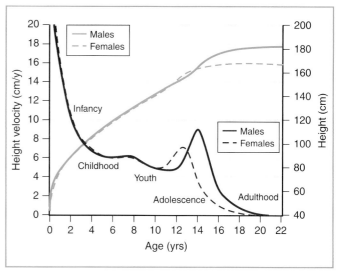

Figure 16-9. The rate of height growth is greatest in infancy and during puberty. After a rapid early change, the increase in height is fairly constant through childhood until a final growth spurt that accompanies puberty leads to attainment of adult height.

male average height being about 6 inches taller than the female average. Height remains stable throughout adult life until there is a small loss of height (1 to 2 inches) in the elderly.

The rate of organ growth varies among tissues (Fig. 16-10). Most brain and head growth occur before age 8, with only small changes through the adolescent years. While height growth is attained early, weight growth is more evenly spaced throughout childhood and adolescence and continues at a much slower rate through the late adult years. In contrast, the reproductive organs experience the majority of their growth during and after puberty.

One consequence of the differing rates of tissue growth is that body composition changes throughout life (Fig. 16-11). In newborns, extracellular fluid volume accounts for the majority of body weight, with the remainder spread across muscle mass, organ weight, and fat. During childhood, fat-free body mass increases in both sexes. By 5 years of age, muscle mass accounts for 35% of total body weight. Muscle accumulation is more pronounced in boys than in girls, particularly after puberty, and this proportion increases until in adulthood, muscle mass accounts for 50% of total body weight in males and 40% in females.

Body mass index (BMI) is calculated as (height in meters)^2/weight in kilograms and is an estimation of body fat. More accurate estimations of body fat involve determining skin-fold thickness or body density. The percentage of adipose and, to a lesser degree, muscle, can vary dramatically based on the diet and exercise patterns.

BMI changes throughout the life span. The median BMI is 16 for a 2-year-old and decreases to 15 by age 5 years. The BMI increases gradually from 15 to 21 by age 18. During this time, there is little average difference between sexes, although the variability is much greater for girls. Body fat continues to accumulate in girls, but not boys, after puberty. The median BMI in both men and women increases gradually from age 20 to age 60 and decreases slightly after age 60 (Fig. 16-12).

Cardiovascular System

Cardiac muscle growth is due primarily to hypertrophy of the cardiac muscle fibers. The cardiac ventricular muscle adapts throughout life in response to the pressure load. In utero, pulmonary artery pressure is approximately equal to aortic pressure, and neonate ventricles are of equal thickness. However, the vascular changes associated with birth lead to a decrease in pulmonary vascular resistance and pressure and an increase in systemic vascular resistance and pressure. During childhood, the greater work of the left ventricle to eject its cardiac output into the high-pressure systemic circulation causes hypertrophy of the left ventricular muscle, which is characteristic of the adult heart.

Arterial blood pressure increases throughout life. At birth, the median blood pressure is 85/37 mm Hg. By age 5, it is 95/53, and by age 10 it has increased to 102/61. During the adult years, blood pressure increases only slightly, remaining close to 120/80 mm Hg. The gradual increase in arterial pressure that occurs with aging contributes to continuing hypertrophy of the left ventricle. Large arteries also lose compliance (arteriosclerosis), causing a more pronounced increase in systolic pressure than diastolic pressure (Table 16-1).

With advancing age, myocardial performance and maximum heart rate gradually decrease. The heart muscle undergoes changes that lead to dilation of the cardiac chambers and lessening of contractility. This has little effect on stroke volume, but it reduces cardiac reserve. Coronary arteries become thickened and rigid. In the elderly, these changes decrease the ability of the heart to respond to additional demands and increase the likelihood of coronary artery disease. The cardiac valves lose compliance and are more prone to calcification. These cardiac changes limit exercise performance in the elderly and increase the likelihood of cardiac valvular abnormalities.

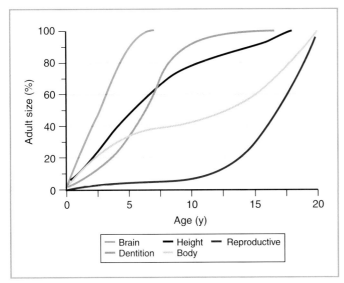

Figure 16-10. Different organs show very different age-dependent growth patterns. By age 8 years, the brain and the head have reached 90% of adult size, and the child has attained 75% of adult height. In contrast, most organs are at 45% of their adult size and the reproductive organs at 10% of their adult size by age 8.

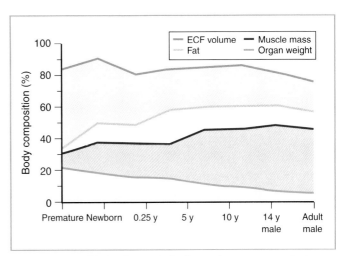

Figure 16-11. Skeletal muscle is the major component of body mass in an adult. In a newborn, extracellular fluid volume is the major contributor to body mass. With age, the proportion attributed to extracellular fluid volume decreases, and the proportion attributed to muscle mass increases.

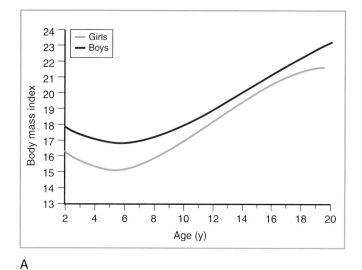

A

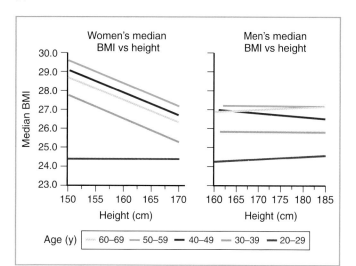

B

Figure 16-12. Body mass index is low at age 6 years but increases through age 60. There is a slight drop to a low point of an average BMI of 15 at age 6, and a gradual increase thereafter, reaching a peak of 27 in males and 28 in females by age 55.

Age	Blood Pressure (mm Hg)
1	88/37
2	88/42
3	91/46
4	93/50
5	95/53
6	96/55
7	97/57
8	99/59
9	100/60
10	102/61

TABLE 16-1. Median Arterial Blood Pressure in Children

PATHOLOGY

Aortic Valve Calcification

Aortic valve calcification can result from an inflammatory process or impaired Ca^{++} regulation; it causes the valve to become rigid and often results in stenosis. Elevated cholesterol, hypertension, and diabetes are risk factors for the disease. Aortic valve calcification also may occur in patients with end-stage renal disease.

Respiratory System

The neonate has approximately 60 million alveoli, or less than 20% of the adult complement. The number of alveoli increases rapidly during the first 2 years of life. Alveolar growth rate then slows, and the adult complement of 360 million is reached by age 12.

In advanced age, the major change in the respiratory system is a reduction in O_2 uptake, both from diminished gas exchange and diminished ventilation. The number of functioning alveoli decreases with age, which limits the surface area available for exchange. The loss in compliance of the lungs reduces alveolar ventilation, especially in the lower portion of the lung. Since this is the area of highest perfusion, a ventilation/perfusion mismatch develops.

There is a progressive loss of elastic recoil with aging. The loss of elastic recoil causes the lungs to be more susceptible to trapping of air during expiration. Consequently, an increase in residual volume and an increase in functional residual capacity are characteristic of aging.

Reduction in strength in the accessory muscles of respiration also limits ventilation. All these changes result in a decreased vital capacity and an increase in the residual volume. These changes do not impair normal function but do limit maximum exertion.

Gastrointestinal System

The GI system is constantly being remodeled throughout life, with little apparent age-related change. In middle age, there is a reduction in pepsin production. This change, however, is not progressive, and it stabilizes.

Diminished colonic motility can occur in the elderly. Decreased colonic peristalsis combines with diminished abdominal wall muscle tone, leading to difficulty in defecation. The decreased ability to defecate is often compounded by a decreased sensation to defecate, leading to constipation.

Renal System

Glomerular filtration rate (GFR) in neonates is low and poorly regulated. After age 2, GFR regulation is established, and when adjusted for body surface area, GFR is constant. In middle age, there is a gradual reduction in renal blood flow and GFR. The decline in kidney function is progressive but highly variable. There is a vast reserve in normal renal function, so the age-related decline does not usually present a problem. There is a loss of compliance of the bladder, which reduces the ability of the bladder to store as large a volume of urine as before. In addition, the ability to empty the bladder completely during micturition is diminished. Consequently, the elderly may need to urinate more frequently.

Endocrine System

The major endocrine change occurring in the young is puberty (see Chapters 14 and 15) and for adult women, menopause (see Chapter 14). With advancing age, there is a decrease in the number of receptors for many hormones and also a decrease in the actual hormone concentration. This includes estrogens, androgens, insulin, cortisol, thyroid hormone, and growth hormone. The increased resistance to insulin that accompanies aging may be secondary to obesity and body fat accumulation.

Integument

Newborn skin is elastic, is thin, and has a limited amount of subcutaneous fat. Skin remains thin through much of childhood.

During puberty, sex hormone secretion stimulates the maturation of hair follicles, sebaceous glands, and apocrine and eccrine units in certain body areas. Hair follicles on the face (males), pubic region, and axillae activate to produce coarse terminal hairs. The rate of the increase in skin thickness can outpace the growth of the glandular secretory ducts, leading to duct blockage and the development of skin blemishes.

The majority of changes in adult skin are tied to sun exposure, but there is an age-related loss of elastin fibers that contributes to the development of wrinkles. Temporary hormonal changes can also account for some adult skin changes. Pregnancy and birth control pills may alter hormonal status and thus change skin structures that are hormonally linked. Pregnancy may cause changes in hair growth patterns, and postpartum there can be a temporary thinning of hair. Heredity and exposure to environmental factors, such as sun, tobacco, alcohol, and chemicals, play a major role in many of the skin changes that occur in adults.

The skin of elders reflects the cumulative influence of environmental insults, decreased circulation, and diminished function of various skin structures. In the elderly, skin becomes more fragile and thinner due to loss of both the dermal and epidermal layers. The number of secretory glands, both sweat and sebaceous, are decreased, leading to dry skin.

As the stratum corneum becomes thinner, the skin reacts more readily to minor changes in humidity, temperature, and other irritants. Skin may be leathery from overexposure to ultraviolet light, and the skin also becomes more transparent. Hair loss is often noticeable on the trunk, pubic area, axillae, and limbs. Loss of pigment causes gray hair. Nails become brittle and may yellow or thicken.

Skeletal System

Aging affects bone, muscle, and tendons. Bone is resorbed, and new bone is added to the skeleton throughout the life span. During childhood and the teenage years, bones become larger, heavier, and denser because new bone is added faster than old bone is removed. Bone formation outpaces resorption until peak bone mass (maximum bone density and strength) is reached around age 30. After that time, bone resorption slowly begins to exceed bone formation. The haversian systems in compact bone can erode. The lacunae enlarge, and cortical bone becomes thin and porous. Osteoporosis, a condition of decreased Ca^{++} in bone, leads to weak and brittle bones and increased risk of fracture.

For women, bone loss is fastest in the first few years after menopause, and it continues into the postmenopausal years. Women can lose 30% of their bone mass over their lifetime, whereas men lose about 15%. Osteoporosis develops when bone resorption occurs too quickly or when replacement occurs too slowly. Osteoporosis can be delayed by formation of strong bones before the mid-twenties. The rate of bone loss with aging can be diminished by appropriate nutrition and by estrogen replacement therapy.

Muscle/Exercise Performance

Skeletal muscle is a plastic organ that remodels to meet sustained levels of physical activity. This remodeling is due to hypertrophy of individual muscle cells, not to hyperplasia. In contrast, injury can stimulate hyperplasia in skeletal muscle.

Physical activity and training can be categorized as either endurance training or strength training. The major muscular adaptation to endurance training is biochemical. Aerobic endurance training increases the numbers of mitochondria as well as the concentration and activities of enzymes that support oxidative metabolism.

PATHOLOGY

Osteoporosis

Osteoporosis is a disease characterized by low bone density and structural deterioration of bone tissue, leading to bone fragility and an increased risk of fractures. Risk is higher for women, the elderly, and individuals with low levels of androgens or estrogens, of white or Asian ancestry, and with a positive family history. Bone density can be increased by appropriate dietary calcium and vitamin D intake, good nutrition, and exercise.

Muscle Fiber Types

Red skeletal muscle fibers contain numerous mitochondria, have high myoglobin levels, and depend on aerobic glycolysis for energy production. Red muscle fibers contract slowly but can maintain contractions for long period of time. White muscle fibers have fewer mitochondria and contract more rapidly. Human skeletal muscle is usually a mixture of red, white, and some intermediate muscle fibers.

Inactivity leads to atrophy of muscle. Atrophy involves the loss of myofibrils but not a decrease in the total number of muscle cells. The effects of atrophy are more prominent in muscles having a high proportion of anaerobic type II fibers. Atrophy from inactivity is completely reversible in healthy young adults.

Skeletal muscle is a major metabolic tissue. The increase in skeletal muscle mass during childhood and young adulthood accounts for a significant increase in BMR. Beginning around age 30 years, the skeletal muscle mass gradually decreases, reducing basal metabolic rate and also reducing the number of calories needed. This progressive loss in muscle mass continues in spite of training and activity. For women, there is a sharp increase in the rate of muscle loss in the three years following menopause. The rate at which muscle is lost, however, can be diminished by continuing training. The amount of adipose tissue in the body remains constant, so the percentage of body fat shows a gradual increase (see Fig. 16-11).

Peak athletic performance declines with aging. Maximal strength can decline by 50% between the ages of 20 and 50 years. For aerobic activities, the decline is gradual and only begins in the third or fourth decade of life. For anaerobic activities, the decline is more prominent and often begins in the middle of the second decade of life. Several theories have been offered to explain these changes, including changes in activity, reduced circulation, cardiovascular disorders, and nutritional problems.

●●● TOP 5 TAKE-HOME POINTS

1. In utero, the placenta serves as the site of gas exchange, nutrient absorption, and waste elimination.
2. At birth, the gas exchange function shifts to the lungs, nutrient absorption shifts to the GI tract, and waste elimination shifts to the GI and renal systems.
3. The major organ systems continue to mature through childhood, and the reproductive systems develop during puberty.
4. With advancing age, there is a gradual loss of organ system function, but no individual organ system ceases to function.
5. Growth and development are under the control of a variety of hormones, including growth hormone, insulin-like growth factors, thyroid hormone, insulin, and the sex steroids.

Integration

17

Integration is the blending of multiple pieces into a larger, coherent picture. Physiology is by nature an integrative science, since the function of each of the organ systems described in this book has an impact on all other organ systems. Two instances illustrate the extremes of physiologic regulation. Acid-base regulation utilizes body proteins and the respiratory, metabolic, and renal systems to maintain a constant pH. Homeostasis is the dominant regulatory goal. In contrast, exercise utilizes the metabolic, respiratory, and cardiovascular systems to adapt to a new physiologic situation. Adaptation to new metabolic needs, rather than homeostasis, underlies the physiologic changes.

●●●● INTEGRATED ACID-BASE REGULATION

Enzymatic activity in the body is dependent on pH. Consequently, body $[H^+]$ must be maintained within very narrow limits for survival. Normal $[H^+]$ is 0.00004 mEq/L, and an increase in $[H^+]$ above 0.00016 mEq/L or a decrease below 0.000016 mEq/L is fatal.

Hydrogen concentration is normally expressed as pH units to make it easier to track the very small changes in $[H^+]$. pH is the negative logarithm of $[H^+]$. The consequence of the "negative" is that pH falls as $[H^+]$ increases, and pH rises as $[H^+]$ decreases (Table 17-1). Normal pH is 7.4, and a pH below 7.35 is an acidosis because of the high $[H^+]$, and a pH above 7.45 is an alkalosis as a result of the low $[H^+]$. A pH below 6.8 or above 7.8 is often fatal.

The body has multiple pH buffering and regulatory systems to assist in the maintenance of pH (Fig. 17-1). The amino acids of the extracellular proteins have a large buffering capacity and provide immediate buffering of pH. This buffering capacity, however, is not regulated, since protein synthesis is

not altered as a result of pH disturbances. By the time plasma pH changes, the buffering capacity of the body protein pool has been exceeded.

The HCO_3^- buffer is physiologically important because it is regulated. The HCO_3^- reaction is

$$H_2O + CO_2 \rightleftharpoons H_2CO_3 \rightleftharpoons H^+ + HCO_3^-$$

with a pKa of 6.1. The combination of H^+ and HCO_3^- to form CO_2 and H_2O is a reversible reaction catalyzed by the enzyme carbonic anhydrase. Because this reaction proceeds to equilibrium, adding new H^+ or new HCO_3^- will shift the reaction to the left, generating more CO_2. Adding more CO_2 will shift the reaction to the right, generating more H^+ and HCO_3^-.

The HCO_3^- levels are expressed in mEq/L. CO_2 concentration is estimated based on the arterial blood gas partial

TABLE 17-1. Plasma pH

$[H^+]$ (mEq/L)	pH	Acid-Base Status
0.00006	7.22	Acidosis
0.00004	7.40	Neutral
0.00002	7.70	Alkalosis

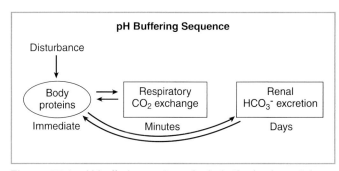

Figure 17-1. pH buffering systems include the body proteins, the respiratory system, and the renal system. Body proteins and other buffers prevent large, sudden shifts in body pH. Once the buffer systems are overwhelmed, respiratory elimination of CO_2 and renal excretion of H^+ or HCO_3^- provide control of body pH.

pressure (P_{CO_2}), normally measured in mm Hg. CO_2 partial pressure is converted to mEq/L by multiplying by 0.03. If both HCO_3^- and P_{CO_2} are known, pH can be calculated as

$$pH = 6.1 + \log \frac{[HCO_3^-]}{0.03\ P_{CO_2}}$$

The bicarbonate buffer is significant because HCO_3^- excretion can be varied by the kidney, and CO_2 exchange can be varied by the lungs. Consequently, both the numerator and the denominator in the equation can change.

Respiratory CO_2 elimination provides acute (minutes) control of pH. Expired CO_2 is proportionate to alveolar ventilation. Acidosis stimulates respiration via both central and peripheral chemoreceptors. An increase in CO_2 causes an acidosis, which stimulates respiration to increase the rate at which CO_2 is eliminated from the body.

Renal acid or base excretion allows long-term balance of pH. Plasma acidosis stimulates renal HCO_3^- reabsorption and the production of acidic urine. Chronic acidosis causes ammonia production, resulting in an additional net H^+ loss in urine. Conversely, alkalosis causes net HCO_3^- loss in urine.

The renal and respiratory changes in acid-base elimination can oppose each other. pH disturbances of renal or metabolic origin usually initiate a respiratory compensation. Conversely, respiratory pH disturbances usually initiate a renal compensation.

Acidosis can be associated with an increase in CO_2 or a decrease in HCO_3^-. Alkalosis can be associated with a decrease in CO_2 or an increase in HCO_3^-. However, increases in CO_2 occur in acidosis by adding CO_2, and also in alkalosis by adding HCO_3^-. Increases in HCO_3^- can occur in alkalosis caused by adding HCO_3^- or in acidosis caused by adding CO_2. For clinical acid-base interpretation, the pH, CO_2, and HCO_3^- values have to be tracked together (Fig. 17-2).

Acid-Base Disturbances

Acid-base disturbances are first characterized by the initial change in pH. There are four major classes of acid-base disturbances: respiratory acidosis, respiratory alkalosis, metabolic acidosis, and metabolic alkalosis. The acid-base disturbances are further categorized as compensated or uncompensated. Compensation attenuates the acid-base disturbance and returns the pH toward normal. There can be a respiratory compensation for an initial metabolic disorder, and there can be a renal (metabolic) compensation for an initial respiratory disorder.

Respiratory Acidosis

Respiratory acidosis results from inadequate ventilation (hypoventilation). P_{CO_2} rises, leading to a drop in pH (acidosis). If the acidosis persists for more than 12 hours, the acidosis may be partially compensated by increased renal H^+ loss. During respiratory acidosis, HCO_3^- may rise slightly due to equilibration with excess CO_2. There is a 1 mEq/L increase in HCO_3^- per 10 mm Hg increase P_{CO_2} that represents chemical equilibrium and is not part of a renal compensation.

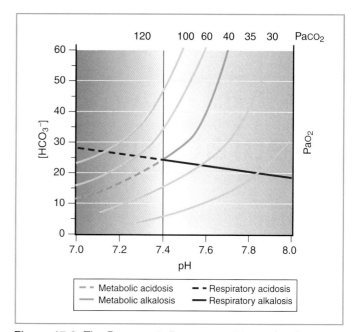

Figure 17-2. The Davenport diagram provides a visual representation of acid-base disturbances. This diagram allows simultaneous plotting of pH, plasma HCO_3^-, and P_{CO_2} and rapid determination of acid-base disorder.

PHARMACOLOGY

Barbiturates

Barbiturates depress the activity of all excitable tissue by enhancing the activity of the inhibitory $GABA_A$ receptor. Cells in the central nervous system are particularly sensitive to barbiturate depression, and barbiturate overdose impairs respiration, leading to a respiratory acidosis.

Respiratory acidosis is often accompanied by hypoxia. Common causes include ventilation/perfusion mismatch or a central respiratory depression from a barbiturate overdose.

Respiratory Alkalosis

Respiratory alkalosis results from excessive ventilation (hyperventilation). In respiratory alkalosis, P_{CO_2} falls, leading to an increase in pH (alkalosis). If the alkalosis persists for more than 12 hours, the alkalosis may be partially compensated by decreased renal H^+ excretion. During respiratory alkalosis, HCO_3^- may fall acutely owing to equilibration with depleted CO_2. There is a 2 mEq/L decrease in HCO_3^- per 10 mm Hg decrease P_{CO_2} that is chemical and not part of the renal compensation. Common causes of respiratory alkalosis include hyperventilation from voluntary effort (anxiety) or stimulation of central respiratory centers secondary to meningitis or a fever.

Metabolic Acidosis

Metabolic acidosis results from a loss of HCO_3^- or a gain of non-CO_2 acid. The acidosis may be acutely attenuated by increased respiratory loss of CO_2 because of the much more rapid response time of the respiratory system. If the kidneys are also functioning, the renal compensation for acidosis is to excrete acidic urine. Chronically, the renal excretion of H^+ is enhanced as the renal ability to produce ammonium from glutamine is induced. Common causes of metabolic acidosis include renal failure, uncontrolled diabetes (ketoacidosis), and diarrhea.

Metabolic Alkalosis

Metabolic alkalosis results from a gain of HCO_3^- or loss of a non-CO_2 acid. In metabolic acidosis, HCO_3^- accumulates, binding H^+ and causing pH to rise (alkalosis). The alkalosis may be acutely attenuated by decreasing respiratory loss of CO_2. If the kidneys are working properly, renal compensation for alkalosis is to excrete HCO_3^-, making the urine alkaline. Common causes of metabolic acidosis include ingestion of antacids, loss of gastric acid (vomiting), and enhanced renal H^+ loss in hyperaldosteronism.

Determination of Acid-Base Disturbances

An acid-base algorithm allows the determination of the acid-base disturbance (Fig. 17-3). The first step is to assess the pH. A pH of less than 7.35 is acidotic. A pH of greater than 7.45 is alkalotic. If either pH disturbance exists, the next step is to examine the CO_2 and HCO_3^- levels to identify the cause.

In acidosis, determine if the cause is excess CO_2. If so, it is at least a respiratory acidosis. Then assess the HCO_3^-. If the HCO_3^- is normal (after accounting for the 1 mEq HCO_3^- increase per 10 mm Hg P_{CO_2} increase), then it is a simple respiratory acidosis. If the HCO_3^- is higher than expected, there has been some renal compensation for the respiratory acidosis. If the HCO_3^- is lower than expected, the acidosis has two causes: a combined respiratory and metabolic acidosis.

If the acidosis is not associated with an increase in CO_2, it is not a respiratory acidosis. The next step is to assess the HCO_3^-. If the HCO_3^- is lower than expected, it is a metabolic acidosis. Then assess the CO_2 (again, adjusting expectations for the 1 mEq HCO_3^- increase per 10 mm Hg P_{CO_2}). If the CO_2 is normal, it is a simple metabolic acidosis. If the CO_2 is lower than expected, there has been a respiratory compensation for the metabolic acidosis. If the CO_2 is elevated, it is a combined metabolic and respiratory acidosis.

The "error" box is reached when an acidosis is not associated with either an increase in CO_2 or a decrease in HCO_3^-. In this case, an error in reporting of the values is a likely possibility. The equivalent steps can be used to identify the cause of alkalosis, as indicated in Figure 17-3.

Anion Gap

The anion gap is clinically useful in the differential diagnosis of acid-base disorders. The anion gap is due to the presence

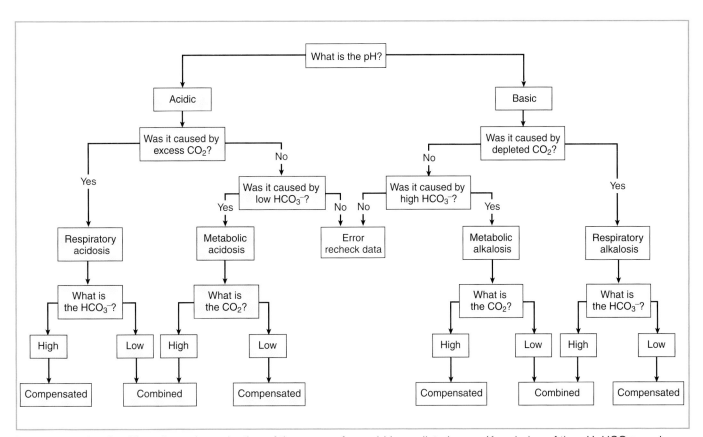

Figure 17-3. An algorithm allows determination of the cause of an acid-base disturbance. Knowledge of the pH, HCO_3^-, and P_{CO_2} allows identification of the acid-base disturbance based on a decision tree.

of anions that are not measured in a standard plasma analysis, such as the negative charges associated with proteins. It is calculated as

$$Plasma\ [Na^+] - ([Cl^-] + [HCO_3^-])$$

and a normal anion gap is approximately 10–16 mEq/L. An anion gap of 17 or higher represents an increased anion gap, and an anion gap of 9 or lower represents a decreased anion gap.

Acid-base disturbances that are characterized by an increased, normal, or decreased anion gap have little mechanistically in common. However, the anion gap is useful in the differential diagnosis, since it eliminates some possible causes of the acid-base disturbance.

An increased anion gap can come from an increase in the unmeasured anions (hyperalbuminemia, lactic acidosis, ketoacidosis) or a decrease in the unmeasured cations (hypocalcemia, hypokalemia, hypomagnesemia). If the decrease in HCO_3^- is offset by an increase in Cl^-, there is a hyperchloremic acidosis but a normal anion gap.

●●● EXERCISE

Participation in exercise represents a physiologic stress to which the body must adapt. Adaptations to a single aerobic exercise event include increases in cardiac output, alveolar minute ventilation, metabolism, and heat transfer. Sustained exercise training leads to structural remodeling of skeletal muscle, cardiac muscle, and bone. Physiologic adjustments to the cardiovascular and respiratory systems complement the normal "homeostatic" control mechanisms to allow the body to adapt to meet a changing environment.

Aerobic Exercise

Aerobic exercise is a sustained activity in which O_2 and nutrient consumption are increased to support metabolic activity. A sustained increase in the workload of skeletal muscle requires increased O_2 and nutrient delivery and increased removal of waste products. Consequently, exercise is associated with an increase in skeletal muscle blood flow. The increase in cardiac output supports the increased skeletal muscle blood flow while causing only a small change in arterial pressure. The pumping ability of the heart normally limits aerobic exercise, but respiratory gas exchange can become limiting if any gas exchange deficiency exists.

PATHOLOGY

Hyperchloremic Acidosis

Diarrhea causes intestinal loss of bicarbonate. The decrease in plasma HCO_3^- is accompanied by an increase in plasma chlorite concentration, and consequently there is a normal anion gap.

Resting cardiac output is approximately 5 L/min, achieved by heart rate of 72 beats/min and a stroke volume of 70 mL/beat. Cardiac output increases in proportion to the intensity of the exercise, reaching up to 25 L/min in an untrained individual. At intensities below 50% of the maximum, the increase in cardiac output is due to increases in both heart rate and stroke volume. At exercise intensity greater than 60% of the maximum, the increases in cardiac output are due to increases in heart rate only (Fig. 17-4).

The increase in cardiac output is directed preferentially to the exercising muscle as a result of local metabolic control of the microcirculation. Increase in cardiac work also results in an increase in myocardial blood flow during exercise. Sustained exercise generates excessive heat, and an increase in cutaneous blood flow assists thermal transfer. Blood flow to the GI tract and kidney may be diminished, particularly

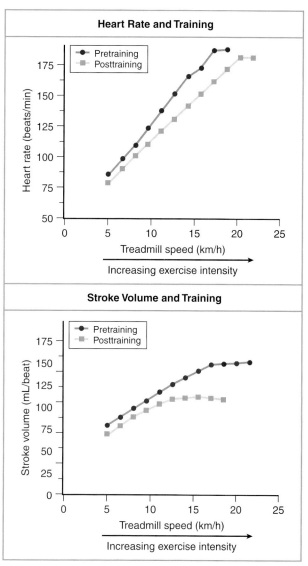

Figure 17-4. The increasing cardiac output during exercise is due to increases in heart rate and stroke volume. Cardiac output increases as workload increases. The increasing heart rate is also proportionate to workload; however, increases in stroke volume plateau at about 60% of the maximal workload.

during heavy exercise. Blood flow to the brain is generally unchanged during exercise.

An elevated cardiac output must be accompanied by an increase in venous return. Venous return during exercise is enhanced by the vasodilation in the exercising skeletal muscle, by sympathetic nervous system–mediated constriction of venules and veins, and by the negative intrathoracic pressure that accompanies active breathing. For activities such as running, the rhythmic compression of the veins in the exercising skeletal muscle also assists venous return.

Skeletal muscle blood flow during exercise can increase tenfold. In skeletal muscle, only 25% of the capillaries are perfused at rest. Opening of all precapillary sphincters results in a fourfold increase in skeletal muscle blood flow. The remainder of the increase is due to arteriolar dilation. In addition to enhancing O_2 and nutrient delivery to the tissues, perfusion of all the capillaries enhances diffusion by decreasing the distance between the skeletal muscle cells and a functioning capillary.

Exercise causes a moderate increase in arterial blood pressure that is proportionate to exercise intensity. Most of this increase is due to an increase in systolic pressure, with the drop in total peripheral resistance preventing an increase in diastolic pressure.

Alveolar ventilation increases in proportion to the exercise load during aerobic exercise. The increased alveolar ventilation allows increased O_2 uptake across the pulmonary capillaries as well as increased CO_2 elimination. The increase in ventilation is mediated by descending nerves from the CNS motor cortex to the pons and medulla. The increase in ventilation is a learned response, beginning during infancy and constantly being fine-tuned. Arterial blood gas concentrations do not change with moderate exercise, and peripheral and CNS chemoreceptors do not play a significant role in stimulating ventilation during exercise.

Increased O_2 delivery to the tissues is accomplished by an increase in perfusion. Oxygen extraction by the exercising skeletal muscle is enhanced during exercise. The increased mitochondrial consumption of exercise drops the tissue P_{O_2}, and O_2 extraction is increased threefold over normal. This results in a drop in venous O_2 levels and an increase in venous CO_2 levels (Fig. 17-5).

Stopping exercise represents a signficant physiologic challenge. Decreased activity in the motor cortex removes the stimulus that had been driving the increased alveolar ventilation and increased sympathetic traffic to the cardiovascular system. Local control maintains the dilation of the skeletal muscle microcirculation. The loss of sympathetic drive causes venous return (and therefore cardiac output) to fall, and consequently blood pressure to fall. The hypotension elicits a baroreceptor reflex, which elevates the heart rate and maintains the blood pressure until the vasodilation abates. The high rate of cutaneous heat loss continues after exercise, and hypothermia can occur.

A single maximal contraction, such as produced by athletes participating in a power weightlifting competition, causes a very different set of changes. Blood pressure during this resistance exercise can increase to over 400 mm Hg. There is a voluntary stopping of ventilation. The sustained muscle contraction prevents any blood flow to the muscles, so O_2 delivery is halted and the exercise cannot be maintained.

Adaptations to Training

Aerobic training increases endurance and performance. Training causes an increase in cardiac performance, tissue blood flow, and tissue O_2 consumption. The minute oxygen consumption is used to estimate cardiac output based on the Fick equation:

$$\text{Cardiac output} = \frac{\text{minute } O_2 \text{ consumption}}{\text{arteriovenous } O_2 \text{ difference}}$$

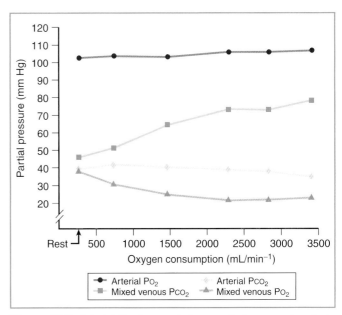

Figure 17-5. Arterial O_2 does not change during exercise, but mixed venous O_2 falls because of the enhanced extraction in the capillaries. Arterial blood gas values reflect the efficiency of pulmonary gas exchange, which is normal during exercise. The increased mitochondrial consumption of O_2 causes a drop in the tissue P_{O_2}, which facilitates the diffusion of O_2 from the capillaries. Consequently, the arteriovenous O_2 gradient increases during exercise.

HISTOLOGY

Cutaneous Microcirculation

The vascular supply of the skin forms two plexuses—one between the papillary and reticular layers and another between the dermis and the subcutaneous hypodermis tissue. The vascular layer of the skin is specialized to facilitate heat exchange and is under strong sympathetic nervous system control.

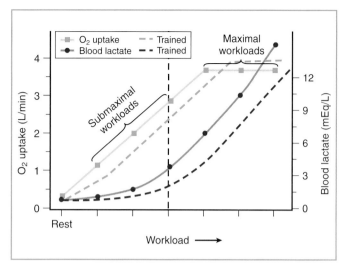

Figure 17-6. Lactate threshold and peak workload increase with training. Lactate threshold represents a shift from aerobic to anaerobic glycolysis. Aerobic training increases mitochondrial O_2 utilization, and consequently lactate production does not begin until workloads are greater.

Peak exercise performance is estimated by the Vo_{2max}, the highest rate of O_2 consumption. Vo_{2max} represents a maximal amount of O_2 consumption by an exercising individual using both aerobic and anaerobic energy production. Sustained aerobic exercise is at a lower Vo_2, usually about 70% of Vo_{2max}.

Aerobic training causes remodeling of the cardiac muscle. This leads to both dilation and hypertrophy of the left ventricle. The dilation increases the chamber diameter and enhances ventricular filling. The hypertrophy increases the strength generated during myocardial contraction. At rest, trained athletes have an elevated stroke volume and therefore can maintain a normal cardiac output at much lower heart rates.

The maximal heart rate is not changed by exercise training. The maximal heart rate for an individual declines slightly with age and often is predicted as (220 − age in years). Because the peak heart rate is not changeable, starting from a lower resting heart rate allows a trained athlete to achieve a larger increase in cardiac output during exercise.

The increase in tissue blood flow caused by training is due to both angiogenesis in the trained muscles and a greater vasodilatory response during exercise. Endurance training

Glycolysis

During moderate exercise, sufficient oxygen is available to completely oxidize glucose and form NADH. When energy demand exceeds the oxygen supply, NADH cannot be processed through the respiratory chain and lactic acid is formed from pyruvic acid.

also causes an increase in the number and density of mitochondria in the skeletal muscle cell, enhancing aerobic capacity.

Endurance training increases circulating blood volume, both plasma volume and red cell mass. Plasma volume increases more than red blood cell mass, and consequently the hematocrit falls. The decrease in hematocrit causes the decrease in blood viscosity, contributing to the decrease in resistance to blood flow in athletes.

Resting arterial blood pressure is decreased by endurance training. This decrease is small in individuals with normal blood pressure but more prominent in individuals with elevated blood pressure. Endurance training can normalize blood pressure in individuals with borderline or moderate hypertension (Fig. 17-6).

The lactate threshold is the level of exercise intensity at which an individual shifts from aerobic to anaerobic metabolism. Endurance training increases the lactate threshold by improving O_2 delivery to the exercising skeletal muscle as well as improving the ability of the exercising muscle to consume O_2.

● ● ● TOP 5 TAKE-HOME POINTS

1. Acid-base regulation results from the interaction of the metabolic, renal, and respiratory systems.
2. Primary acid-base disturbances are characterized by the pH change (acidosis vs alkalosis) and the organ system responsible for the shift (metabolic vs respiratory).
3. Acid-base alterations can be compensated by the actions of the uninvolved organ system, such as a respiratory compensation for a metabolic acidosis.
4. Cardiac output increases during exercise owing to a CNS-mediated increase in heart rate and contractility.
5. In healthy individuals, aerobic exercise performance is limited by the ability of the heart to pump blood.

Case Studies

Chapter 1: Hot Tub Hyperthermia

A 35-year-old man is brought to an emergency department by the rescue squad. He was found unconscious in a hot tub, and there was evidence that he had been drinking. Hot tub water temperature was 40°C. The patient's body core temperature was elevated at 41°C, blood pressure was 100/70 mm Hg, heart rate was 85 beats/min, and respiratory rate was 18 breaths/min. Ice packs were placed on the extremities and groin and under the armpits. After 15 minutes, body temperature was reduced to 38°C. The patient regained consciousness but remained groggy. The patient admitted to consuming 2 L of wine earlier in the evening.

1. What caused the severe elevation in body core temperature?

2. How could the alcohol consumption have contributed to the development of hyperthermia?

3. What is the significance of the locations of the ice packs that were placed on this patient?

4. Why would placing ice packs on the skin of the hands, arms, and legs not be equally effective?

Chapter 2: Poison Ivy Contact Dermatitis

A 12-year-old boy is brought to the pediatrician because of a rash covering both arms and one leg. The rash appeared on one leg 2 days ago when the child returned from an overnight camping trip and has recently appeared on both arms. The rash is characterized by papules or vesicles on an erythematous bed. Patient's past history includes contact dermatitis following exposure to poison ivy. The patient was advised to not scratch the area, and a topical corticosteroid was prescribed.

1. What component of poison ivy is responsible for initiating the contact dermatitis?

2. How does the allergen in poison ivy cross the epidermal barrier?

3. Why is the rash only now appearing on the arms?

4. What is the advantage of treating the area with topical corticosteroids?

Chapter 3: Ethanol Intoxification

A 25-year-old male comes to the office complaining of headaches, nausea, and fatigue. Blood pressure is 100/70, heart rate is 80 beats/min, and respirations are 16/min. Physical examination shows signs of dehydration, and the patient says he is thirsty but the nausea prevents him from drinking. History reveals that he accompanied a group of friends last night celebrating a birthday, and he remembers drinking a number of shots of whiskey during the evening but confesses that he does not remember getting to bed that night. Remember that ethanol inhibits ADH release.

1. Contrast the changes in body water balance caused by ingesting 1 L of pure water with the changes caused by ingesting 1 L of water containing ethanol.

2. What changes in plasma osmolarity are expected to occur during an evening of ethanol drinking?

3. Contrast the effects of body fluid regulation the next morning with the disordered regulation occurring the previous night.

Chapter 4: Calcium Channel Blocker Toxicity

A 3-year-old boy is brought to the emergency department by his grandparents because of suspected ingestion of a Ca^{++} channel blocker. He was found at his grandparent's house playing with an open pill bottle that contained verapamil, a drug that blocks voltage-sensitive Ca^{++} channels. The patient is hypotensive and bradycardic. An intravenous line is started, and glucagon is administered, followed by calcium chloride (20 mg/kg, IV push). Activated charcoal is administered orally. The patient's blood pressure and heart rate gradually recover. The patient is transferred to the ICU for monitoring.

1. What is the normal function of Ca^{++} channels in the heart and vascular smooth muscle?

2. What is the rationale for administering glucagon? Would a β-adrenergic agonist also be effective?

3. What is the rationale for administering calcium chloride?

4. For verapamil overdose in an adult, inamrinone often is administered. What is the rationale for using this agent, and how does its mechanism differ from that of glucagon?

Chapter 5: Duchenne's Muscular Dystrophy

A 3-year-old boy is brought to the clinic for a physical examination. His mother reports that the child has difficulty walking and running and appears clumsier than other boys of the same age. He learned to walk 8 months after most of the boys in his play group who were born around the same time. On physical examination, the boy is of normal height and weight. His calf muscles however appear hypertrophied. The child was placed on the floor and asked to stand up. The child got up on his hands and knees. He then walked his hands up his legs for support as he arose to a standing position. There was no history of musculoskeletal problems on the father's side of the family. The mother was adopted, and consequently no information is available about her family of origin. A blood test reveals elevated creatinine kinase levels. A muscle biopsy confirms the diagnosis of Duchenne's muscular dystrophy.

1. What is the name and normal function of the protein that is abnormal in this patient?

2. What accounts for the observed increase in the size of the patient's calf muscle?

3. Diseases affecting striated muscle cells are uncommon but are devastating and characteristically lethal. Why?

4. What is the significance of the elevated serum creatinine kinase?

5. What type of genetic history would be expected in the mother's family of origin? Why does Duchenne's muscular dystrophy appear almost exclusively in boys?

6. What are the current treatment options for an individual diagnosed early with Duchenne's muscular dystrophy?

Chapter 6: Idiopathic Thrombocytopenia Purpura

A mother brings her 3-year-old son to the pediatrician because of persistent, frequent nosebleeds during the past month. The nosebleeds occur twice a week and continue for 2 hours before stopping. On physical examination, the child shows petechiae and bruising on the skin. Analysis of the stool is positive for blood. Complete blood count shows normally formed red blood cells and white blood cells. The platelet count is 25,000 platelets/mL (abnormally low), and hematocrit is low. Partial thromboplastin time and prothrombin time are both normal. The patient is started on a short treatment of prednisone, and the symptoms disappear after 3 weeks.

1. What mechanism underlies the appearance of the petechiae?

2. What is the relationship between the bruising, blood in the stool, and persistent nosebleed to the appearance of petechiae?

3. Why are the partial thromboplastin time and prothrombin time normal in an individual with a clotting problem?

4. What is the mechanism of action of prednisone treatment for this disease?

Chapter 7: Atrial Fibrillation

A 35-year-old female comes to the ER complaining of "palpitations." Blood pressure is 90/70, and heart rate is 170 beats/min and irregular. ECG shows atrial fibrillation, characterized by an absence of a clear P wave and an irregular but extremely rapid Q-Q interval. The patient is treated with an anticoagulant and a calcium channel blocker. Cardioversion is attempted with the electrical discharge timed to occur immediately after the QRS complex.

1. Why has the fibrillation been confined to the atria and not spread to the ventricles?

2. Why is the Q-Q interval irregular?

3. Why is the patient's blood pressure so low?

4. What is the rationale for treatment with an anticoagulant and a calcium channel blocker?

5. Why is the cardioversion timed to the ventricular QRS complex?

Chapter 8: Hemorrhagic Shock

While camping, a 28-year-old male suffers a laceration to the right leg and loses an estimated 1 L of blood. Shortly after the accident, his pulse rate is 105 beats/min, respiratory rate is 23 breaths/min, and blood pressure is 100/80 mm Hg, his skin is pale and sweaty, and he is mildly anxious. Transport from the scene of the accident is not possible for 24 hours. In the 4 hours following the injury, his pulse rate decreases to 90 beats/min, respiratory rate decreases to 20 breaths/min, and blood pressure increases to 110/80 mm Hg and the hematocrit falls from 42% to 36%.

1. What nervous system mechanism accounts for the increase in heart rate seen shortly after the accident?

2. What accounts for the drop in pulse pressure seen shortly after the accident?

3. What mechanism causes the loss in skin color and the increase in sweating?

4. What accounts for the drop in hematocrit in the 4 hours following hemorrhage?

Chapter 9: Pericardial Tamponade

A 65-year-old male is transported by rescue squad to the emergency department following a motor vehicle collision. He was not wearing a seat belt, and the steering wheel impacted his chest . Blood pressure was normal at the accident scene

but is progressively falling. No external bleeding is evident. Jugular venous pressure is rising, and Kussmaul's sign (a rise in jugular venous pressure during inspiration) is present. Cardiac sounds are faint. Aspiration of pericardial fluid revealed blood, and removal of 50 mL blood caused an increase in arterial pressure and a decrease in jugular venous pressure.

1. What accounts for the progressive decrease in blood pressure?

2. What is the basis for Kussmaul's sign?

3. Why are the heart sounds difficult to detect?

4. What pressure in the pericardium is sufficient to impair cardiac output?

Chapter 10: Carbon Monoxide Poisoning

A 42-year-old man is brought to the emergency department complaining of headache, vertigo, dizziness, and nausea. He was cooking outdoors with charcoal briquettes and moved the grill indoors because of the threat of rain. Blood pressure is 130/90 mm Hg, heart rate 70 beats/min, and respiratory rate 15 breaths/min. Arterial blood gas shows P_{O_2} of 95 mm Hg, P_{CO_2} of 40 mm Hg, pH 7.4, and carboxyhemoglobin level of 25%. Hematocrit is 40%, and arterial O_2 content is estimated at 15 mL O_2/100 mL blood. Mixed venous blood gases are P_{O_2} 25 mm Hg, P_{CO_2} 46 mm Hg, and pH of 7.35.

1. Why does carbon monoxide poisoning cause a drop in the estimated arterial O_2 content?

2. Mixed venous blood gases show that the tissues are hypoxic. Why is there no respiratory stimulation?

3. Why would administering 100% O_2 be beneficial for this patient?

Chapter 11: Urinary Calculi (Kidney Stones)

A 48-year-old male came to the emergency department complaining of a sharp severe pain deep in the lumbar region and radiating around the side and toward the testicle. The pain has now subsided. It appeared suddenly while the man was mowing the lawn. The patient complained of nausea and vomited when the pain first appeared. Blood pressure is 140/110, pulse 80, respirations 24 and shallow. The patient is pale and diaphoretic. Upon questioning, the patient indicated a past history of kidney stones, and he has not been maintaining adequate hydration. The patient is given oral fluids and an NSAID for pain relief, and he is admonished to ingest at least 4 L of water each day and to limit protein ingestion.

1. What is the significance of the location of the pain?

2. How does dehydration promote kidney stone formation?

3. What is the consequence of complete ureteral obstruction by a kidney stone?

4. What is the basis for the dietary recommendations?

Chapter 12: Lactose Intolerance

A 14-year-old Chinese-American male comes to the clinic at a summer camp complaining of an upset stomach and abdominal cramping. The symptoms began shortly after he arrived at camp and have persisted for 4 days. His stool is loose and watery. Dietary history reveals that he's eating the normal camp meals, which includes yogurt for breakfast. The nurse recommends that he eliminate dairy products from his diet, and the symptoms disappear. The nurse recommends that the boy be tested for lactase deficiency upon returning home from camp and that he avoid all dairy products until the determination can be made.

1. What is the normal role of lactase in carbohydrate digestion?

2. Why does the absence of lactase cause abdominal cramping?

3. What is the significance of the age and ethnic heritage of the patient for this deficiency?

4. What type of tests can be used to determine if an individual is lactase deficient?

Chapter 13: Subacute Granulomatous Thyroiditis

A 35-year-old woman comes to the physician complaining of tiredness, a sore throat, and the abrupt onset of left-sided anterior neck pain that radiates to the left ear. She has a fever that has persisted for 3 weeks that began during a respiratory infection. Physical examination reveals an enlarged thyroid gland. Plasma studies show elevated T_3 and T_4 levels and borderline low TSH levels. Treatment is begun with NSAIDs. One week later, the goiter and the pain are diminished, and plasma studies reveal hypothyroid levels and elevated TSH levels. Therapy is continued. One month later, the thyroid is of normal size, and the plasma levels reveal euthyroid status.

1. Did TSH cause the initial goiter? If not, what did?

2. What is the rationale for using NSAIDs to treat the thyroid problem?

3. At the one-week follow-up, what accounts for the hypothyroid status?

Chapter 14: Endometriosis

A 38-year-old unmarried woman comes to the physician complaining of recurring lower abdominal pain. Her pain usually begins shortly before her menstrual period, reaches a peak during the first day, and lasts until the end of menstruation. The pain has become progressively more severe for the last three menstrual cycles; until recently, menstruation was not significantly painful. A pelvic examination was unremarkable. Laparoscopic examination reveals endometriosis in the dependent portion of the pelvic peritoneum. The patient is treated with danazol, a testosterone derivative that inhibits gonadotropin release.

1. What endocrine changes are causing the onset of pain?

2. What is the significance of the endometrial tissue being localized to an extrauterine area?

3. Why was danazol effective in relieving this patient's symptoms?

4. Why is infertility often associated with endometriosis?

Chapter 15: Benign Prostatic Hyperplasia

A 51-year-old male comes to the physician complaining of urinary frequency, urgency, change in stream, and nocturia. Physical examination reveals a symmetrically enlarged prostate gland with an obliterated central sulcus. The patient was started on a 5α-reductase inhibitor, which decreased the rate of prostate growth, and an α_1-adrenergic blocker. At the one-week follow-up, the patient reported a lessening of the urinary symptoms.

1. Why does hypertrophy of the prostate lead to impaired urination?

2. What is the importance of the symmetric enlargement of the prostate in making the diagnosis of benign prostatic hyperplasia?

3. What is the mechanism of action of the 5α-reductase inhibitor?

4. Why does the α_1-adrenergic blocker improve the ability to urinate?

Chapter 16: Patent Ductus Arteriosus

A 2-week old female of 32 weeks' gestational age exhibits a continuous murmur that peaks during the second heart sound. She was in the 10th percentile for gestational age at birth, and growth remains below normal. There is no evidence of cyanosis. A patent ductus arteriosus is confirmed by echocardiography. Indomethacin treatment is begun, resulting in closure of the ductus arteriosus.

1. What is the normal role of the ductus arteriosus in fetal circulation?

2. Why is the cardiac murmur continuous?

3. What is the significance of the absence of cyanosis in this patient?

4. What is the mechanism of indomethacin treatment?

Chapter 17: Salicylate Overdose Acid-Base Disturbance

A 3-year-old child is brought to the emergency department. The only pertinent history is that he was found playing with a bottle of aspirin tablets. An arterial blood gas analysis showed

$$\text{Arterial pH} = 7.47$$
$$P_{CO_2} = 20 \text{ mm Hg}$$
$$[HCO_3^-] = 14 \text{ mEq/L}$$

During the next 30 minutes, the child becomes less responsive to stimuli, and respiratory rate is decreased.

1. Identify the initial acid-base disturbance.

2. What action of aspirin accounts for the low P_{CO_2}?

3. What accounts for the decrease in HCO_3^-?

4. If the child is not treated, which acid-base disturbance will occur next?

Case Study Answers

Chapter 1: Hot Tub Hyperthermia

1. Normal body core temperature is 98.6°F, or 37°C. The body produces excess heat from metabolic processes. Normally 97% of this excess heat is transferred through the skin by a combination of conduction, convection, radiation, and evaporation. Immersion in a hot tub disrupts all these processes. Radiation and conduction require gradient between the body core temperature and the environmental temperature. In this case, the environmental temperature was not sufficiently low to allow significant heat transfer. Evaporation normally assists heat unloading when environmental temperature is high. Because the patient was immersed in water, evaporation was not an option, nor was convection. In the absence of any effective mechanism to unload heat, body core temperature increased.

2. Alcohol consumption increases cutaneous blood flow, but as described above, an increase in blood flow does not assist dissipation of the heat load. In the absence of the normal physiologic heat control mechanisms, the only remaining mechanism to assist thermoregulation is behavioral. As an individual's core temperature rises, the person needs to move from the hot tub to a cooler location. Alcohol impairs judgment, diminishing the effectiveness of behavioral responses to hyperthermia.

3. Decreasing body core temperature requires the transfer of a significant heat load. The groin and armpits are areas where large blood vessels pass close to the surface of the body. Consequently, cooling these areas will more effectively dissipate body core heat.

4. There are two reasons why cooling the extremities is not as effective a mechanism for heat dissipation. First, cutaneous blood flow is regulated by both the hypothalamus and cutaneous temperature sensors. Placing ice on the extremities will cool the extremities. The local cooling will result in decrease of blood flow to those areas. Heat transfer depends on a continuing high rate of blood flow, and the reduction in blood flow to the extremities will diminish the effectiveness of the cooling. Second, the arteries and veins of the extremities are arranged to permit counter-current exchange of heat. This would allow the warm blood flowing in the arteries away from the body core to lose heat to the cooler venous blood returning from the extremities. Counter-current heat exchange minimizes the heat transfer in the extremities, so cooling of the extremities does not provide as effective a mechanism for unloading the heat.

Chapter 2: Poison Ivy Contact Dermatitis

1. Poison ivy and plants of the *Rhus (Toxicodendron)* genus produce an oily compound (urushiol) on their leaves and sap.

2. The urushiol is lipid soluble and slowly penetrates the epithelia of the skin. Washing the affected area immediately with cold water can limit the quantity of urushiol remaining and prevent an allergic outbreak. Exposures of 15 minutes or longer provide time for the allergen to penetrate the skin. Once urushiol penetrates the skin, further washing with detergent (which remains on the surface of the skin) has minimal effect.

3. The appearance of the allergic reaction depends on the quantity of urushiol on the skin surface and the thickness of the epithelial layer. It is likely that some urushiol still remaining on the surface of the leg was moved to the arms by scratching.

4. The corticosteroids will reduce the intensity of the immune reaction to the allergen. Topical treatment will limit the high corticosteroid concentration to the area where the immune response is most intense.

Chapter 3: Ethanol Intoxification

1. Ingestion of pure water causes a decrease in plasma osmolarity. This decrease in osmolarity causes a drop in the release of antidiuretic hormone (ADH) and consequently an increase in urine volume. If these mechanisms are working correctly, there will be no net change in body water, since an increase in urine volume will completely offset the increase in body fluid volume caused by the water ingestion. Normally, the body will excrete most of a load of ingested water within the first 60 to 90 minutes. In contrast, consumption of a fluid

containing ethanol has a different effect. There is a drop in plasma osmolarity as the volume is absorbed. However, now in addition to the decreased osmolarity, ethanol as a drug blocks ADH release. Consequently, the increase in urine volume is greater than the volume of fluid ingested, and there is a net decrease in total body water.

2. The net negative body water balance leads to an increase in plasma osmolarity, which stimulates thirst. Continued ethanol ingestion, however, introduces new ethanol into the body, further inhibiting ADH release. The ingestion of salty foods would further increase plasma osmolarity and stimulate thirst. Urine volume remains high because of the inhibition of ADH. Consequently, the individual remains in negative body water balance in spite of the continued ingestion of fluids. This positive feedback cycle continues whereby strong thirst encourages fluid consumption, but the choice of fluid consumed results in a net loss of fluid from the body.

3. By the next morning, the ethanol has been metabolized and is no longer present in the system. Now there can be a physiologically appropriate response of both the thirst and the ADH systems to the increase in plasma osmolarity. The increase in ADH causes a drop in urine production and hopefully will combine with thirst to reestablish normal body fluid balance. It is important to note that the increase in osmolarity will also draw water from the intracellular spaces, causing a shrinking of the cells, which is often perceptible in the brain as a headache.

Chapter 4: Calcium Channel Blocker Toxicity

1. The influx of extracellular calcium is an early step in myocardial contraction. The extracellular Ca^{++} stimulates additional calcium release from the sarcoplasmic reticulum, and the strength of contraction of both the heart and vascular smooth muscle is tied to the rise in intracellular Ca^{++}. Calcium channel blockers diminish the entry of extracellular calcium. Consequently, they reduce the contractility of the heart and decrease the contraction of vascular smooth muscle. These effects combine to produce a drop in blood pressure from the drop in both total peripheral resistance and cardiac output.

2. Physiologically, glucagon is not a regulator of myocardial contractility. Glucagon does work through cAMP, however, just as do norepinephrine and epinephrine when bound to the β_1-adrenergic receptor. Given the existing hypotension, sympathetic activity is likely already high, and the β_1-adrenergic receptors are being stimulated. Glucagon receptors are found on myocardial cells. Consequently, glucagon administration provides a second pathway to activate adenylyl cyclase and increase cAMP.

3. Calcium entry is driven by a concentration gradient. The regulation of Ca^{++} entry is accomplished by the opening and closing of a channel that is (relatively) specific for Ca^{++}. Increasing the extracellular Ca^{++} increases the

gradient, so that more Ca^{++} is likely to enter the cells during the period when the remaining functional Ca^{++} channels are open.

4. Inamrinone is a phosphodiesterase inhibitor and exerts its biological actions by preventing the degradation of cAMP. Agents that release cAMP stimulate sarcoplasmic Ca^{++} release and consequently have a positive inotropic effect. While glucagon increases cAMP synthesis, inamrinone prevents the degradation. Both ultimately increase the amount of cAMP in the cell.

Chapter 5: Duchenne's Muscular Dystrophy

1. The protein that is abnormal is dystrophin. It is a cytoskeleton protein that attaches F-actin to the β-subunit of dystroglycan. The β-subunit is intracellular, and the α-subunit is extracellular and attaches to laminin and the basal lamina. Dystrophin anchors contractile muscle filaments to the membrane of the muscle cell. As the contractile elements shorten, dystrophin allows the entire cell to shorten and to generate the force needed to move the skeleton. Abnormalities in dystrophin diminish the force generated by the contracting muscle.

2. Cell injury elicits an immune response and replacement of injured tissue with connective tissue. This leads to pseudohypertrophy in which muscles (particularly of the calf) appear much larger than normal. This increase in muscle mass does not reflect an increase in strength, since most of the mass is connective rather than contractile tissue. Pseudohypertrophy is an early clinical indicator of Duchenne's muscular dystrophy.

3. Any disease that causes complete malfunction of skeletal muscle will also affect the diaphragm and will be immediately fatal. Muscular dystrophies develop more gradually and cause only a partial loss of skeletal muscle function in their early stage.

4. Creatinine kinase is usually only found within the striated cells. In patients with Duchenne's muscular dystrophy, the stress on the cell membrane during muscle contraction causes the membrane to rupture and lose intracellular contents. The elevated serum creatinine kinase is a clinical indicator of damage to the skeletal muscle cells. A myocardial isoform of creatinine kinase is elevated following myocardial damage and is a clinical indicator of myocardial infarction.

5. Duchenne's muscular dystrophy is passed from mother to son through X-linked recessive inheritance. Boys inherit an X chromosome from their mother and a Y chromosome from their father. The defective gene that causes Duchenne's muscular dystrophy is located on the X chromosome. Women who have the defective gene are carriers and exhibit no signs or symptoms of the disease. The father's genetic history is unimportant for this diagnosis except to rule out other causes.

6. There is currently no cure for any form of muscular dystrophy. Current treatment is designed to help prevent or reduce deformities in the joint and spine and to allow people with muscular dystrophy to remain mobile for as long as possible.

Chapter 6: Idiopathic Thrombocytopenia Purpura

1. Petechiae are tiny red dots on the surface the skin. Small blood vessels frequently are damaged and need to be repaired. If the injury is small and localized, formation of a platelet plug is sufficient to seal the damage. If the platelet plug does not form, small, localized areas of hemorrhage occur and appear on the surface of the skin as the tiny red dots.

2. All the symptoms are related to impaired blood clotting ability. The platelets contribute to the formation of a blood clot and also contribute factor VIII to the clotting cascade. Severely depressed platelet function impairs the ability of blood to clot, leading to the symptoms described above.

3. The individual has a deficiency in only the platelet component of the clotting pathway. The plasma concentration and function of the enzymes involved in the clotting cascade are normal. Deficiency in platelets alone is sufficient to impair clotting enough to allow the symptoms to appear.

4. The cause of idiopathic thrombocytopenia purpura is not known. It is an autoimmune disease in which individuals develop antibodies against the normal blood platelets. The antibodies destroy the blood platelets at an accelerated rate, leading to thrombocytopenia. Prednisone treatment causes a general suppression of the immune system, which may diminish the production of antibodies.

Chapter 7: Atrial Fibrillation

1. The atria are fibrillating, exhibiting an uncoordinated depolarization of individual atrial myocytes. The atrioventricular node cells represent the only normal electrical pathway for an impulse to pass from the atria to the ventricles. These cells have not fibrillated, so they are unable to transmit an electrical signal until they have passed out of their refractory period.

2. The Q-Q interval represents depolarization of the ventricles from an impulse originating in the atrioventricular node. Once the AV nodal cells pass out of the absolute refractory period, the next impulse from the fibrillating atria that reaches the AV node will be transmitted. There is no fixed time interval for this event, so the interval between QRS complexes is at least 0.25 seconds (the refractory period of the atrioventricular nodal cells) and can extend longer.

3. Blood pressure is low for two reasons. The fibrillating atria do not generate any forward pumping into the ventricles, decreasing the cardiac output by 5% to 25%. In addition, as heart rate increases above 200 beats/min, the rapid ventricular heart rate impairs the diastolic filling of the ventricles, and the decreased filling interval impairs cardiac output.

4. The lack of atrial pumping of blood results in blood pooling in the atria. Blood remaining immobile has an increased tendency to clot. The clot formed in the atrial chamber can then pass through the ventricles and become lodged in a capillary bed. Clots formed in the right atrium will become lodged in the pulmonary circulation, and clots formed in the left atrium become lodged in the systemic circulation. The calcium channel blocker decreases the automaticity of myocardial cells, hopefully interrupting the fibrillation.

5. Cardioversion is the external addition of a strong depolarizing electrical charge. The application is timed to the QRS complex to ensure that the ventricles are in their absolute refractory period, reducing the chance that the cardioversion for atrial fibrillation will generate ventricular fibrillation.

Chapter 8: Hemorrhagic Shock

1. Hemorrhage causes a drop in cardiac output and therefore blood pressure. The drop in blood pressure reduces the stretch on the arterial baroreceptors and reduces their rate of firing. As a result of the decreased nerve traffic from the arterial baroreceptors, the cardiovascular centers in the medulla mediate an increase in sympathetic nervous system activity and a decrease in parasympathetic nervous system activity. The pacemaker region of the heart responds to the withdrawal of parasympathetic tone and the increase in sympathetic tone by increasing the frequency with which it depolarizes and therefore increasing heart rate.

2. Multiple mechanisms account for the drop in pulse pressure. Hemorrhage causes a drop in stroke volume, causing a drop in both systolic arterial pressure and pulse pressure. The increase in heart rate causes an increase in diastolic arterial pressure and a decrease in pulse pressure. The increase in total peripheral resistance also causes an increase in diastolic arterial pressure and a decrease in pulse pressure.

3. Increased sympathetic nervous system activity to the cutaneous blood vessels causes vascular constriction and reduces cutaneous blood flow. This causes the skin to appear pale in individuals with light skin tone. The sympathetic cholinergic nerve fibers innervate the sweat glands and cause an increase in sweating. The

combination of reduced vascular flow and sweating produces the "cold and clammy" (diaphoretic) skin appearance.

4. The drop in hematocrit is due to reabsorption of interstitial fluid in the capillaries. The drop in arterial blood pressure combined with the increase in total peripheral resistance causes a drop in the capillary blood pressure. The drop in capillary pressure favors the reabsorption of fluid from interstitial space. Interstitial fluid does not contain red blood cells or plasma proteins, so the addition of interstitial fluid to the circulation dilutes the red blood cell and plasma protein concentration.

Chapter 9: Pericardial Tamponade

1. The progressive decrease in arterial pressure and the increase in venous pressure are both caused by impairment of cardiac pumping. As blood accumulates in the pericardial space, diastolic ventricular filling is impaired. In the absence of preload, cardiac output is diminished. The decrease in blood pressure is progressive because the bleeding into the pericardial space is continuing.

2. The rise in jugular venous pressure during inspiration is caused by enhanced flow into the thoracic vena cava caused by the negative thoracic pressures of inspiration. Normally, this increased venous return passes into the right side of the heart. In pericardial tamponade, the right heart is unable to expand to accommodate the increased volume, and the volume accumulates in the vena cava and large veins.

3. Cardiac sounds are difficult to detect because the fluid in the myocardium does not transmit sound well. The heart is also "small" because the fluid in the pericardium is impairing filling of the atria and ventricles.

4. Cardiac systolic pressures are high (120 for the left ventricle, 25 for the right ventricle). Ventricular filling, however, occurs at low pressures (<10 mm Hg). The pericardium is a nondistensible fibrous pouch. Any free fluid accumulating in the pericardial space can impair cardiac filling during diastole, even though the pressure in the pericardial space remains low (<10 mm Hg)

Chapter 10: Carbon Monoxide Poisoning

1. Carbon monoxide preferentially binds to hemoglobin with an affinity 200 times greater than that of O_2. The carboxyhemoglobin cannot bind O_2 and is effectively removed from O_2 transport capability. Consequently, the arterial O_2 content is decreased much as would be seen in anemia.

2. The reduction in arterial O_2 content causes reduced O_2 delivery to the tissues. There should be some increase in blood flow from local regulation, but this may not be sufficient to restore normal O_2 delivery. In spite of the reduced arterial O_2 content, the arterial dissolved O_2 is normal. Consequently, there is no respiratory stimulus from the peripheral chemoreceptors. This is not a design flaw, since increased ventilation would not improve O_2 delivery because the hemoglobin that is capable of binding O_2 is already 100% saturated.

3. Administering 100% O_2 would have two benefits. First, the increased alveolar PO_2 would increase the amount of O_2 dissolved in the plasma and partially compensate for the loss of the carboxyhemoglobin ability to bind O_2. Secondly, administering 100% O_2 will shorten the biological half-life of carboxyhemoglobin to 80 minutes, about one quarter of the normal half-life of 320 minutes.

Chapter 11: Urinary Calculi (Kidney Stones)

1. Pain from urinary stones is localized to the lumbar region and radiates around the side. Pain from ureteral stones radiates toward the thigh, along the dermatomes of sensory innervation. The visceral pain causes a pronounced activation of the sympathetic nervous system, resulting in the elevated heart rate, blood pressure, respiratory rate, and sweating.

2. The majority of kidney stones contain calcium phosphate or calcium oxalate. In both cases, the stone forms around a crystal nucleus and continues to grow. Dehydration reduces the amount of urine excreted and, consequently, increases the concentration of calcium and phosphate in the urine. This increased concentration causes stones to develop more rapidly.

3. In addition to severe pain, blockade of the ureter prevents outflow of urine from the kidney. The involved kidney will increase in size and become nonfiltering as the pressure moves back through the renal tubule system and increases the pressure in Bowman's capsule. This results in unilateral renal failure.

4. Fluid ingestion helps wash out any existing stones that can pass through the ureter before they grow large enough to become symptomatic. Reduced protein intake is effective in delaying the recurrence of calcium oxalate kidney stones.

Chapter 12: Lactose Intolerance

1. Lactase is an intestinal brush border enzyme that digests the disaccharide lactose, or milk sugar, into glucose and galactose. The disaccharide cannot be absorbed across the intestinal epithelia; however, the products of digestion

(glucose and galactose) are transported by apical sodium-coupled transport and basolateral GLUT2-facilitated diffusion transport.

2. Normally, carbohydrates are digested into one of three monosaccharides: glucose, galactose, and fructose. In the absence of lactase, lactose remains a nonabsorbable disaccharide. The lactose remains in the lumen of the GI tract and enters the colon. Within the colon, the colonic microflora digest the lactose and metabolize it, producing intestinal gas.

3. Newborn mammals use lactase to break down the lactose consumed while nursing. After weaning, most mammals lose the ability to metabolize lactose. Some human populations, including individuals of northern European descent, inherit a dominant gene that provides lactase activity into adulthood. This gene is very rare in individuals of Chinese descent.

4. The definitive test is an intestinal biopsy and analysis for the presence of the brush border enzyme. More frequently, lactose is removed from the diet. If the symptoms disappear, lactose is reintroduced to the diet, and the patient is monitored for the return of symptoms.

Chapter 13: Subacute Granulomatous Thyroiditis

1. The increased size of the thyroid gland was not caused by TSH. TSH levels were low and physiologically appropriate for the elevated thyroid hormone levels. The increase in thyroid gland size is due to inflammation and an immune response. The bacterial inflammation resulted from the earlier respiratory infection and by the continuing elevated body core temperature.

2. The patient's problem is the enhanced immune response rather than a true thyroid problem. The NSAIDs diminished the immune response and relieved the symptoms.

3. The bacterial infection damaged the thyroid gland cells. The initial elevation in thyroid hormone is due to thyroid hormone release from the damaged tissue. After that initial release, the ability of the thyroid gland to synthesize thyroid hormone is impaired. This results in the drop in circulating thyroid hormone and elevation in TSH.

Chapter 14: Endometriosis

1. The patient's symptoms are caused by endometrial tissue that is located in the pelvic peritoneum. In spite of the extrauterine location, the endometrial tissue responds to estrogen and progesterone just as does the normal uterine endometrium. Estrogen stimulates proliferation and growth of the tissue during the first half of the menstrual cycle. Progesterone from the corpus luteum causes

vascular congestion in the tissue during the second half of the menstrual cycle. As the corpus luteum involutes and progesterone levels fall, the endometrial tissue undergoes necrosis and inflammation, causing pain. The onset of pain occurs during the onset of normal menstruation.

2. Menstruation results in the loss of the outer layer of the uterine endometrium and expulsion through the vagina as menses. The extrauterine endometrial tissue does not have a route through which it can easily be expelled from the body. Consequently, the necrotic extrauterine endometrial tissue serves as a site of inflammation.

3. Danazol inhibits hypothalamic GnRH release and consequently diminishes anterior pituitary FSH and LH release. In the absence of FSH and LH, the ovaries do not produce sufficient estrogen or progesterone to support the menstrual cycle. This ovarian suppression results in the cessation of menstruation. The extrauterine endometrial tissue similarly is no longer subjected to hormone-induced growth or necrosis.

4. Endometriosis often causes scarring and inflammation at the extrauterine site. The fallopian tubes are fragile structures that often are destroyed by the scarring.

Chapter 15: Benign Prostatic Hyperplasia

1. The urethra passes through the center of the prostate gland shortly after exiting the urinary bladder. Enlargement of the prostate gland decreases the lumen of the urethra, impairing the flow of urine exiting the bladder.

2. Prostatic enlargement can result from numerous causes. The tumor of the prostate would not cause symmetric enlargement of the gland. Prostatic infection is associated with symmetric enlargement, but it causes discomfort on palpation.

3. Enlargement of the prostate is stimulated by the testosterone metabolite dihydrotestosterone. Within the target tissue, testosterone is converted to dihydrotestosterone by the enzyme 5α-reductase. Dihydrotestosterone has a much stronger biological activity than does testosterone. Inhibition of 5α-reductase prevents the conversion of testosterone to a more biologically active form.

4. α₁-Adrenergic blockers relax the smooth muscle of the prostate, bladder neck, and proximal urethra. Relaxation of the smooth muscle diminishes the resistance to urine flow through the prostate and reduces the symptoms associated with impaired urination.

Chapter 16: Patent Ductus Arteriosus

1. The ductus arteriosus allows blood pumped by the right ventricle to bypass the fetal pulmonary circulation. The

ductus arteriosus carries blood from the pulmonary artery into the aorta after the arch of the aorta. The fetal pulmonary arterial blood is poorly oxygenated. In the aorta, the pulmonary arterial blood mixes with O_2-rich blood pumped by the fetal left ventricle.

2. In the adult, cardiac murmurs associated with valvular disorders are usually limited to only a portion of cardiac cycle. The narrowed, or stenotic, valves generate a murmur during the portion of the cardiac cycle when the valve is normally open. Valves that fail to seal properly on closure generate a murmur from the retrograde flow of blood during the portion of the cardiac cycle when they are normally closed. In the neonate, aortic blood pressure is always higher than pulmonary artery blood pressure. Consequently, the murmur is continuous throughout the cardiac cycle. The intensity of the murmur increases during ventricular ejection, because the pressure gradient between the aorta and the pulmonary artery is greatest during this time.

3. A patent ductus arteriosus represents a left-to-right shunt. This brings oxygenated blood into the pulmonary artery. Cyanosis results from a right-to-left shunt, in which poorly oxygenated blood enters the systemic circulation. Patients with a patent ductus arteriosus do not exhibit cyanosis but can exhibit right-sided heart failure.

4. In utero, the ductus arteriosus remains open because of the production of prostaglandin E. Prostaglandin E is a vasodilator. The presence of oxygenated blood in the ductus arteriosus inhibits the production of prostaglandin E. In this patient, prostaglandin E production is continuing despite the presence of oxygenated blood. Indomethacin is used to biochemically inhibit prostaglandin production. Interruption of the synthesis of the vasodilator should result in constriction of the ductus, closing the connection between the aorta and pulmonary artery. In the adult, the remnants of the ductus arteriosus persist as the ligamentum arteriosum.

Chapter 17: Salicylate Overdose Acid-Base Disturbance

1. There is a mild alkalosis. Based on the algorithm, it was caused by a low CO_2, so it is at least a respiratory alkalosis. The predicted HCO_3^- is 22 mEq/L (normal 24 mEq) diminished to 2 mEq/L because of the decrease in P_{CO_2}. The actual HCO_3^- is lower, so it is a partially compensated respiratory alkalosis.

2. Salicylates stimulate the respiratory center directly, increasing alveolar minute ventilation. This causes a decrease in P_{CO_2}, and respiratory alkalosis is an early finding in salicylate overdose.

3. The drop in HCO_3^- is a result of metabolic compensation of the respiratory alkalosis. Toxic doses of salicylates cause a drop in renal function and an accumulation of acids normally excreted by the kidney. Salicylates also alter carbohydrate metabolism, causing the production of lactic and pyruvic acids. Finally, salicylates are themselves acids, but the amount of salicylates in the blood during salicylate poisoning is sufficient to drop HCO_3^- by only 2 to 3 mEq.

4. The metabolic acidosis will proceed and become more pronounced. The respiratory depression will cause an accumulation of CO_2, which in the presence of an already depressed HCO_3^-, will cause a combined metabolic acidosis and respiratory acidosis.

Index

Note: Page numbers followed by f indicate figures; those followed by t indicate tables; and those followed by b indicate boxed material.

GHIH (growth hormone–inhibiting hormone). *See* Somatostatin (SS).
GHRH (growth hormone–releasing hormone), 160, 162f, 162t
GI. *See* Gastrointestinal (GI).
Glans penis, 190, 194f
Globulins, in arterial blood, 61t
Glomerular blood flow, 124
Glomerular capillaries, 119f
Glomerular capillary blood pressure, 123, 124f, 124t
Glomerular capillary filtration, 124f
Glomerular capillary hydrostatic pressure, 124, 124f
Glomerular capillary oncotic pressure, 124, 124f
Glomerular filtrate, 117, 120
  osmolarity of, 132–133, 133f
Glomerular filtration barrier, 125f
Glomerular filtration rate (GFR)
  estimation of, 122, 123f
  factors determining, 123–124, 124f
  feedback control of, 4t, 134–135, 134f
  over life span, 207
Glomerular tuft, 117, 119f
Glomerulonephrosis, poststreptococcal, 125b
Glomerulotubular balance, 134–135
Glomerulus, 117, 119f
Glucagon, 159t, 170, 171, 172f
  for calcium channel blocker toxicity, 216, 222
Glucagon-like peptide 1, 143t
Glucoamylase, 152
Glucocorticoids, 165
  biosynthesis of, 166f–167f
  and plasma glucose, 171, 172f
  during pregnancy, 199
  secretion of, 168
Gluconeogenesis, 171, 172f–173f
Glucose
  blood
    fasting, 171
    neonatal, 203
  carbohydrate metabolism and, 170–174, 172f–173f
  insulin and, 169b, 170f–172f, 171
  plasma
    feedback control of, 4t, 5
    hormonal regulation of, 158, 170–174, 172f–173f
  serum, 61t
Glucose consumption, 171
Glucose reabsorption, 125, 126, 127f
Glucose tolerance test, 171f
Glucose uptake, 171
GLUT4 transporter, 169, 170f
Glycogen synthesis, 171, 172f–173f
Glycogenolysis, 171, 172f–173f
Glycolysis, 214b
  in muscle contraction, 50
GnRH. *See* Gonadotropin-releasing hormone (GnRH).
Goblet cells, 101, 141f, 151
Golgi apparatus, 28f
Gonadal differentiation, 177, 189, 191f
Gonadotropin-releasing hormone (GnRH), 160, 162t
  in female reproductive system, 178f, 181
    during menstrual cycle, 185, 185f
    during puberty, 177–178
  in male reproductive system, 190, 193, 193f
Graafian follicle, 179–180, 180b, 183, 183f, 186f
Gradient, movement against, 2
Granulosa cells, 183, 185, 185f

Graphs, 5–6, 6f
Gravity
  and cardiovascular function, 96
  and pulmonary blood flow, 110, 110f
Growth, 204–208
  in body mass, 205, 205f, 206f
  of cardiovascular system, 205–206, 206t
  endocrine control of, 204, 204f
  of endocrine system, 207
  of gastrointestinal system, 206–207
  in height, 204, 204f
  of integument, 207
  organ, 205, 205f
  of renal system, 207
  of respiratory system, 206
  of skeletal system, 207–208, 207b, 208b
Growth hormone (GH), 160–161, 162t, 204, 204f
  and plasma glucose, 171, 173f
  release of, 162f
Growth hormone–inhibiting hormone (GHIH). *See* Somatostatin (SS).
Growth hormone–releasing hormone (GHRH), 160, 162f, 162t

H
H+ (hydrogen), plasma, and potassium balance, 25
H+ (hydrogen) concentration, 209
H zone, 46f, 51f
H_2O. *See* Water (H_2O).
Hair, 13–14
Hair bulb, 13
Hair follicles, 13, 14, 14b, 14f, 15
Haldane effect, 111–112
Haptocorrin, 142f, 155
Haptoglobin, 61
Hard palate, 144f
HCl (hydrochloric acid), 148, 150f
HCO_3^-. *See* Bicarbonate (HCO_3^-).
Heart, 65–75
  blood flow through, 65, 66f
  electrophysiology of, 65–69, 67b, 67f–69f, 69t
  endocrine function of, 159t
  mechanical activity of, 71–74, 71t, 72f–74f
  myocardial physiology of, 69–71, 70f, 71f
  neural and hormonal regulation of, 74–75
  structure of, 65, 66f
Heart failure, congestive, 71b
Heart murmurs, 73, 73b, 81b
Heart rate
  control of, 67, 68f, 74–75, 91
  during exercise, 212, 212f, 214
Heart sounds, 73
Heartburn, 145
Heat conservation, 8
Heat gain, mechanisms of, 8b
Heat loss, mechanisms of, 8, 8b
Heat-shock proteins (HSPs), in signal transduction, 41f
Height, 204, 204f
Helicobacter pylori, 149b
Hematocrit, 60, 60f, 64t
Hematopoiesis, 57–59, 58f
  fetal, 200
Hematopoietic stem cells, 57, 58f
Hemodynamics, 79–82, 81f, 82f, 82t
Hemoglobin, 59, 111b
  fetal, 198, 201b
  in O_2 and CO_2 transport, 110–112, 111f, 112f
  total, 64t
Hemoglobin affinity, of oxygen, 111–112, 112f

Hemoglobin concentration, 60
Hemopexin, 61
Hemorrhage, volume depletion due to, 22
Hemorrhagic shock, 23b, 93, 217, 223–224
Hemostasis, 57, 58f, 61–63, 62f, 63t
Heparin, 63
Hepatic acinus, 151b
Hepatic artery, 88, 89f
Hepatic circulation, 88, 89f
Hepatic function, neonatal, 204
Hepatic secretions, 139, 151–152, 153f
Hepatic vein, 88, 89f
Hering-Breuer reflex, 112
Heterometric G protein target kinases, 39t
HIF-1 (hypoxia-inducible factor 1), 79b
Hirschsprung's disease, 147
Histamine, 86
  in gastric secretion, 149, 150f
  in respiratory control, 99
Homeostasis, 1
Hormone(s), 157, 159t. *See also* Endocrine system.
  synthesis of, 157, 160f
  trophic, 159t, 161, 162t, 163t
Hormone response elements, 41b
Hormone signaling pathways, modulation of, 41–42, 42f
Hormone-receptor interactions, and enzyme kinetics, 33b
Hot tub hyperthermia, 215, 221
HSPs (heat-shock proteins), in signal transduction, 41f
Human somatomammotropin, 198
Hydrochloric acid (HCl), 148, 150f
Hydrogen (H+), plasma, and potassium balance, 25
Hydrogen (H+) concentration, 209
17α-Hydroxylase, 166f–167f, 181f
18-Hydroxylase, 166f–167f
21-Hydroxylase, 166f–167f
17-Hydroxypregnenolone, 167f
17α-Hydroxypregnenolone, 182f
17-Hydroxyprogesterone, 167f
17α-Hydroxyprogesterone, 182f
17β-Hydroxysteroid dehydrogenase, 182f
Hymen, 179f
Hyperaldosteronism, 25
Hypercalcemia, 165
Hypercapnia
  and cardiac function, 75
  and ventilation, 113, 114f
Hyperchloremic acidosis, 212b
Hyperemia
  active, 84
  reactive, 84, 85f
Hyperglycemia, 171
Hyperkalemia, 25, 26
Hypernatremia, 25
Hyperplasia, 29
Hyperpolarization, 36f, 37f
Hypertension, malignant, 124b
Hyperthermia, 8
  hot tub, 215, 221
Hypertonic fluid depletion, 22f, 23
Hypertonic fluid gain, 22f
Hypertonic saline, intravenous infusion of, 23
Hypertrophy, 27
Hypocalcemia, 165
Hypodermis, 14f, 15
Hypogastric artery, 180
Hypoglycemia, 171
Hypokalemia, 26
Hyponatremia, 25
Hypophyseal stalk, 158, 161f
Hypophysis, 158–161, 161f